Certification Review for Nurse Anesthesia

Second Edition

Shari M. Burns, CRNA, Ed.D.
Professor with Tenure
Doctor of Nurse Anesthesia
Practice Program
Midwestern University, Glendale, Arizona

With Contributors
Rodney L. Fisher, CRNA, Ph.D.
Director
Associate Professor with Tenure
Doctor of Nurse Anesthesia
Practice Program
Midwestern University, Glendale, Arizona

David Good, CRNA, DNP
Assistant Professor
Doctor of Nurse Anesthesia
Practice Program
Midwestern University, Glendale, Arizona

Deanna Villalino, CRNA, DNAP
Assistant Professor
Doctor of Nurse Anesthesia
Practice Program
Midwestern University, Glendale, Arizona

New York Chicago San Francisco Athens London Madrid Mexico City
Milan New Delhi Singapore Sydney Toronto

Certification Review for Nurse Anesthesia, Second Edition

1 2 3 4 5 6 7 8 9 LWI 28 27 26 25 24 23

ISBN 978-1-265-21096-0
MHID 1-265-21096-9

Notice

Medicine is an ever-changing science. As new research and clinical experience broaden our knowledge, changes in treatment and drug therapy are required. The author and the publisher of this work have checked with sources believed to be reliable in their efforts to provide information that is complete and generally in accord with the standards accepted at the time of publication. However, in view of the possibility of human error or changes in medical sciences, neither the author nor the publisher nor any other party who has been involved in the preparation or publication of this work warrants that the information contained herein is in every respect accurate or complete, and they disclaim all responsibility for any errors or omissions or for the results obtained from use of the information contained in this work. Readers are encouraged to confirm the information contained herein with other sources. For example and in particular, readers are advised to check the product information sheet included in the package of each drug they plan to administer to be certain that the information contained in this work is accurate and that changes have not been made in the recommended dose or in the contraindications for administration. This recommendation is of particular importance in connection with new or infrequently used drugs.

This book was set in Adobe Garamond Pro by MPS Limited.
The editors were Timothy Y. Hiscock and Kim J. Davis.
The production supervisor was Catherine H. Saggese.
Project management was provided by Karan Singh Rana of MPS Limited.
This book is printed on acid-free paper.

Library of Congress Cataloging-in-Publication Data

Names: Burns, Shari, author. | Fisher, Rodney L., contributor. | Good,
    David (David B.), contributor. | Villalino, Deanna, contributor.
Title: Certification review for nurse anesthesia / Shari M. Burns; with
    contributors, Rodney L. Fisher, David Good, Deanna Villalino.
Description: Second edition. | New York : McGraw Hill, [2024] | Includes
    bibliographical references and index. | Summary: "The purpose of this
    book is to provide a strong updated resource for graduating student
    nurse anesthetists that assists in preparation for the National
    Certification Examination and to offer current, comprehensive review
    material for seasoned Certified Registered Nurse Anesthetists"—
    Provided by publisher.
Identifiers: LCCN 2023007010 (print) | LCCN 2023007011
    (ebook) | ISBN 9781265210960
    (paperback; alk. paper) | ISBN 1265210969
    (paperback; alk. paper) | ISBN 9781265212308
    (ebook) | ISBN 1265212309 (ebook)
Subjects: MESH: Anesthesia—nursing | Nurse Anesthetists | Examination Questions
Classification: LCC RD82 (print) | LCC RD82
    (ebook) | NLM WY 18.2 | DDC 617.96—dc23/eng/20230602
LC record available at https://lccn.loc.gov/2023007010
LC ebook record available at https://lccn.loc.gov/2023007011

Contents

First Edition Contributors

Jacob D. Hantla, CRNA, MS

F. Scott Imus, CRNA, MS

Shaun Mendel, CRNA, MS

Michael MacKinnon, CRNA, MSN

Christol Williams, CRNA, DNAP

Preface

Building a solid foundation of knowledge is pivotal for practice as a Certified Registered Nurse Anesthetist (CRNA). Continuous changes in science, pharmacology, and technology necessitate the need to consistently strive to build upon material learned through classroom, simulation, and clinical rotations. Even with years of practice, seasoned CRNAs strive to consistently update knowledge to improve anesthetic care. The purpose of this book is twofold: to provide a strong updated resource for graduating student nurse anesthetists that assists in preparation for the National Certification Examination (NCE); and to offer current, comprehensive review material for seasoned CRNAs.

The review book is based upon the 2018 content areas tested by the National Board of Certification and Recertification of Nurse Anesthetists (NBCRNA). The NBCRNA's quest to promote patient safety is laudable. The review questions foster knowledge acquisition providing a foundation for safe anesthetic practice. Basic Science; Equipment, Instrumentation, and Technology; and Basic and Advanced Principles serve as the focus for each chapter.

The second edition contributors poured over each question editing, making corrections, and updating references to reflect current information. New questions were added to each chapter. The intent of the content-based questions provides you with the ability to identify strengths and gaps in your knowledge base. Rationale for the correct responses is provided along with current anesthesia references. The questions are intentionally not grouped according to specific topics to provide a review that mirrors a real test environment. Enjoy the review!

Acknowledgments

Many thanks to nurse anesthesia colleagues, faculty, and students who reviewed items contained in this review book. Contributions by clinical and academic faculty foster a comprehensive review for students and practicing nurse anesthetists. Thank you to the contributors from the first edition who laid a strong foundation for the review items. The second edition represents a labor of love by CRNAs Dr. Rodney Fisher, Dr. Deanna Villalino, and Dr. David Good. Their diligence underscores a keen passion for excellence in nurse anesthesia education and the profession.

Appreciation is also extended to SRNAs who discovered questions that needed revision. Kudos to you for your due diligence and professionalism!

Special thanks to Jacquelyn Smith, Ph.D., Dean (now retired), College of Health Sciences, Glendale and the Midwestern University Nurse Anesthesia Program faculty for unwavering support and encouragement. This work is dedicated to the nurse anesthesia profession and today's students who aspire to continue the tradition of providing safe anesthetic care. Finally, thank you to my dear Pa, Monica, Mary Catherine, and their families.

SMB

CHAPTER 1

Basic Sciences
Questions

1. What results when alpha-1 receptors are activated?

   (A) Presynaptic nerve terminals are stimulated.
   (B) Adenylate cyclase activity is inhibited.
   (C) Negative feedback loop inhibits norepinephrine release.
   (D) Intracellular calcium ion concentration increases.

2. Which initial intervention is correct if pulmonary embolism is suspected?

   (A) Discontinue intravenous fluids
   (B) Increase FiO_2
   (C) Extubate the patient
   (D) Discontinue inotropic support

3. Which anticholinergic increases heart rate the most?

   (A) Scopolamine
   (B) Glycopyrrolate
   (C) Atropine
   (D) Pyridostigmine

4. What is the normal V/Q ratio?

   (A) 1
   (B) 0.8
   (C) 2
   (D) 0.5

5. What is the underlying pathology of cor pulmonale?

   (A) Pulmonary hypertension
   (B) Decreased pulmonary vascular resistance
   (C) Systemic hypertension
   (D) Orthostatic hypotension

6. What is the blood to gas partition coefficient of halothane?

   (A) 0.47
   (B) 0.65
   (C) 1.4
   (D) 2.4

7. Which inhalational agent is a halogenated alkane?

   (A) Halothane
   (B) Nitrous oxide
   (C) Desflurane
   (D) Sevoflurane

8. How would you classify a patient with repeated blood pressure measurements ranging from 160/100 to 179/109?

   (A) High normal
   (B) Stage 1 hypertension
   (C) Stage 2 hypertension
   (D) Stage 3 hypertension

9. Which condition is not associated with precipitating unstable angina?

   (A) Polycythemia
   (B) Anemia
   (C) Thyrotoxicosis
   (D) Emotional stress

10. Which neuromuscular blocking drug is contraindicated during the care of a patient with Guillain-Barré syndrome?

    (A) Succinylcholine
    (B) Rocuronium
    (C) Atracurium
    (D) Pancuronium

11. Which lung pathology is a form of COPD?

   (A) Asthma
   (B) Cystic fibrosis
   (C) Aspiration pneumonitis
   (D) Emphysema

12. Which is a normal functional residual capacity?

   (A) 500 mL
   (B) 1,200 mL
   (C) 2,300 mL
   (D) 1,100 mL

13. What are the three most used pharmacological agents for treating ischemic heart disease?

   (A) Nitrates, alpha-blockers, and ACE-inhibitors
   (B) Nitrates, beta-blockers, and calcium channel blockers
   (C) Beta-blockers, calcium channel blockers, and ACE-inhibitors
   (D) Calcium channel blockers, nitrates, and ARBs

14. Which narcotic does not cause histamine release?

   (A) Fentanyl
   (B) Morphine
   (C) Hydromorphone
   (D) Meperidine

15. Which of the following occurs following administration of morphine?

   (A) Increased hypoxic drive
   (B) Decreased apneic threshold
   (C) Decreased hypoxic drive
   (D) Decreased $PaCO_2$

16. The patient is shivering in the postanesthesia care unit. Which intravenous medication will you use?

   (A) Meperidine 10 to 25 mg
   (B) Fentanyl 25 μg
   (C) Morphine 5 mg
   (D) Hyromorphone 5 mg

17. A patient with mitral valve stenosis is asymptomatic with occasional mild symptoms upon exertion. Which mitral valve area is associated with these symptoms?

   (A) 0.2 to 0.5 cm^2
   (B) 0.5 to 1.0 cm^2
   (C) 1.5 to 2.0 cm^2
   (D) 2.0 to 2.5 cm

18. Which term describes full drug activation of a receptor?

   (A) Antagonist
   (B) Partial agonist
   (C) Agonist
   (D) Noncompetitive Antagonist

19. A 60-year-old female with mitral valve stenosis has the following post-induction vital signs: HR-125, B/P-70/45 followed by sudden supraventricular tachycardia (SVT). What will you do first?

   (A) Cardioversion
   (B) Ephedrine
   (C) Phenylephrine
   (D) Vasopressin

20. Which adrenergic agonist has the greatest effect on the heart rate?

   (A) Norepinephrine
   (B) Dobutamine
   (C) Ephedrine
   (D) Isoproterenol

21. What is the onset of analgesia following administration of epidural morphine 5 mg?

   (A) 30 to 60 minutes
   (B) 15 to 30 minutes
   (C) 5 to 15 minutes
   (D) >60 minutes

22. Which of the following local anesthetics and dosages are used for cesarean section with spinal anesthesia?

   (A) Lidocaine (100 mg)
   (B) Tetracaine (14 mg)
   (C) Bupivacaine (12 mg)
   (D) Mepivacaine (16 mg)

23. Which anticholinergic is classified as a quaternary amine?

    (A) Scopolamine
    (B) Atropine
    (C) Neostigmine
    (D) Glycopyrrolate

24. Which anticholinergic cannot cross the blood–brain barrier?

    (A) Glycopyrrolate
    (B) Atropine
    (C) Scopolamine
    (D) Scopolamine and Atropine

25. Which variable increases minimal alveolar concentration (MAC)?

    (A) Hypernatremia
    (B) Hyperthermia
    (C) Acute intoxication
    (D) Ketamine

26. Which factors will exacerbate mitral regurgitation?

    (A) Tachycardia and acute increases in afterload
    (B) Tachycardia and acute decreases in afterload
    (C) Bradycardia and acute increases in afterload
    (D) Bradycardia and acute decreases in afterload

27. Which volumes are included in vital capacity?

    (A) Tidal volume and residual volume
    (B) Residual volume and expiratory reserve volume
    (C) Expiratory reserve volume and inspiratory capacity volume
    (D) Inspiratory capacity volume and residual volume

28. Your patient's hemodynamic profile is as follows: HR = 100 beats/min, cardiac output (CO) = 5.0 L/min, end-diastolic volume (EDV) = 100 mL. **Calculate the ejection fraction and write answer in the box below:**

    [   ]   %

29. What classic triad of symptoms is associated with aortic stenosis with a valve area <1 cm^2?

    (A) Hypotension, dyspnea on exertion, and pulmonary congestion
    (B) Hoarseness, chest pain, and pulmonary emboli
    (C) Chest pains, arrhythmias, and embolic events
    (D) Dyspnea on exertion, angina, and exertional syncope

30. How does the elimination half-time of remifentanyl differ from alfentanil?

    (A) Elimination half-time is longer for remifentanyl.
    (B) Elimination half-time is shorter for alfentanil.
    (C) Elimination half-time is similar for alfentanil and remifentanyl.
    (D) Elimination half-time is shorter for remifentanyl.

31. One goal during a general anesthetic is to decrease the neuroendocrine stress response to surgical stimulation. Which medication will be helpful?

    (A) Vecuronium
    (B) Midazolam
    (C) Lidocaine
    (D) Fentanyl

32. You administered meperidine IV. Immediately following administration, the patient developed profound hypotension, hyperpyrexia, and respiratory arrest. What drug interaction do you suspect?

    (A) Interaction with monoamine oxidase inhibitors (MAOs)
    (B) Interaction with erythromycin
    (C) Interaction with sodium pentathol
    (D) Interaction with etomidate

33. What is the normal aortic valve area?

    (A) 0.5 to 1.0 cm^2
    (B) 1.0 to 1.5 cm^2
    (C) 1.5 to 2.5 cm^2
    (D) 2.5 to 3.5 cm^2

34. For which severity of aortic stenosis is spinal anesthesia contraindicated?

    (A) 0.5 to 1.0 cm^2

    (B) 1.0 to 1.5 cm^2

    (C) 1.5 to 2.5 cm^2

    (D) 2.5 to 3.5 cm^2

35. Which agent results in an increased heart rate during inhalational anesthesia?

    (A) Desflurane 0.75 MAC

    (B) Sevoflurane >1.5 MAC

    (C) Desflurane 0.5 MAC

    (D) Sevoflurane <1 MAC

36. The anesthetic plan includes an inhalational induction. Which inhalational agent is the least desirable for a patient with chronic bronchitis and a 50-pack year history of smoking?

    (A) Desflurane

    (B) Sevoflurane

    (C) Halothane

    (D) Nitrous oxide

37. Which local anesthetic is metabolized by *0*-toluidine?

    (A) Nesicaine

    (B) Cocaine

    (C) Prilocaine

    (D) Mepivacaine

38. Which local anesthetic is linked to methemoglobinemia?

    (A) Prilocaine

    (B) EMLA

    (C) Lidocaine

    (D) Cocaine

39. Which risk factor contributes to myocardial ischemia in a patient with aortic regurgitation?

    (A) Heart rate 40 to 50 beats/min

    (B) Heart rate 50 to 70 beats/min

    (C) Heart rate 80 to 100 beats/min

    (D) Heart rate 110 to 120 beats/min

40. Prior to general anesthesia the patient reports taking daily imipramine. What is your most serious concern for this patient?

    (A) Dry mouth

    (B) Sedation

    (C) Orthostatic hypotension

    (D) Sympathomimetic activity

41. Where is the primary location of hepatic microsomal enzymes?

    (A) Hepatic smooth endoplasmic reticulum

    (B) Kidneys

    (C) Gastrointestinal system

    (D) Small intestine

42. In which valvular disease is the pulmonary capillary wedge pressure (PCWP) an overestimation of the left ventricular end-diastolic pressure (LVEDP)?

    (A) Mitral stenosis

    (B) Mitral regurgitation

    (C) Aortic stenosis

    (D) Aortic regurgitation

43. Which of the following medications block alpha- and beta-receptors?

    (A) Phentolamine

    (B) Isoproterenol

    (C) Propanolol

    (D) Labetolol

44. The patient arrives in the operating room following a motor vehicle accident. Forty percent of the body is burned. When is it permissible to use succinylcholine?

    (A) There is no time parameter.

    (B) Succinylcholine is used within 48 hours of injury.

    (C) Succinylcholine is used after 48 hours of injury.

    (D) No succinylcholine is used for patients with burns.

45. What variables are needed to calculate systemic vascular resistance (SVR)?

    (A) Body surface area, cardiac output, and central venous pressure
    (B) Mean arterial pressure, heart rate, and pulmonary capillary wedge pressure
    (C) Mean arterial pressure, cardiac output, and pulmonary capillary wedge pressure
    (D) Mean arterial pressure, cardiac output, and central venous pressure

46. The patient is scheduled for a tympanoplasty. Which inhalational agent will you avoid?

    (A) Sevoflurane
    (B) Nitrous oxide
    (C) Desflurane
    (D) Isoflurane

47. Which agent increases the cerebral metabolic rate for oxygen ($CMRO_2$)?

    (A) Halothane
    (B) Isoflurane
    (C) Sevoflurane
    (D) Nitrous oxide

48. Which hemodynamic event will decrease coronary perfusion pressure the most?

    (A) Decreased systolic blood pressure
    (B) Decrease in left ventricular end-diastolic pressure (LVEDP)
    (C) Increase in pulmonary capillary wedge pressure (PCWP)
    (D) Increase in diastolic blood pressure

49. Which antibiotic is not classified as a beta-lactam?

    (A) Penicillin
    (B) Gentamicin
    (C) Erythromycin
    (D) Ciprofloxin

50. To avoid hypotension and possible cardiac arrest what is the best method for administering IV vancomycin?

    (A) >60 minutes
    (B) <30 minutes
    (C) >20 minutes
    (D) <10 minutes

51. What is the most common cause of myocardial remodeling?

    (A) Congenital heart disease
    (B) Myocardial ischemic injury
    (C) Chronic lung disease
    (D) Cardiomyopathy

52. A 55-year-old male with congestive heart failure, status post-cardiac transplantation is now undergoing elective surgery for hernia repair. Thirty minutes into the case, his heart rate drops to 28. What medication will you give for bradycardia?

    (A) Atropine
    (B) Ephedrine
    (C) Isoproterenol
    (D) Dexmedetomidine

53. The patient with renal disease is scheduled for an exploratory laparotomy. What muscle relaxant is the best choice for this patient?

    (A) Vecuronium
    (B) Pancuronium
    (C) Rocuronium
    (D) Cisatracurium

54. The patient's glomerular filtration rate is 20 mL/min. What condition most likely exists?

    (A) Acute glomerulonephritis
    (B) Uremia
    (C) Renal calculi
    (D) Acute kidney failure

55. What arterial line waveform might you observe in a patient with severe aortic regurgitation?

    (A) Pulsus paradoxus
    (B) Pulsus alternans
    (C) Pulsus bisferiens
    (D) Anacrotic pulse

56. Which characteristic describes a typical patient with diastolic heart failure?

    (A) Left ventricular ejection fraction less than 40%
    (B) Dilated left ventricular cavity size
    (C) Persistent atrial fibrillation
    (D) Fourth heart sound

57. How does the mechanism of action of methylxanthines affect patients with asthma?

    (A) Blocks degranulation of mast cells
    (B) Bronchodilates via beta-2 receptors
    (C) Bronchodilates via beta-1 receptors
    (D) Inhibits phosphodiesterase

58. A 42-year-old female with multiple sclerosis is scheduled for major surgery with general anesthesia. She has been taking corticosteroid therapy. Which approximate equivalent dose achieves the anti-inflammatory potency of prednisone 50 mg?

    (A) 8 mg dexamethasone
    (B) 100 mg methylprednisone
    (C) 25 mg prednisolone
    (D) 300 mg cortisone

59. A patient with rheumatoid arthritis has been receiving long-term corticosteroid therapy and infliximab. Which statement best describes the major anesthetic implication for this drug regimen?

    (A) Avoiding anesthetic drugs that are excreted via kidneys
    (B) Administering po dose of infliximab via NGT intraoperatively
    (C) Paying meticulous attention to sterile techniques
    (D) Monitoring intraoperative labs for hypoglycemia

60. A patient with a prosthetic heart valve presents for a scheduled total abdominal hysterectomy with a heparin infusion. How far in advance of surgery will you recommend this heparin be discontinued?

    (A) 2 to 4 hours
    (B) 4 to 6 hours
    (C) 24 hours
    (D) 48 hours

61. What is the predicted FEV_1/FVC ratio for a patient whose history includes a 55-pack year history of smoking with wheezing on auscultation?

    (A) FEV_1/FVC ratio of >0.7
    (B) FEV_1/FVC ratio equal to 0.08
    (C) FEV_1/FVC ratio equal to >0.9
    (D) FEV_1/FVC ratio of <0.7

62. Where do local anesthetics exert their primary mechanism of action?

    (A) Sodium channel alpha subunit
    (B) Calcium channel
    (C) Vanilloid 1 channel
    (D) Potassium channel

63. Which neuromuscular blocker is considered an acetylcholine (ACh) receptor agonist?

    (A) Vecuronium
    (B) Rocuronium
    (C) Cisatracurium
    (D) Succinylcholine

64. When administering neuromuscular blockers to patients with myasthenia gravis, what do you expect?

    (A) Up-regulation
    (B) Profound response to succincylcholine
    (C) Down-regulation
    (D) Decreased sensitivity to vecuronium

65. Which fibers are most sensitive to local anesthetics?

    (A) A-alpha fibers
    (B) Small unmyelinated fibers C fibers
    (C) A-gamma
    (D) C fibers

66. Which ratio of the forced expiratory volume in the first second of exhalation (FEV_1) to the total forced vital capacity (FVC) would signify the greatest degree of obstruction?

    (A) FEV_1/FVC ratio of 80%
    (B) FEV_1/FVC ratio of 40%
    (C) FEV_1/FVC ratio of 20%
    (D) FEV_1/FVC ratio of 60%

67. What compensatory mechanism is commonly seen with aortic regurgitation?

    (A) Eccentric hypertrophy
    (B) Dilated annulus of aortic valve
    (C) Concentric hypertrophy
    (D) Elevated brain natriuretic peptide

68. Which pharmacological agent is contraindicated in the patient with Wolff-Parkinson-White (WPW) syndrome exhibiting atrial fibrillation?

    (A) Atropine
    (B) Diltiazem
    (C) Verapamil
    (D) Metoprolol

69. Your patient has mitral valve prolapse. What is the most common arrhythmia associated with this disease?

    (A) Paroxysmal supraventricular tachycardia
    (B) Atrial fibrillation
    (C) Premature ventricular contraction
    (D) Junctional tachycardia

70. From where do the cardiac sympathetic fibers originate?

    (A) T_1–T_4
    (B) T_2–T_4
    (C) T_3–T_6
    (D) T_4–T_8

71. Which statement about coronary blood flow is incorrect?

    (A) At rest, approximately 4 to 5% of the cardiac output passes through the coronary vessels.
    (B) The left ventricle is perfused almost entirely during diastole.
    (C) The right ventricle is perfused during systole and diastole.
    (D) Increases in the aortic pressure can reduce coronary perfusion pressure.

72. What is indicated by a V/Q ratio that is equal to infinity?

    (A) Dead space
    (B) Shunting
    (C) Normal V/Q ratio
    (D) Inadequate ventilation

73. As compared to other anticholinergics, what are scopolamine's sedative effects?

    (A) Less than atropine
    (B) Greater than glycopyrrolate
    (C) Same as atropine
    (D) Same as atropine and glycopyrrolate

74. Who studied the relationship between volume and temperature when pressure remains constant?

    (A) Boyle
    (B) Charles
    (C) Gay-Lussac
    (D) Dalton

75. Which factor most negatively affects myocardial oxygen consumption?

    (A) Cardiac volume work
    (B) Electrical activity
    (C) Heart rate
    (D) Wall stress

76. What is the functional residual capacity for an adult patient in the supine position following induction of general anesthesia?

    (A) 500 mL
    (B) 800 mL
    (C) 1,300 mL
    (D) 2,300 mL

77. What is the normal coronary blood flow at rest?

    (A) 175 to 200 mL/min
    (B) 200 to 225 mL/min
    (C) 225 to 250 mL/min
    (D) 250 to 275 mL/min

78. If a 64-kg woman receives a standard initial dose of dantrolene during malignant hyperthermia crisis, how many grams of mannitol have been administered?

    (A) 12
    (B) 16
    (C) 20
    (D) 24

79. Which statement about protamine is incorrect?

    (A) A hypotensive reaction can be treated with incremental doses of phenylephrine.
    (B) Administering protamine over 10 to 15 minutes will decrease risk of hypotension reaction.
    (C) The normal dose is 10 mg of protamine for every 100 units of heparin.
    (D) Supplementary doses of 50 to 100 mg can be administered to reverse residual anticoagulation.

80. What pathology can increase alveolar dead space?

    (A) Mucous plug
    (B) Pulmonary embolism
    (C) Hyperventilation
    (D) Hypoventilation

81. How is residual volume defined?

    (A) Maximum volume of air expired from resting end-expiratory level
    (B) Maximum volume of air inspired from the resting end inspiratory level
    (C) Normal breath
    (D) Volume remaining after maximal exhalation

82. Which patient does not pose an increased risk for an allergic reaction to protamine sulfate?

    (A) A patient who has a history of two previous cardiac catheterizations
    (B) A patient who is currently undergoing aortic valve replacement
    (C) A diabetic patient on maintenance of NPH insulin therapy
    (D) A patient who is maintained on a weekly hemodialysis regimen

83. Compared to neostigmine, what is the onset of action of pyridostigmine?

    (A) Longer than neostigmine
    (B) Same as neostigmine
    (C) Slower than neostigmine
    (D) Clinically inconsequential

84. Which condition potentiates neuromuscular blockade?

    (A) Hypomagnesemia
    (B) Hypercalcemia
    (C) Hyperkalemia
    (D) Hypothermia

85. What is the result of acetylcholine acting on the muscarinic receptor (M2) in the sinoatrial node?

    (A) Positive dromotropic effects
    (B) Negative dromotropic effects
    (C) Positive chronotropic effects
    (D) Positive inotropic effects

86. Which paradoxical cardiac wall motion, when diagnosed with transesophageal echocardiography (TEE) is indicative of myocardial infarction?

    (A) Dyskinesia
    (B) Hypokinesia
    (C) Akinesia
    (D) Hyperkinesia

87. You plan a standard induction for an 80-kg patient scheduled for cholecystecomy. What induction dose of cisatracurium will you use?

    (A) 16 mg
    (B) 8 mg
    (C) 1.6 mg
    (D) 0.8 mg

88. Following topical administration of a local anesthetic you note erythema, skin blanching, and edema. Which local anesthetic did you apply?

    (A) Chloroprocaine
    (B) Tetracaine
    (C) Ropivacaine
    (D) EMLA

89. Which rate of systemic absorption of local anesthetics is true?

    (A) Intravenous > tracheal > intercostals > para-cervical > epidural > brachial plexus > sciatic > subcutaneous

    (B) Tracheal > intercostals > intravenous > para-cervical > epidural > brachial plexus > sciatic > subcutaneous

    (C) Intravenous < tracheal < intercostals < para-cervical < epidural < brachial plexus < sciatic < subcutaneous

    (D) Tracheal < intercostals < intravenous < para-cervical < epidural < brachial plexus < sciatic < subcutaneous

90. What do you expect when adding epinephrine to local anesthetic?

    (A) Vasodilation at the site of injection
    (B) Increased absorption
    (C) Decreased duration of action
    (D) Vasoconstriction at the site of injection

91. During surgery for a bowel obstruction, you note persistent tachycardia and hypertension. What neuromuscular blocker was most likely used?

    (A) Rocuronium
    (B) Cisatracurium
    (C) Atracurium
    (D) Pancuronium

92. Which factor is a relative contraindication to pulmonary artery (PA) catheterization?

    (A) Left bundle branch block
    (B) Right bundle branch block
    (C) A patient in septic shock
    (D) A patient undergoing thoracic aortic aneurysm repair

93. Which statement about the central venous waveform *a* wave is correct?

    (A) It is produced by the passive filling of the right atrium.
    (B) It is produced by right atrial contraction.
    (C) It is produced by the closure of the tricuspid valve.
    (D) It is produced by the venous return against a closed tricuspid valve.

94. Which statement is false regarding nitric oxide (NO)?

    (A) NO regulates pulmonary vascular resistance.
    (B) NO inhibits platelet activation.
    (C) NO regulates systemic vascular resistance.
    (D) NO is an exogenous neurotransmitter.

95. The patient is taking gabapentin. In which patient would you decrease the dose?

    (A) Hepatic compromised patients
    (B) Cardiac compromised patients
    (C) Renal compromised patients
    (D) Respiratory compromised patients

96. Which statement about monitoring the CVP waveform in a patient with atrial fibrillation is correct?

    (A) There are large *v* waves.
    (B) The *v* waves are absent.
    (C) There are giant, "cannon" *a* waves.
    (D) The *a* waves are absent.

97. Which pathologic state will not cause giant, "cannon" *a* waves on the CVP waveform?

    (A) Tricuspid stenosis
    (B) Tricuspid regurgitation
    (C) Mitral stenosis
    (D) Ventricular hypertrophy

98. The patient received streptokinase. When is surgery permitted?

    (A) 3 days following administration
    (B) 5 days following administration
    (C) 7 days following administration
    (D) 10 days following administration

99. Where does acetazolamide exert its action?

    (A) Proximal convoluted tubule
    (B) Ascending Loop of Henle
    (C) Distal Convoluted Tubule
    (D) Collecting ducts

100. Which hemodynamic profile is consistent with pulmonary embolism?

	CVP	PCWP
(A)	High	High
(B)	High	Normal
(C)	High	Low
(D)	Normal	High

101. Which antibiotic would you avoid in patients with myasthenia gravis?

    (A) Chloramphenicol
    (B) Amphotercin B
    (C) Ciprofloxin
    (D) Gentamicin

102. Which chemotherapeutic agent is strongly associated with pulmonary fibrosis?

    (A) 5-FU
    (B) Cyclophosphamide
    (C) Doxorubicin
    (D) Bleomycin

103. Which hemodynamic profile reflects chronic left ventricular failure?

	CVP	PCWP
(A)	High	High
(B)	High	Normal
(C)	High	Low
(D)	Normal	High

104. In which West zone must the tip of the pulmonary artery catheter lie for the pulmonary artery wedge pressure (PAWP) measurement to be accurate?

    (A) I
    (B) II
    (C) III
    (D) IV

105. How do codeine and morphine differ?

    (A) Codeine undergoes O-demethylation.
    (B) Codeine is less antitussive than morphine.
    (C) Codeine undergoes 2-glucuronide conjugation.
    (D) Codeine's equipotent dose is 1.5 mg.

106. What is the characteristic pulmonary artery catheter (PAC) pressure waveform that tells you the catheter has entered the pulmonary artery?

    (A) A sharp, upstroke/down stroke waveform with the highest point reaching the 10 mmHg point
    (B) A brisk upstroke followed by a steep down stroke returning to mean central venous pressure levels
    (C) A brisk upstroke followed by a notched, sloping down stroke with acute rise in diastolic pressure
    (D) An undulating waveform that occurs near the 10 mmHg point

107. Which statement about correlation of the CVP waveform and the EKG waveform is incorrect?

    (A) The *a* wave follows the P wave on the ECG.
    (B) The *c* wave immediately follows the start of the QRS complex on ECG.
    (C) The *v* wave appears shortly after the start of the T wave on the ECG.
    (D) The *y* descent occurs during the QRS complex on the ECG.

108. During induction of anesthesia you note the inability to ventilate the patient. The chest wall appears rigid. Which medication did you administer?

    (A) Sufentanil
    (B) Versed
    (C) Etomidate
    (D) Methohexital

109. Which of the following is false regarding the mechanism of action of opioids?

    (A) Coupling to G proteins
    (B) Binding to Mu receptors
    (C) Inhibition of voltage gated sodium channels
    (D) Inhibition of adenylyl cyclase

110. How do COX-1 and COX-2 enzymes differ?

   (A) COX-1 responds to inflammation.

   (B) COX-1 inhibition increases thrombosis.

   (C) COX-2 inhibition increases heart attack risk.

   (D) COX-1 sites attract large molecules.

111. If amiodarone is not available, what antiarrhythmic will you use to treat unsuccessful defibrillation?

   (A) Lidocaine

   (B) Diltiazem

   (C) Dobutamine

   (D) Magnesium

112. What is the mechanism of action of aspirin?

   (A) Irreversible inhibition of COX-2

   (B) Low binding to plasma proteins

   (C) Plasma esterase hydrolysis

   (D) Irreversible inhibition of COX-1

113. Which central line site has the shortest distance to the junction of the vena cava and the right atrium?

   (A) Left internal jugular

   (B) Right internal jugular

   (C) Subclavian vein

   (D) Right median basilic vein

114. What is the hallmark sign of a catheter-induced pulmonary artery rupture?

   (A) Hypotension

   (B) Hypoxemia

   (C) Hemoptysis

   (D) Arrhythmias

115. Which law of physics explains why an increase in left ventricular wall thickness will reduce ventricular wall tension?

   (A) LaPlace's law

   (B) Ohm's law

   (C) Poiseuille's law

   (D) Fick's law

116. Which cardiovascular reflex does not result in an efferent vagal response?

   (A) Baroreceptor reflex

   (B) Bainbridge reflex

   (C) Valsalva maneuver

   (D) Oculocardiac reflex

117. Which herbal remedy does not delay awakening from anesthesia?

   (A) Valerian

   (B) Kava kava

   (C) St. John's wort

   (D) Garlic

118. While floating a pulmonary artery catheter via the right internal jugular, the patient monitor shows a run of ventricular tachycardia. Which insertion depth is most likely to induce this arrhythmia?

   (A) 15 cm

   (B) 22 cm

   (C) 28 cm

   (D) 45 cm

119. At what dose is the onset of action of rocuronium like that of succinylcholine for rapid sequence intubation?

   (A) 0.9 to 1.2 mg/kg

   (B) 1.5 to 2.0 mg/kg

   (C) 2.0 to 2.5 mg/kg

   (D) >2.5 mg/kg

120. What is the primary neurotransmitter of the parasympathetic nervous system?

   (A) Norepinephrine

   (B) Acetylcholine

   (C) Acetylcoenzyme A

   (D) Muscarine

121. Which is correct about the CVP waveform in a patient with tricuspid regurgitation?

   (A) Decreasing CVP pressure implies worsening right ventricular dysfunction.

   (B) The *x* descent is usually absent.

   (C) Giant, "cannon" *a*-waves are apparent.

   (D) The *v*-waves become diminished.

122. Which sympathomimetic amine structurally related to amphetamine may cause cardiac arrhythmias, myocardial infarction, and stroke?

(A) Echinacea
(B) Ma Huang
(C) Ginkgo biloba
(D) Genseng

123. How does hydromorphone differ from morphine?

(A) Hydromorphone is more potent.
(B) Hydromorphone has a shorter duration of action.
(C) Hydormorphone is less potent.
(D) Hydromorphone is less lipid soluble.

124. What should be used to reconstitute a standard vial of dantrolene?

(A) 60 mL normal saline
(B) 100 mL normal saline
(C) 60 mL sterile water
(D) 100 mL sterile water

125. Preoperatively you learn that the patient is taking warfarin. Which herbal remedy poses the potential for bleeding?

(A) Ginkgo biloba
(B) Evening primrose
(C) Kola nut
(D) Goldenseal

126. Which antibiotic should not be administered during pregnancy?

(A) Penicillin
(B) Aminoglycosides
(C) Tetracycline
(D) Erythromycin

127. How is emphysema characterized?

(A) Narrowing of small airways by inflammation and mucus
(B) Destruction of parenchyma that leads to loss of surface area, elastic recoil, and structural support to maintain the airway
(C) Antigen binding to immunoglobulin E on the surface of mast cells causing degranulation
(D) Reversible enlargement of the airways distal to terminal bronchioles with damage of the alveolar septa

128. Preoperatively, the patient shares that they were treated with vincristine for Hodgkin's disease. What side effect would you expect?

(A) Paresthesias
(B) Coagulopathy
(C) Magnesium wasting
(D) Arthralgias

129. A 70-kg adult patient with mitral valve prolapse is scheduled for an exploratory laparotomy. If the patient has history of anaphylaxis to penicillin, what antibiotic prophylaxis will you administer?

(A) Cefazolin 1 g IV
(B) Clindamycin 600 mg IV
(C) Ampicillin 2 g IV
(D) Amoxicillin 2 g IV

130. A 70-year old female is undergoing a large bowel resection when the following hemodynamic profile is obtained: B/P 100/80, cardiac output 6 L/min, and central venous pressure 3 mmHg. What is the systemic vascular resistance?

(A) 504 dynes/s/cm^5
(B) 1,120 dynes/s/cm^5
(C) 1,160 dynes/s/cm^5
(D) 2,200 dynes/s/cm^5

131. What has been firmly established as the primary environmental risk factor associated with emphysema and bronchitis?

(A) Homozygous α_1-antitrypsin
(B) Cigarette smoking
(C) Antigen binding to immunoglobulin E
(D) Drug toxicity with bleomycin and nitrofurantoin

132. What is the most significant precipitating factor leading to obstructive sleep apnea (OSA)?

   (A) History of stroke
   (B) History of type II diabetes
   (C) Obesity
   (D) Hypertension

133. By what mechanism do local anesthetics depress cardiac contractility?

   (A) By increasing Ca^{2+} influx and release into the myocardial cell
   (B) By decreasing Ca^{2+} influx and release into the myocardial cell
   (C) By enhancing the intracellular levels of cAMP of the myocardial cell
   (D) By enhancing the intracellular levels of cGMP of the myocardial cell

134. Which local anesthetic agent depresses cardiac contractility the least?

   (A) Bupivacaine
   (B) Tetracaine
   (C) Ropivacaine
   (D) Lidocaine

135. A patient is scheduled for a general anesthetic. You plan to induce with propofol. What is the best dose for a 70-kg male?

   (A) 350 mg
   (B) 100 mg
   (C) 250 mg
   (D) 200 mg

136. What clinical sign is not consistent with Cushing syndrome?

   (A) Hypoglycemia
   (B) Hypertension
   (C) Hyperglycemia
   (D) Hypokalemia

137. What are the electrophysiologic effects of diltiazem on the myocardial cells?

   (A) Binding to calcium channels in their resting active state
   (B) Binding to T-type calcium channels
   (C) Binding to L-type calcium channels
   (D) Inhibiting potassium efflux during cardiac repolarization

138. Which is an appropriate initial intervention to correct intraoperative bronchospasm?

   (A) Deepen the level of anesthesia with a volatile agent
   (B) Give 10 mg morphine IV
   (C) Administer intravenous corticosteroids
   (D) Give Labetalol 10 mg IV

139. What is the correct classification of asthma symptoms that limit daily activity and require daily use of a short-acting beta agonist?

   (A) Mild persistent asthma
   (B) Severe persistent asthma
   (C) Moderate persistent asthma
   (D) Intermittent asthma

140. What are the two strongest predictors of postoperative pulmonary complications?

   (A) Operative site and well-controlled asthma
   (B) Operative site and history of dyspnea
   (C) Obesity and operative site
   (D) History of dyspnea and abnormal chest exam

141. Which intervention lessens air trapping in a COPD patient?

   (A) Increase respiratory rate
   (B) Decrease respiratory rate
   (C) Increase I:E ratio
   (D) Increase tidal volume

142. What is the leading cause of cor pulmonale?

   (A) Obesity
   (B) Asthma
   (C) Sleep apnea
   (D) COPD

143. Which statement is false concerning anesthetic management of OSA patients?

    (A) Patients who use CPAP at home should be encouraged to bring device from home for use in PACU.
    (B) The anesthetist should anticipate a difficult intubation.
    (C) Increased doses of benzodiazepines and opioids may be needed preoperatively.
    (D) The anesthetist should anticipate a reduced FRC.

144. What type of pulmonary disease demonstrates an FEV_1/FVC ratio that is normal with a reduction in vital capacity?

    (A) Asthma
    (B) COPD
    (C) Emphysema
    (D) Pulmonary fibrosis

145. What diagnosis of a patient could be made with a pulmonary function test that revealed an FEV_1/FVC ratio that is 0.6 of predicted valve?

    (A) Pulmonary fibrosis
    (B) COPD
    (C) Pulmonary edema
    (D) Aspiration pneumonia

146. What clinical feature of a pulmonary embolism is false?

    (A) Hypoxemia
    (B) Tachycardia
    (C) Decreased pulmonary vascular resistance
    (D) Hypocapnia

147. Which I:E ratio is most appropriate in a patient with severe restrictive disease?

    (A) I:E of 1:4
    (B) I:E of 1:2
    (C) I:E of 1:1
    (D) I:E of 1:3

148. Deficiency in which protease inhibitor is linked to early-onset emphysema?

    (A) Beta-1 antitrypsin
    (B) Alpha-2 antitrypsin
    (C) Alpha-1 antitrypsin
    (D) Beta-2 antitrypsin

149. What is the hallmark sign of aspiration pneumonitis?

    (A) Hypertension
    (B) Pulmonary edema
    (C) Arterial hypoxemia
    (D) Tachycardia

150. Which statements regarding emphysema are true?

    (A) Emphysema is a restrictive lung disease
    (B) Elevated hematocrit
    (C) Copious sputum
    (D) Hyperinflation of the lungs on chest x-ray

151. Which mechanical ventilation modalities would be most appropriate for a patient with COPD?

    (A) Increasing respiratory rate and an I:E ratio of 1:1
    (B) Decreasing respiratory rate and an I:E ratio of 1:1
    (C) Increasing respiratory rate and an I:E ratio of 2:1
    (D) Decreasing respiratory rate and an I:E ratio of 1:3

152. Which four criteria are consistent with the diagnoses of Adult Respiratory Distress Syndrome?

    (A) Acute onset, PaO_2 to FiO_2 ratio < 200 regardless of the level of peep applied, bilateral infiltrates on chest x-ray, and a PA wedge pressure less than or equal to 18 mmHg
    (B) Acute onset, PaO_2 to FiO_2 ratio < 200 regardless of the level of peep applied, normal chest x-ray, and a PA wedge pressure less than or equal to 18 mmHg
    (C) Acute onset, PaO_2 to FiO_2 ratio < 300 regardless of the level of peep applied, bilateral infiltrates on chest x-ray, and a PA wedge pressure less than or equal to 18 mmHg
    (D) Slow onset, PaO_2 to FiO_2 ratio < 200 regardless of the level of peep applied, bilateral infiltrates on chest x-ray, and a PA wedge pressure less than or equal to 18 mmHg

153. Which criteria are consistent with the diagnoses of pulmonary hypertension?

    (A) A mean pulmonary artery pressure 14 mmHg with a pulmonary capillary occlusion pressure of no more than 15 mmHg
    (B) A mean pulmonary artery pressure at least 25 mmHg with a pulmonary capillary occlusion pressure of no more than 15 mmHg
    (C) A mean pulmonary artery pressure at least 10 mmHg with a pulmonary capillary occlusion pressure of no more than 15 mmHg
    (D) A mean pulmonary artery pressure at least 12 mmHg with a pulmonary capillary occlusion pressure of no more than 15 mmHg

154. Which of the following statements about chronic bronchitis is true?

    (A) Patients with chronic bronchitis display hyperinflation on the chest x-ray.
    (B) Patients with chronic bronchitis display decreased elastic recoil.
    (C) Patients with chronic bronchitis display a normal hematocrit.
    (D) Patients with chronic bronchitis display an elevated $PaCO_2$.

155. How long should a patient discontinue smoking to decrease secretions and reduce pulmonary complications?

    (A) 1 to 2 weeks
    (B) 2 to 4 weeks
    (C) 3 to 5 days
    (D) 4 to 6 weeks

156. What is the acid-base interpretation for a patient with the following ABG, pH 7.29, $PaCO_2$ 52, HCO_3 24?

    (A) Uncompensated respiratory alkalosis
    (B) Compensated respiratory acidosis
    (C) Compensated respiratory alkalosis
    (D) Uncompensated respiratory acidosis

157. When giving neostigmine, what is the resultant muscarinic effect?

    (A) Bradycardia
    (B) Tachyarrhythmias
    (C) Improved contractility
    (D) Increased conduction

158. Which anticholinesterase crosses the blood–brain barrier?

    (A) Edrophonium
    (B) Neostigmine
    (C) Pyridostigmine
    (D) Physotigmine

159. Your patient's Train-of-Four is ¼. You decide to use neostigmine to reverse neuromuscular blockade. What drug combination and doses will you use?

    (A) Neostigmine 0.04 mg/kg and glycopyrrolate 0.2 mg per 1 mg of neostigmine
    (B) Neostigmine 0.08 mg/kg and glycopyrrolate 0.2 mg per 1 mg of neostigmine
    (C) Neostigmine 0.02 mg/kg and atropine 0.014 mg per 1 mg of neostigmine
    (D) Neostigmine 0.01 mg/kg and atropine 0.1 mg per 1 mg of neostigmine

160. What is the acid-base interpretation for a patient with the following ABG, pH 7.49, $PaCO_2$ 22, HCO_3 24?

    (A) Uncompensated respiratory alkalosis
    (B) Compensated respiratory acidosis
    (C) Compensated respiratory alkalosis
    (D) Uncompensated respiratory acidosis

161. Which cardiovascular effect would you expect when stimulating beta-1 receptors?

    (A) Decreased heart rate
    (B) Decreased conduction
    (C) Increased heart rate
    (D) Decreased contractility

162. What statement is true regarding internal cardioverter defibrillators (ICD)?

    (A) ICDs are indicated for left ventricular ejection fractions >35%.
    (B) Placement of ICDs requires general anesthesia.
    (C) ICDs are indicated for intraoperative ventricular fibrillation.
    (D) ICDs are indicated for patients with an ejection fraction <35%.

163. How does beta-2 receptor stimulation affect insulin levels?

    (A) Increases insulin
    (B) No change in insulin level
    (C) Decreases insulin
    (D) Alpha-1 decreases insulin

164. What is the acid-base state of a patient with the following ABG, pH 7.35, $PaCO_2$ 50, HCO_3 44?

    (A) Uncompensated respiratory alkalosis
    (B) Compensated respiratory acidosis
    (C) Compensated respiratory alkalosis
    (D) Uncompensated respiratory acidosis

165. What is the classification of metoclopramide?

    (A) Antacid
    (B) H_1-receptor antagonist
    (C) Gastrointestinal prokinetic
    (D) H_2-receptor antagonist

166. Which of the following physiological effects is not associated with serotonin?

    (A) Arteriolar and venous vasoconstrictor
    (B) Bronchoconstrictor
    (C) Increase bleeding time
    (D) Decreased peristalsis

167. Which of the following is a serotonin receptor antagonist?

    (A) Droperidol
    (B) Decadron
    (C) Aprepitant
    (D) Dolansetron

168. Which ABG result is indicative of acute hyperventilation?

    (A) pH 7.25, $PaCO_2$ 20, HCO_3 24
    (B) pH 7.35, $PaCO_2$ 50, HCO_3 44
    (C) pH 7.35, $PaCO_2$ 40, HCO_3 24
    (D) pH 7.45, $PaCO_2$ 30, HCO_3 14

169. What is the physical structure of succinylcholine?

    (A) Two joined acetylcholine molecules
    (B) Benzylisoquinoline
    (C) Steroid ring with two modified Ach molecules
    (D) Monoquaternary steroid

170. Which of the following factors produces 4 to 8 hours of succincylcholine induced neuromuscular blockade?

    (A) Homozygous atypical enzyme
    (B) Hyperthermia
    (C) Heterozygous atypical enzyme
    (D) Reduced pseudocholinesterase levels

171. During a general anesthesia case with mechanical ventilation the ABG results are: pH 7.29, $PaCO_2$ 52, HCO_3 24. What intervention is appropriate?

    (A) Decrease respiratory rate
    (B) Decrease tidal volume
    (C) Give 150 mEq sodium bicarbonate
    (D) Increase respiratory rate

172. What is the primary anesthetic goal for patients with second- and third-degree burns?

    (A) Pain management
    (B) Restoring circulating volume
    (C) Administration of platelets
    (D) Administration of colloids

173. Hypoxic pulmonary vasoconstriction (HPV) will cause which action in the lungs?

    (A) Increase blood flow to nonventilated lung
    (B) Decrease blood flow to ventilated lung
    (C) Decrease blood flow to nonventilated lung
    (D) Increase ventilation to the nonperfused lung

174. Calculate the oxygen content given the following values: Hb = 14; $PaCO_2$ = 60; SaO_2 = 90%?

(A) 4 mL O_2

(B) 14 mL O_2

(C) 17 mL O_2

(D) 40 mL O_2

175. The Haldane effect is best described by which statement below?

(A) The Haldane effect explains why deoxygenated blood can carry more CO_2.

(B) The Haldane effect explains the influence of pH, PCO_2, and PO_2 on the oxyhemoglobin dissociation curve.

(C) The Haldane effect governs the diffusion of O_2 at the capillary level.

(D) The Haldane effect accounts for the difference in lung volume at inspiration versus expiration.

176. A 22-year-old male emerges from a laparoscopic appendectomy under general endotracheal anesthesia still intubated. The patient is without an oral airway. During emergence, the patient sits up bucking with teeth clamped down occluding the endotracheal tube. He forcefully attempts to breathe. Which respiratory phenomenon could occur based on this scenario?

(A) Pulmonary embolism

(B) Pulmonary edema

(C) Aspiration pneumonia

(D) Acute asthma attack

177. In which lung region are the alveoli most compliant in an upright healthy person?

(A) Apex

(B) Middle

(C) Base

(D) Pleura

178. A ventilation:perfusion (V:Q) ratio of zero (0) may be seen in which disorder?

(A) Pulmonary embolism

(B) Low cardiac output

(C) Emphysema

(D) Mucous plug

179. In what form is the majority of CO_2 transported in the blood?

(A) Carbonic acid

(B) Bicarbonate

(C) Dissolved

(D) Attached to hemoglobin

180. Following repeated doses of meperidine, your patient begins to experience tremors, muscle twitches, and seizures. What is the probable cause?

(A) Delta receptor activation

(B) Meperidine's anticholinergic properties

(C) Normeperidine

(D) Kappa agonism

181. Which anticholinergic possesses the least antisialogogue effect?

(A) Atropine

(B) Glycopyrrolate

(C) Scopolamine

(D) Neostigmine

182. The patient presents for outpatient surgery with a history of asthma. When using glycopyrrolate, what do you expect?

(A) Constriction of bronchial smooth muscle

(B) Increased gastric acid secretion

(C) Decreased body temperature

(D) Relaxation of bronchial smooth muscle

183. How is the action of a single IV bolus dose of Fentanyl terminated?

(A) Metabolism

(B) Redistribution

(C) Distribution

(D) Elimination

184. Which type of pneumocytes in the pulmonary epithelium contains surfactant?

(A) Type I pneumocytes

(B) Pulmonary alveolar macrophages

(C) Type II pneumocytes

(D) Mast cells

185. Which is the origin of the phrenic nerves?

(A) T_{10}

(B) C_2

(C) $C_3–C_5$

(D) $T_4–T_6$

186. What two lung volumes comprise the functional residual capacity?

(A) Residual volume and tidal volume

(B) Tidal volume and expiratory reserve volume

(C) Residual volume and inspiratory reserve volume

(D) Residual volume and expiratory reserve volume

187. What is vital capacity?

(A) Volume remaining after maximal exhalation

(B) Maximal additional volume that can be inspired above tidal volume

(C) Maximal volume that can be expired below tidal volume

(D) Maximum volume of gas that can be expired following maximal inspiration

188. Prior to rapid sequence induction of general anesthesia you plan to administer ranitidine. When is the best time to administer the medication?

(A) 0.5 to 1 hour preoperatively

(B) 1.0 to 1.5 hours preoperatively

(C) 1 to 2 hours preoperatively

(D) 1.5 to 2.5 hours preoperatively

189. Which H_2 receptor antagonist affects the metabolism of warfarin?

(A) Cimedtidine

(B) Ranitidine

(C) Diphenhydramine

(D) Hydroxyzine

190. Which drug affects the absorption of digoxin?

(A) Cimetidine

(B) Bicitra

(C) Metoclopramide

(D) Omeprazole

191. What is the normal ratio of forced expiratory volume to the total forced vital capacity?

(A) Less than 60%

(B) Greater than 50%

(C) Greater than or equal to 80%

(D) Greater than or equal to 20%

192. In the standard 70-kg patient, what is the functional residual capacity in the supine position?

(A) 2,300 mL

(B) 1,300 mL

(C) 1,200 mL

(D) 500 mL

193. Which structure classifies local anesthetics?

(A) Lipophilic group

(B) Benzene ring

(C) Hydrophilic group

(D) Intermediate chain

194. Lipid solubility is greatest with which local anesthetic?

(A) Tetracaine

(B) Procaine

(C) Cocaine

(D) Chloroprocaine

195. Which of these factors most influences the duration of action for local anesthetics?

(A) pKa

(B) Ionization

(C) Lipid solubility

(D) Minimum concentration

196. What factor shifts the hemoglobin dissociation curve to the right?

(A) Normothermia

(B) Hypoventilation

(C) Hyperthermia

(D) Decrease in 2,3-DPG

197. What is the anatomic dead space in a 75-kg healthy adult patient?

   (A) 75 mL
   (B) 100 mL
   (C) 150 mL
   (D) 200 mL

198. What law applies when determining blood flow through an intravenous catheter?

   (A) Poiseuille's law
   (B) Bernoulli's principle
   (C) LaPlace's law
   (D) Van der Waal's principle

199. During a general anesthetic, fentanyl and versed are administered. The interaction of the drugs produces a greater effect than the sum of the two medications. What is the interaction called?

   (A) Addition
   (B) Synergism
   (C) Tolerance
   (D) Tachyphylaxis

200. Which of the following is not a Phase I reaction?

   (A) Oxidation
   (B) Reduction
   (C) Conjugation
   (D) Hydrolysis

201. Which inhalational agent's metabolism produces Compound A?

   (A) Sevoflurane with low flow
   (B) Desflurane with low flow
   (C) Sevoflurane with high flow
   (D) Desflurane with high flow

202. How is propofol classified?

   (A) Alkylphenol
   (B) Barbituric acid
   (C) Phencyclidine
   (D) Carboxylated imidazole

203. What induction agent is least protein bound?

   (A) Ketamine
   (B) Propofol
   (C) Methohexital
   (D) Etomidate

204. Clearance of which benzodiazepine is greatest?

   (A) Diazepam
   (B) Lorazepam
   (C) Midazolam
   (D) Zaleplon

205. Following administration of a beta-lactam antibiotic, the patient exhibits urticaria, hypotension, and arrhythmias. What is the most likely cause?

   (A) Tachyphylaxis reaction
   (B) Anaphylaxis reaction
   (C) Atopic reaction
   (D) Anaphylactoid reaction

206. Which would be best in the care of a patient in myxedema coma needing emergent surgery?

   (A) Propylthiouracil
   (B) Liothyronine
   (C) Thyroxine
   (D) Thyroid stimulating hormone

207. Which indicates primary hypothyroidism?

   (A) Decreased thyroid stimulating hormone with decreased triiodothyronine and thyroxine
   (B) Increased thyroid stimulating hormone with decreased triiodothyronine and thyroxine
   (C) Decreased thyroid stimulating hormone with increased triiodothyronine and thyroxine
   (D) Increased thyroid stimulating hormone with increased triiodothyronine and thyroxine

208. Which statement is true regarding phenytoin?

(A) Chronic treatment with phenytoin leads to prolonged neuromuscular blockade.

(B) Lower doses of neuromuscular blockers are required.

(C) Elimination of neuromuscular blockers is decreased.

(D) Higher doses of neuromuscular blockers are required.

209. Which antiemetic will you avoid for patients with Parkinson's disease?

(A) Dolasetron

(B) Metoclopramide

(C) Odansetron

(D) Diphenhydramine

210. During surgery for breast cancer, the patient receives isosulfan blue dye. What will you expect?

(A) Increased SaO_2

(B) Tachycardia

(C) Decreased SaO_2

(D) Cardiac arrhythmias

211. Which analgesic for labor is not associated with significant respiratory depression affecting the mother or fetus?

(A) Morphine

(B) Nalbuphine

(C) Fentanyl

(D) Demerol

212. Why are benzodiazepines avoided during labor and delivery?

(A) Pain on injection

(B) Prolonged neonatal depression

(C) High Apgar Scores

(D) Nausea and vomiting

213. Which inhalational agent affects the blood pressure the least?

(A) Sevoflurane

(B) Halothane

(C) Isoflurane

(D) Desflurane

214. Which analgesic given to renal failure patients results in prolonged respiratory depression?

(A) Remifentanil

(B) Demerol

(C) Sufentanil

(D) Morphine

215. Which COX-2 selective agent is linked to hepatic failure?

(A) Acetominophen

(B) Aspirin

(C) Ketorolac

(D) Celecoxib

216. Your patient suffers from chronic renal failure. Which nondepolarizer will you avoid?

(A) Vecuronium

(B) Rocuronium

(C) Mivacron

(D) Anectine

217. What is the mechanism of action for reversal of succinylcholine?

(A) Metabolism by acetylcholinesterase

(B) Hydrolyzed pseudocholinesterase

(C) Complex formation with steroidal nondepolarizers

(D) Chemical degradation by L-cysteine

218. The patient undergoing cataract extraction takes echothiophate for glaucoma. If given succinylcholine, what will you expect?

(A) Duration <5 minutes

(B) Duration <10 minutes

(C) Duration >10 minutes

(D) No effect on duration of action

219. You administered propofol 2 mg/kg, succinylcholine 1.5 mg/kg, and fentanyl 2 μg/kg to a 70-kg patient undergoing emergent appendectomy. Following the 45-minute case you observe no respiratory effort. What is the best choice for this patient?

(A) Administer naloxone
(B) Maintain ventilatory support with sedation
(C) Administer neostigmine
(D) Check the ventilator settings

220. Considering hyperkalemia, rhabdomyolysis, and cardiac arrest which neuromuscular blocking agent will you avoid in children?

(A) Rocuronium
(B) Succinylcholine
(C) Atracurium
(D) Cisatracurium

221. Which medication blocks muscarinic receptors?

(A) Atropine
(B) Rocuronium
(C) Pyridostigmine
(D) Neostigmine

222. What part of the structure of glycopyrrolate is responsible for binding to acetylcholine receptors?

(A) Organic base
(B) Ester linkage
(C) Aromatic base
(D) Benzene ring

223. What manifestation occurs as a result of anticholinergic overdose?

(A) Tachycardia
(B) Oral secretions
(C) Bradycardia
(D) Cutaneous vasoconstriction

224. How is EMLA cream formulated?

(A) 1:1 mixture of 0.5% lidocaine and 0.5% prilocaine
(B) 2:1 mixture of 1.5% lidocaine and 2.5% prilocaine
(C) 1:1 mixture of 0.75% benzocaine and 0.5% lidocaine
(D) 2:1 mixture of 0.75% benzocaine and 1.5% lidocaine

225. During an inguinal hernia repair, the surgeon asks how much bupivacaine is allowed for local infiltration. What is the correct maximum dose?

(A) 12 mg/kg
(B) 8 mg/kg
(C) 4.5 mg/kg
(D) 3 mg/kg

226. How does the duration of epidural ropivacaine differ from lidocaine?

(A) The duration of lidocaine is shorter than ropivacaine.
(B) The duration of lidocaine and ropivacaine is similar.
(C) The duration of lidocaine is longer than ropivacaine.
(D) Ropivacaine is similar to all amides.

227. Which local anesthetic is metabolized by pseudocholinesterase?

(A) Lidocaine
(B) Bupivacaine
(C) Ropivacaine
(D) Tetracaine

228. Prolong neurological deficits have been associated with which local anesthetic?

(A) Epidural chloroprocaine
(B) EMLA
(C) Topical chloroprocaine
(D) Intrathecal lidocaine

229. What part of the body houses the greatest concentration of histamine?

(A) Parietal cells

(B) Circulating basophils and mast cells

(C) Gastric mucosa

(D) Peripheral tissues

230. Which cardiovascular effect occurs when administering diphenhydramine?

(A) Hypertension

(B) Peripheral arterioloar constriction

(C) Coronary vasoconstriction

(D) Hypotension

231. When administering promethazine, how long will sedative effects last?

(A) 3 to 6 hours

(B) 4 to 12 hours

(C) 8 to 24 hours

(D) 24 hours

232. Which of the following medications is potentiated by hydroxyzine?

(A) Midazolam

(B) Claritin

(C) Fexofenadine

(D) Metoclopramide

233. You include dexmedetomidine as an adjunct to general anesthesia. Which drug requirements will most likely decrease?

(A) Vecuronium

(B) Propofol

(C) Ephedrine

(D) Methoxamine

234. What is the primary receptor for phenylephrine?

(A) Beta-1

(B) Alpha-1

(C) Beta-2

(D) Alpha-2

235. How do direct and indirect adrenergic agonists differ?

(A) Indirect agonists bind to the receptor.

(B) Ephedrine binds to the receptor.

(C) Direct agonists bind to the receptor.

(D) Neosynephrine increases neurotransmitter activity.

236. What is the primary effect of phenylephrine?

(A) Peripheral vasoconstriction

(B) Decreased vascular resistance

(C) Increased heart rate

(D) Increased cardiac output

237. Which of the following halogenated agents potentiates the effects of epinephrine the most?

(A) Desflurane

(B) Sevoflurane

(C) Isoflurane

(D) Halothane

238. You plan to administer ephedrine for hypotension following spinal anesthesia. What do you expect?

(A) Decreased heart rate

(B) Decreased cardiac output

(C) Increased heart rate

(D) Short duration of action

239. How is ephedrine classified?

(A) Indirect beta-1 and beta-2 agonists

(B) Direct beta agonist

(C) Direct alpha agonist

(D) Indirect alpha-1, beta-1, and beta-2 agonists

240. What cardiac effect do you expect following administration of norepinephrine?

(A) Decreased heart rate

(B) Decreased mean arterial pressure

(C) Increased heart rate

(D) Decreased peripheral vascular resistance

241. You are planning to use clonidine during a general anesthetic. Primary receptor selectivity for clonidine includes which of the following?

(A) Alpha-2
(B) Beta-1
(C) Beta-2
(D) Alpha-1

242. Your patient is taking phenelzine. What is your primary concern when administering epinephrine to this patient?

(A) Profound increase in heart rate
(B) Lowered heart rate
(C) Increased heart rate
(D) Profound decrease in heart rate

243. You are administering an infusion of dopamine (0.5-3 mcg/kg/min). What do you anticipate?

(A) Beta-1 stimulation
(B) DA$_1$ stimulation
(C) Alpha-1 stimulation
(D) Beta-2 stimulation

244. A patient scheduled for an open bowel resection presents with congestive heart failure and well-documented coronary artery disease. You note the patient's heart rate is 98. Which of the following adrenergic agonists would be the best choice for this patient?

(A) Dobutamine
(B) Esmolol
(C) Phentolamine
(D) Norepinephrine

245. A patient presents for removal of a pheochromocytoma. Preoperatively, which medication is most useful?

(A) Phenoxybenzamine
(B) Labetolol
(C) Esmolol
(D) Norepinephrine

246. During metabolism of nitrates (nitroglycerin and sodium nitroprusside), what substance is released?

(A) Guanylyl cyclase
(B) cGMP
(C) Nitric oxide
(D) Nitrate

247. You are infusing sodium nitroprusside at 3 μg/kg/min. What condition is likely to result?

(A) Cyanide toxicity
(B) Adsorption of polyvinylchloride
(C) Increased afterload
(D) Cerebral vessel constriction

248. During esophageal surgery, the endotracheal tube catches fire. What will you do first?

(A) Call for help
(B) Remove the endotracheal tube
(C) Stop the gas flow and remove the endotracheal tube
(D) Remove the surgical drapes

249. The patient with rheumatoid arthritis complains of long-term throbbing joint pain. Which fibers are activated?

(A) Efferent A and C fibers
(B) Alpha and beta efferent fibers
(C) Afferent A and C fibers
(D) Alpha and beta afferent fibers

250. Why is the primary metabolite of tramadol significant?

(A) Greater potency than the parent drug
(B) Shorter elimination half-life than the parent drug
(C) Respiratory depression is not reversible with naloxone
(D) Safety profile when using MAO inhibitors

251. Following general anesthesia for right shoulder arthroscopy, the patient complains of pain. The patient's history includes congestive heart failure. Which analgesic will you avoid?

(A) Butorphanol

(B) Morphine

(C) Demerol

(D) Nalbuphine

252. Which drug would you avoid in an asthmatic patient?

(A) Volatile anesthetics

(B) Nitrous oxide

(C) Morphine

(D) Lidocaine

253. You decide to give butorphanol 2 mg to the patient postoperatively. What is the equipotent dose of morphine?

(A) 100 mg

(B) 8 mg

(C) 10 mg

(D) 80 mg

254. Your patient has a history of asthma. Which opioid will you avoid?

(A) Fentanyl

(B) Morphine

(C) Remifentanil

(D) Tramadol

255. How is remifentanil metabolized?

(A) Hepatic cytochrome P

(B) Hydrolysis by esterase enzymes

(C) Hepatic conjugation

(D) Conjugation with glucuronic acid

256. How does digoxin control atrial arrhythmias?

(A) Enhancing vagal tone

(B) Addition of calcium

(C) Decreased intracellular sodium

(D) Decreasing vagal tone

257. Your patient is undergoing a cholecystecomy with general endotracheal anesthesia. The patient takes digoxin for chronic congestive heart failure. What is the first sign of digitalis toxicity under anesthesia?

(A) Bradycardia

(B) Hypotension

(C) Arrhythmias

(D) Hypertension

258. What medication is indicated for treatment of ventricular fibrillation?

(A) Vasopressin

(B) Verapamil

(C) Ibutilide

(D) Adenosine

259. Why is terbutaline preferred for the treatment of asthma over bronkosol?

(A) Bronkosol's beta-1 adrenergic activity is less than terbutaline.

(B) Both bronchodilators are acceptable.

(C) Terbutaline's beta-1 adrenergic activity is less than bronkosol.

(D) Bronkosol's beta-2 activity is greater than terbutaline.

260. During the preoperative interview, you learn the patient takes daily lithium. How will lithium affect drugs used for general anesthesia?

(A) Shorten the duration of action of vecuronium

(B) Increase the MAC of isoflurane

(C) Increase the duration of action of vecuronium

(D) No interaction with lithium exists for drugs used during general anesthesia.

261. In reviewing the patient's record, you note daily use of lithium and hydrochlorothiazide. What do you expect?

(A) Hypernatremia

(B) Therapeutic lithium levels

(C) Decrease lithium levels

(D) Hyponatremia

262. You are called for an emergency exploratory laparoscopy. The patient was involved in a motor vehicle accident and appears intoxicated. What do you expect?

   (A) Increased requirements for fentanyl
   (B) Decreased requirements for midazolam
   (C) Increased requirements for sodium pentathol
   (D) Decreased requirements for amphetamines

263. Why do patients who take tranylcypromine need to avoid eating cheese?

   (A) Hypotensive crisis due to tyramine
   (B) Decreased agitation
   (C) Hypertensive crisis due to tyramine
   (D) Jaundice

264. Which narcotic will you avoid in patients taking MAO inhibitors?

   (A) Demerol
   (B) Fentanyl
   (C) Morphine
   (D) Sufentanil

265. Which of the following medications does not prolong the QT interval?

   (A) Fluoxetine
   (B) Sertraline
   (C) Azithromycin
   (D) Gentamicin

266. When treating hypotension for a patient taking doxepin what will you use?

   (A) Neosynephrine 10 μg IV
   (B) Ephedrine 5 mg IV
   (C) Neosynephrine 100 μg IV
   (D) Ephedrine 10 mg IV

267. Your patient is taking amitriptyline. What will you tell your patient about taking this drug?

   (A) Continue taking amitriptyline preoperatively.
   (B) Stop taking amitryptyline 24 hours before surgery.
   (C) Stop taking amitryptyline 1 week before surgery.
   (D) Stop taking amitryptyline 2 weeks before surgery.

268. Contractions weaken despite use of oxytocin. Prostaglandin is administered. What do you expect?

   (A) Constipation
   (B) Hypotension
   (C) Headache
   (D) Bronchodilation

269. The patient is scheduled for a cesarean section. You plan to use sevoflurane. How will this choice affect the uterus?

   (A) Increase uterine constriction
   (B) Decrease uterine bleeding
   (C) Increase uterine relaxation
   (D) Inhalational agents have no effect on the uterus.

270. Dantrolene was administered for malignant hyperthermia. What is the most serious complication?

   (A) Respiratory insufficiency
   (B) Aspiration pneumonia
   (C) Hepatic dysfunction
   (D) Generalized muscle weakness

271. What is the result of an excess of glucocorticoids?

   (A) Cushing's syndrome
   (B) Addison's disease
   (C) Conn syndrome
   (D) Pheochromocytoma

272. What is the most effective treatment for moderate to severe Parkinson's disease?

   (A) Levodopa
   (B) Nonergot derivatives
   (C) Levodopa with a decarboxylase inhibitor
   (D) Dopamine receptor agonists

273. The patient is scheduled for a thoracotomy. Upon review of the patient's medical history you note that lovastatin as part of the medical management. What will you tell the patient preoperatively?

   (A) Take the statin as directed prior to surgery.
   (B) Stop the statin immediately.
   (C) Stop the statin 1 week prior to surgery.
   (D) Stop the statin 2 weeks prior to surgery.

274. What is the percent of total body water in the intra-cellular compartment?

    (A) 25%
    (B) 8%
    (C) 100%
    (D) 67%

275. What is the major extracellular cation?

    (A) Sodium
    (B) Potassium
    (C) Magnesium
    (D) Chloride

276. What substance poorly penetrates through the capillary endothelium?

    (A) Oxygen
    (B) Water
    (C) Lipid-soluble substances
    (D) Plasma proteins

277. At what value do serious complications of hyponatremia manifest?

    (A) 150 mEq/L
    (B) 145 mEq/L
    (C) 130 mEq/L
    (D) 120 mEq/L

278. The patient presents for surgery, and you note a potassium level of 6 mEq/L. You choose to administer calcium gluconate. Which drug interaction is most concerning for this patient when administering calcium?

    (A) Digoxin
    (B) Furosemide
    (C) Kayexalate
    (D) Sodium bicarbonate

279. The patient presents with hypercalcemia secondary to a malignancy. What is the most effective means for lower serum calcium?

    (A) A loop diuretic followed by rehydration
    (B) Bisphosphonate
    (C) Rehydration followed by a loop diuretic
    (D) Etidronate

280. What target range is required for therapeutic effects of heparin?

    (A) ACT 200 to 400 seconds
    (B) aPTT 1.5 to 2.5 times the control value
    (C) ACT 100 to 200 seconds
    (D) aPTT 2.5 to 3.5 times the control value

281. Which statement is false regarding low molecular weight heparins (LMWHs)?

    (A) LMWHs prevent formation of prothrombinase.
    (B) Thrombolytic doses do not significantly cross the placenta.
    (C) Bioavailability is greater with LMWHs as compared to heparin.
    (D) Protamine is the antidote of choice for LMWHs.

282. The patient is taking subcutaneous unfractionated heparin. When is the best time to administer a spinal anesthetic?

    (A) 4 to 6 hours after heparin administration
    (B) 2 to 4 hours after heparin administration
    (C) 12 to 24 hours after heparin administration
    (D) 6 to 8 hours after heparin administration

283. What test is used to measure the effect of warfarin on blood coagulation?

    (A) aPTT
    (B) ACT
    (C) AT
    (D) INR

284. How does renal impairment affect insulin requirements?

    (A) Insulin requirements decrease.
    (B) No relationship exists between insulin requirements and renal impairment.
    (C) Insulin requirements increase.
    (D) The kidneys break down insulin to a greater extent.

285. What oral hypoglycemic is relatively contraindicated for patients with renal impairment?

   (A) Glyburide
   (B) Lipizide
   (C) Tolbutamide
   (D) Metformin

286. A patient with preexisting hypertension is undergoing an exploratory laparotomy. The blood pressure increases intraoperatively. What will you do first?

   (A) Give esmolol
   (B) Increase the concentration of isoflurane
   (C) Give labetalol
   (D) Decrease the concentration of isoflurane

287. A patient states they take nitroglycerin for angina. What statement is true regarding nitroglycerin's effect on the heart?

   (A) Decreases preload
   (B) Increases afterload
   (C) Increases preload
   (D) Decreases coronary vasodilatation

288. What patient history represents the greatest risk for cardiac complications?

   (A) Recent angina
   (B) Coronary artery disease involving two vessels
   (C) History of MI 1 year ago
   (D) Coronary artery disease involving three vessels

289. What characterizes a second-degree burn?

   (A) Penetrate epidermis and blisters form
   (B) Replace fluids for burns >10% of the total body surface area
   (C) Full thickness
   (D) Requires debridement

290. An adult male who weighs 100 kg is burned over 50% of his body. Using the Parkland formula, calculate the fluid requirements for the first 24 hours.

291. Which medication decreases the production of aqueous humor in glaucoma patients?

   (A) Pilocarpine
   (B) Solumedrol
   (C) Acetazolamide
   (D) Echothiophate

292. What signs and symptoms are associated with acute opioid intoxication?

   (A) Tachypnea and pinpoint pupils
   (B) Hypotension and pinpoint pupils
   (C) Dilated pupils and hypotension
   (D) Pinpoint pupils and hypertension

293. How does chronic alcohol ingestion affect anesthetic requirements including central nervous system hypnotics?

   (A) Decreases requirements
   (B) Increases requirements
   (C) No effect on anesthetic requirements
   (D) No effect with central nervous system hypnotics

294. Which of the following statements regarding cigarette smoking is true?

   (A) Carbon monoxide's affinity for hemoglobin is 100 times greater than oxygen.
   (B) Carboxyhemoglobin returns to normal following two nights without smoking.
   (C) Smoking cessation within 12 to 48 hours of surgery decreases circulating catecholamines.
   (D) Nicotine causes hypotension and tachycardia.

295. During the preoperative interview, the patient admits to the use of anabolic steroids. What implications for anesthesia are most concerning?

   (A) Impaired liver function and myocardial infarction
   (B) Cardiomyopathy
   (C) Behavioral disturbances
   (D) Atherosclerosis

296. The patient has a history of porphyria. What drug will you avoid?

(A) Methohexital

(B) Propofol

(C) Vecuronium

(D) Nitrous oxide

297. Which risk factor is not related to latex allergy?

(A) Allergy to passion fruit

(B) Greater than five surgical procedures

(C) Spina stenosis

(D) Chronic exposure to latex

298. What statement is true regarding trauma-induced coagulopathy?

(A) Tissue hyperperfusion results in coagulopathy.

(B) Thrombomodulin and activated protein C are released from the endothelium.

(C) Thrombomodulin binds to factor I.

(D) Thrombomodulin binds to protein C.

299. Which statement is false regarding epidural hematomas?

(A) It is typically associated with skull fractures.

(B) Patient may present conscious and then lapse into an unconscious state.

(C) When supratentorial hematomas exceed 30 mL volume, surgical decompression is used.

(D) It is typically associated with blunt force injury.

300. What condition results from a deficiency of Complement 1 esterase inhibitor?

(A) Angioedema

(B) Neutropenia

(C) Chronic granulomatous disease

(D) Chediak-Higashi syndrome

301. What statement is true regarding allergic reactions?

(A) Anaphylaxis is a Type II hypersensitivity reaction.

(B) Type II hypersensitivity include transfusion reactions.

(C) Angioedema is a Type II hypersensitivity reaction.

(D) Anaphylactoid reactions result due to an interaction with IgE.

302. Which classification of anesthetic agents is most linked to anaphylactic reactions?

(A) Thiobarbiturates

(B) Narcotics

(C) Benzodiazepines

(D) Muscle Relaxants

303. What statement about human immunodeficiency virus (HIV) infection and acquired immunodeficiency syndrome (AIDS) is true?

(A) AIDS is caused by a retrovirus.

(B) Seroconversion occurs 2 to 3 months following transmission of the HIV virus.

(C) Seroconversion occurs 4 to 6 weeks following transmission of the HIV virus.

(D) There is no contraindication for the use of spinal anesthesia.

304. What signs and symptoms are linked to the pathophysiology of septic shock?

(A) Hypervolemia and wide pulse pressure

(B) Bounding pulse and hypotension

(C) Bradycardia and narrow pulse pressure

(D) Hypotension and narrow pulse pressure

305. What is the recommended minimum liter flow to avoid renal injury when using Sevoflurane?

(A) 1 L/min

(B) 2 L/min

(C) 3 L/min

(D) 4 L/min

306. What percent of total cardiac output flows through the kidneys?

(A) 10 to 15%

(B) 20 to 25%

(C) 30 to 35%

(D) 40 to 45%

307. What is the normal glomerular filtration rate (GFR)?

(A) 440 mL/min

(B) 660 mL/min

(C) 1,200 mL/min

(D) 120 mL/min

308. What drug is associated with acute kidney injury?

(A) Halothane

(B) Demerol

(C) Radiocontrast dye

(D) Morphine

309. Which narcotic's metabolite is most likely to accumulate in patients with renal dysfunction?

(A) Fentanyl

(B) Demerol

(C) Remifentanil

(D) Morphine

310. What condition is most likely to cause complications during extracorporeal shock wave lithotripsy (ESWL)?

(A) Renal calculi <4 mm

(B) Cardiac arrhythmias

(C) Ecchymosis

(D) Skin blistering

311. What is the normal hepatic blood flow?

(A) 15 to 20%

(B) 25 to 30%

(C) 20 to 5%

(D) 30 to 35%

312. Which coagulation factor is not produced in the liver?

(A) Factor V

(B) Factor I

(C) Factor VIII

(D) Factor II

313. What factors cause a vitamin K deficiency?

(A) VI, IX, X

(B) VII, IX, X

(C) VIII, IX, X

(D) VII, IX, VI

314. What albumin level is associated with chronic liver disease?

(A) 3.5 g/dL

(B) 4.0 g/dL

(C) 4.5 g/dL

(D) 2.5 g/dL

315. Which of the following is false regarding prothrombin time (PT)?

(A) The normal PT range is 11 to 14 seconds.

(B) PT measures factors V, VII, X, finbrinogen, and prothrombin.

(C) PT assists in the evaluation of chronic and acute liver disease.

(D) PT is decreased in vitamin K deficiency.

316. What is the characteristic of hepatitis B?

(A) Incubation period 20 to 37 days

(B) Fecal-oral transmission

(C) Incubation period 60 to 110 days with progression to chronic liver disease

(D) No progression to chronic liver disease

317. What are the risk factors for halothane hepatitis?

(A) >40 years, female, and obese

(B) Male gender and obese

(C) Female gender and <40 years

(D) Obesity and smoker

318. When evaluating a patient with cirrhosis, what laboratory findings are expected?

(A) Increased bilirubin, decreased albumin, hyponatremia

(B) Increased albumin, hyponatremia

(C) Increased prothrombin time, hyponatremia

(D) Decreased albumin, hypernatremia, decreased belirubin

319. The intoxicated patient arrives for an emergent exploratory laparotomy following a motor vehicle accident. What statement is true regarding this scenario?

(A) Anesthetic requirements are increased.

(B) Alcohol increases MAC.

(C) Alcohol decreases GABA receptor activity.

(D) Alcohol inhibits NMDA receptors.

320. Which statement is true regarding the pneumatic tourniquet?

    (A) Hypertension occurs when the tourniquet is released.
    (B) Tissue hypoxia occurs within 2 minutes of application.
    (C) Metabolic alkalosis occurs after tourniquet release.
    (D) Core body temperature increases upon tourniquet release.

321. A 65-year-old patient presents for an open reduction and internal fixation following a hip fracture. The patient is short of breath, confused and you notice petechiae on the chest. What is the most likely cause?

    (A) Fat embolism syndrome
    (B) Mentation changes due to aging
    (C) Deep vein thrombosis
    (D) Thromboembolism

322. Which congenital cardiac malformation may benefit from a modified Blalock-Taussig shunt procedure?

    (A) Tetralogy of Fallot
    (B) Truncus arteriosus
    (C) Bicuspid atresia
    (D) Transposition of the great vessels

323. How does the National Asthma Education and Prevention Program Expert Panel Report 3 define asthma?

    (A) A chronic inflammatory disorder of the airways
    (B) Preventable and treatable disease state characterized by airflow limitation that is not fully reversible
    (C) Mechanical obstruction to breathing that occurs during sleep
    (D) Right heart failure secondary to pulmonary pathology

324. How is the clinical diagnosis of chronic bronchitis made?

    (A) Presence of a productive cough on most days of 3 consecutive months for at least 2 consecutive years
    (B) Presence of an occasional productive cough for 2 consecutive months for at least 1 year
    (C) Presence of a productive cough on most days of 3 consecutive weeks for at least 2 consecutive months
    (D) Presence of a productive cough on 3 consecutive days for at least 2 consecutive weeks

325. Which congenital cardiac malformation includes a right-to-left intracardiac shunt?

    (A) Tetralogy of Fallot
    (B) Atrial septal defect
    (C) Ventricular septal defect
    (D) Patent ductus arteriosus

326. Which disease does not place the patient at increased risk for developing cor pulmonale?

    (A) Adenotonsillar hypertrophy
    (B) Chronic obstructive pulmonary disease
    (C) Obesity
    (D) Eaton-Lambert syndrome

327. What is indicated by an apnea/hypopnea index of 42 occurrences per hour?

    (A) Normal result
    (B) Mild obstructive sleep apnea
    (C) Moderate sleep apnea
    (D) Severe sleep apnea

328. What is the most common cause of obstructive sleep apnea?

    (A) Ondine's curse
    (B) Obesity
    (C) Muscular dystrophy
    (D) Central apnea

329. Which structure is commonly occluded in obstructive hydrocephalus?

   (A) Choroid plexus
   (B) Foramen of Monro
   (C) Aqueduct of Sylvius
   (D) Foramen of Magendie

330. Which state should be avoided during the anesthetic care of a patient with multiple sclerosis?

   (A) Hyperthermia
   (B) Hyperoxia
   (C) Hypercapnia
   (D) Hypertension

331. What causes weakness in myasthenia gravis?

   (A) Autoimmune damage to nerve axons
   (B) Damage to presynaptic calcium channels
   (C) Damage to postsynaptic cholinergic receptors
   (D) Autoimmune damage to type I muscle fibers

332. What would be the effect on muscle strength if a patient with myasthenia gravis were treated with an anticholinesterase?

   (A) No change
   (B) Decreased strength
   (C) Increased strength

333. Is an aneurysm in the brain more likely to occur in a larger vessel or a smaller vessel? Why?

   (A) Equally likely in either a large or small vessel because blood pressure is constant
   (B) More likely in a larger vessel due to increased diameter
   (C) More likely in a smaller vessel due to increased resistance
   (D) More likely in a smaller vessel due to decreased flow

334. Which level of spinal cord injury is most associated with autonomic hyperreflexia?

   (A) T_5–T_8
   (B) T_{10}–L_1
   (C) L_1–L_4
   (D) L_4–S_1

335. What is the most important cervical radiographic finding in a patient with rheumatoid arthritis?

   (A) Cervical stenosis
   (B) Cervical spondylosis
   (C) Atlantoaxial subluxation
   (D) Lordosis

336. What is the most common form of muscular dystrophy?

   (A) Becker
   (B) Limb-girdle
   (C) Myotonic
   (D) Duchenne

337. Which statement is true regarding Duchenne muscular dystrophy?

   (A) The disease is X-linked and occurs more frequently in girls.
   (B) The disease occurs equally in boys and girls and is diagnosed in early childhood.
   (C) The disease is X-linked and symptoms occur only in boys.
   (D) The disease primarily manifests as contractures of the large joints.

338. What is the anesthetic implication of a patient taking tricyclic antidepressants who is scheduled to receive general anesthesia?

   (A) Meperidine will produce skeletal muscle rigidity and hyperpyrexia.
   (B) Tricyclic antidepressants should be discontinued 2 weeks before surgery.
   (C) MAC requirements may be increased for inhaled anesthetics.
   (D) Ephedrine is preferred agent to treat post-induction hypotension.

339. Which characteristic is not shared by malignant hyperthermia and neuroleptic malignant syndrome?

   (A) Generalized muscular rigidity
   (B) Flaccid paralysis after vecuronium administration
   (C) Effectively treated with dantrolene
   (D) Hyperthermia

340. A patient is taking an MAO inhibitor. What anesthetic agent can be safely used in this patient?

(A) Phenylephrine
(B) Ketamine
(C) Bupivacaine with epinephrine
(D) Pancuronium

341. A 25-year-old 50-kg otherwise healthy patient complains of nausea and demonstrates vomiting, refractory to ondansetron and dexamethasone therapy. Which dose of droperidol will achieve a safe therapeutic response?

(A) 1.25 mg IV
(B) 0.625 mg/kg IV
(C) 0.5 mg IV
(D) 12.5 mg IV

342. Which statement about phenytoin is correct?

(A) Chronic phenytoin therapy requires higher dose requirements of vecuronium.
(B) Chronic phenytoin therapy requires lower dose requirements of vecuronium.
(C) Chronic phenytoin therapy requires higher dose requirements of succinylcholine.
(D) Chronic phenytoin therapy requires lower dose requirements of succinylcholine.

343. Which statement about gabapentin is false?

(A) Gabapentin is not bound to plasma proteins.
(B) Gabapentin is an effective monotherapy for partial seizures.
(C) Gabapentin is unable to cross blood–brain barrier.
(D) Gabapentin undergoes no metabolism.

344. For which pathophysiologic state would gabapentin not be prescribed for management?

(A) Postherpatic neuralgia
(B) Diabetic neuropathy
(C) Acute postoperative pain adjuvant
(D) Status epilepticus

345. Which neuromuscular disease is associated with increased resistance to succinylcholine?

(A) Myasthenic syndrome
(B) Myasthenia gravis
(C) Myotonic dystrophy
(D) Muscular dystrophy

346. What is the initial dose of dantrolene for a 74-kg man in acute malignant hyperthermia crisis?

(A) 150 mg
(B) 185 mg
(C) 200 mg
(D) 215 mg

347. Which of the following is a late sign of malignant hyperthermia?

(A) Increased end-tidal carbon dioxide
(B) Increased heart rate
(C) Increased temperature
(D) Masseter rigidity

348. Which disease is least likely to be associated with malignant hyperthermia?

(A) King syndrome
(B) Central-core disease
(C) Multi-minicore myopathy
(D) Duchenne muscular dystrophy

349. Which would be expected in a patient with Graves' disease?

(A) Increased thyroid stimulating hormone with decreased thyroid hormone
(B) Increased thyroid stimulating hormone with increased thyroid hormone
(C) Decreased thyroid stimulating hormone with decreased thyroid hormone
(D) Decreased thyroid stimulating hormone with increased thyroid hormone

350. Which diagnosis indicates adrenal insufficiency?

(A) Addison's disease
(B) Conn syndrome
(C) Cushing's disease
(D) Mendelsohn syndrome

351. Which is secreted from the posterior pituitary?

(A) Antidiuretic hormone

(B) Adrenocorticotropic hormone

(C) Prolactin

(D) Thyroid stimulating hormone

352. What causes acromegaly?

(A) Hypersecretion of adrenocorticotropic hormone

(B) Hypersecretion of thyroid stimulating hormone

(C) Hypersecretion of growth hormone

(D) Hypersecretion of prolactin

353. What condition results from hypersecretion of growth hormone in a child?

(A) Acromegaly

(B) Dwarfism

(C) Osteomalacia

(D) Gigantism

354. Which common anesthetic medication should be avoided during the induction of a patient diagnosed with acute intermittent porphyria?

(A) Sufentanil

(B) Propofol

(C) Etomidate

(D) Fentanyl

355. Which correctly describes acute intermittent porphyria?

(A) Accumulation of delta-aminolevulinic acid and porphobilinogen secondary to porphobilinogen deaminase deficiency

(B) Accumulation of protoporphyrin secondary to protoporphyrinogen oxidase deficiency

(C) Accumulation of delta-aminolevulinic acid and protoporphyrin secondary to ferrochelatase deficiency

(D) Accumulation of delta-aminolevulinic acid and coproporphyrinogen secondary to coproporphyrinogen oxidase deficiency

356. Which are secreted by tumors in carcinoid syndrome?

(A) Ocotreotide

(B) Serotonin, kallikrein, histamine

(C) Interferon alpha

(D) Capecitabine

357. What is the most likely location of a carcinoid tumor?

(A) Kidney

(B) Lung

(C) Ovary

(D) Appendix

358. What is the typical progression of Guillain-Barré syndrome?

(A) Descending paralysis

(B) Unilateral hemiparesis

(C) Ascending paralysis

(D) Concurrent upper and lower extremity weakness

359. Which neuromuscular blocking agent is most appropriate for use in severe cirrhosis?

(A) Cisatracurium

(B) Rocuronium

(C) Vecuronium

(D) Pancuronium

360. Which drugs will be prolonged in the glaucoma patient treated with echothiophate?

(A) Cocaine and succinylcholine

(B) Succinylcholine and chloroprocaine

(C) Glycopyrrolate and succinylcholine

(D) Chloroprocaine and glycopyrrolate

361. What causes Eaton-Lambert syndrome?

(A) Autoimmune destruction of calcium channels

(B) Atypical pseudocholinesterase

(C) Autoimmune destruction of cholinergic receptors

(D) Autoimmune destruction of thyroid tissue

362. Which abnormality is associated with syringomyelia?

    (A) Craniosynostosis
    (B) Crouzon's syndrome
    (C) Arnold-Chiari malformation
    (D) Apert syndrome

363. Which causes Zollinger-Ellison syndrome?

    (A) Gastrinoma
    (B) Pheochromocytoma
    (C) Pituitary adenoma
    (D) Osteosarcoma

364. A patient's cardiac assessment reveals a functional capacity of four metabolic equivalents. What activity can she most likely perform?

    (A) Walk one to two blocks on level ground
    (B) Singles tennis
    (C) Cross-country skiing
    (D) Swimming

365. What factors may cause a flow volume loop to change?

    (A) Pulmonary and airway compliance
    (B) Airway compliance and increased fluid volume
    (C) Increased fluid volume and pulmonary compliance
    (D) Patent airways

366. Meperidine's effectiveness in reducing postoperative shivering is due to its action on _____ receptors in the hypothalamus.

    (A) Kappa
    (B) Delta
    (C) GABA
    (D) Mu_1

367. Which opioid may cause delayed respiratory depression 8 to 12 hours following subarachnoid administration?

    (A) Fentanyl
    (B) Morphine
    (C) Sufentanil
    (D) Alfentanil

368. Which drug provides analgesia at the level of the spinal cord by binding to pre- and postsynaptic alpha-2 receptors?

    (A) Nortriptyl
    (B) Clonidine
    (C) Venlafaxine
    (D) Duloxetine

369. Substance P primarily works on which receptor?

    (A) Neurokinin-1
    (B) 5 HT
    (C) Interleukin-1
    (D) NMDA

370. What type of pain is well localized, sharp in nature, and generally hurts at the point or area of the stimulus?

    (A) Visceral
    (B) Musculoskeletal
    (C) Neuropathic
    (D) Somatic

371. Within the pain pathway, what region of the brain does secondary afferent neurons synapse with third-order neurons?

    (A) Thalamus
    (B) Periaqueductal gray area
    (C) Cerebral cortex
    (D) Amygdala

372. Which fibers are primarily responsible for nociception?

    (A) A-alpha fibers
    (B) Beta fibers
    (C) A-delta and C fibers
    (D) C-delta fibers

373. What is physiologic process where a noxious mechanical, chemical, or thermal stimulus is converted into an electrical impulse called an action potential?

    (A) Transmission
    (B) Transduction
    (C) Perception
    (D) Modulation

Answers and Explanations: Basic Sciences

1. What results when alpha-1 receptors are activated?

   (A) Presynaptic nerve terminals are stimulated.
   (B) Adenylate cyclase activity is inhibited.
   (C) Negative feedback loop inhibits norepineph-rine release.
   (D) Intracellular calcium ion concentration increases.

   Rationale: Alpha-1 receptors activate postsynatptic adrenoceptors. Alpha-2 receptors are located presynaptically. Adenylate cyclase activity is inhibited when alpha-2 receptors are activated. Calcium ion concentration decreases creating a negative feedback loop that inhibits norepinephrine release.
   Reference: Butterworth JF IV, Mackey DC, Wasnick JD, eds. *Morgan & Mikhail's Clinical Anesthesiology.* 7th ed. New York, NY: McGraw Hill; 2022: Chapter 14.

2. Which initial intervention is correct if pulmonary embolism is suspected?

   (A) Discontinue intravenous fluids
   (B) Increase FiO$_2$
   (C) Extubate the patient
   (D) Discontinue inotropic support

   Rationale: Increase intravenous fluids, keep the patient intubated, provide inotropic support, and increase FiO$_2$.
   References: Butterworth JF IV, Mackey DC, Wasnick JD, eds. *Morgan & Mikhail's Clinical Anesthesiology.* 7th ed. New York, NY: McGraw Hill; 2022: Chapter 24.
   Elisha S, Heiner JS, Nagelhout JJ. *Nurse Anesthesia.* 7th ed. St. Louis, MO: Elsevier Saunders; 2023: Chapter 32.

3. Which anticholinergic increases heart rate the most?

   (A) Scopolamine
   (B) Glycopyrrolate
   (C) Atropine
   (D) Pyridostigmine

   Rationale: While all anticholinergics increase heart rate, scopolamine exerts the least effect followed by glycopyrrolate. Pyridostigmine is a cholinesterase inhibitor.
   Reference: Butterworth JF IV, Mackey DC, Wasnick JD, eds. *Morgan & Mikhail's Clinical Anesthesiology.* 7th ed. New York, NY: McGraw Hill; 2022: Chapter 13.

4. What is the normal V/Q ratio?

   (A) 1
   (B) 0.8
   (C) 2
   (D) 0.5

   Rationale: Normally, ventilation (V) is approximately 4 L/min, whereas pulmonary blood flow (Q) is approximately 5 L/min. Therefore, the ventilation-perfusion ratio (V/Q) for the whole lung is 0.8.
   References: Butterworth JF IV, Mackey DC, Wasnick JD, eds. *Morgan & Mikhail's Clinical Anesthesiology.* 7th ed. New York, NY: McGraw Hill; 2022: Chapter 23.
   Elisha S, Heiner JS, Nagelhout JJ. *Nurse Anesthesia.* 7th ed. St. Louis, MO: Elsevier Saunders; 2023: Chapter 29.

5. What is the underlying pathology of cor pulmonale?

   (A) Pulmonary hypertension
   (B) Decreased pulmonary vascular resistance
   (C) Systemic hypertension
   (D) Orthostatic hypotension

   Rationale: The underlying pathology of cor pulmonale is pulmonary hypertension.
   References: Butterworth JF IV, Mackey DC, Wasnick JD, eds. *Morgan & Mikhail's Clinical Anesthesiology.* 7th ed. New York, NY: McGraw Hill; 2022: Chapter 24.
   Elisha S, Heiner JS, Nagelhout JJ. *Nurse Anesthesia.* 7th ed. St. Louis, MO: Elsevier Saunders; 2023: Chapter 29.

6. What is the blood to gas partition coefficient of Halothane?

(A) 0.47

(B) 0.65

(C) 1.4

(D) 2.4

Rationale: The blood to gas partition coefficient of nitrous oxide is 0.47; sevoflurane is 0.65; and isoflurane is 1.4.

TABLE 1-1. Partition coefficients of volatile anesthetics at 37°C.[1]

Agent	Blood/Gas	Brain/Blood	Muscle/Blood	Fat/Blood
Nitrous oxide	0.47	1.1	1.2	2.3
Halothane	2.4	2.9	3.5	60
Isoflurane	1.4	2.6	4.0	45
Desflurane	0.42	1.3	2.0	27
Sevoflurane	0.65	1.7	3.1	48

[1]These values are averages derived from multiple studies and should be used for comparison purposes, not as exact numbers.
(Reproduced with permission from Butterworth JF IV, Mackey DC, Wasnick JD, eds. *Morgan & Mikhail's Clinical Anesthesiology.* 7th ed. New York, NY: McGraw Hill; 2022.)

Reference: Butterworth JF IV, Mackey DC, Wasnick JD, eds. *Morgan & Mikhail's Clinical Anesthesiology.* 7th ed. New York, NY: McGraw Hill; 2022: Chapter 8.

7. Which inhalational agent is a halogenated alkane?

(A) Halothane

(B) Nitrous oxide

(C) Desflurane

(D) Sevoflurane

Rationale: Nitrous oxide is an inorganic anesthetic gas. Desflurane and sevoflurane are halogenated with fluorine.

Reference: Butterworth JF IV, Mackey DC, Wasnick JD, eds. *Morgan & Mikhail's Clinical Anesthesiology.* 7th ed. New York, NY: McGraw Hill; 2022: Chapter 8.

8. How would you classify a patient with repeated blood pressure measurements ranging from 160/100 to 179/109?

(A) High normal

(B) Stage 1 hypertension

(C) Stage 2 hypertension

(D) Stage 3 hypertension

Rationale: Stage two or moderate hypertension is defined as systolic pressure between 160 and 179 mmHg and diastolic pressure between 100 and 109 mmHg.

References: Butterworth JF IV, Mackey DC, Wasnick JD, eds. *Morgan & Mikhail's Clinical Anesthesiology.* 7th ed. New York, NY: McGraw Hill; 2022: Chapter 21.

Elisha S, Heiner JS, Nagelhout JJ. *Nurse Anesthesia.* 7th ed. St. Louis, MO: Elsevier Saunders; 2023: Chapter 21.

9. Which condition is not associated with precipitating unstable angina?

(A) Polycythemia

(B) Anemia

(C) Thyrotoxicosis

(D) Emotional stress

Rationale: Unstable angina can be precipitated by anemia, thyrotoxicosis, emotional stress, or anything that causes myocardial ischemia due to an increased oxygen demand.

References: Butterworth JF IV, Mackey DC, Wasnick JD, eds. *Morgan & Mikhail's Clinical Anesthesiology.* 7th ed. New York, NY: McGraw Hill; 2022: Chapter 21.

Hines RL, Marschall KE. Chapter 1. *Stoelting's Anesthesia and Co-existing Disease.* 7th ed. Philadelphia, PA: Elsevier Saunders; 2018.

10. Which neuromuscular blocking drug is contraindicated during the care of a patient with Guillain-Barré syndrome?

(A) Succinylcholine

(B) Rocuronium

(C) Atracurium

(D) Pancuronium

Rationale: The risk of severe hyperkalemia with succinylcholine is a contraindication.

References: Butterworth JF IV, Mackey DC, Wasnick JD, eds. *Morgan & Mikhail's Clinical Anesthesiology.* 7th ed. New York, NY: McGraw Hill; 2022: Chapter 28.

Gropper MA, Cohen NH, Eriksson LI, et al, eds. *Miller's Anesthesia.* 9th ed. Philadelphia, PA: Churchill Livingstone Elsevier; 2020: Chapter 37.

11. Which lung pathology is a form of COPD?

(A) Asthma

(B) Cystic fibrosis

(C) Aspiration pneumonitis

(D) Emphysema

Rationale: Emphysema and chronic bronchitis provide the prototype of pathological changes in COPD.

References: Butterworth JF IV, Mackey DC, Wasnick JD, eds. *Morgan & Mikhail's Clinical Anesthesiology.* 7th ed. New York, NY: McGraw Hill; 2022: Chapter 24.
Elisha S, Heiner JS, Nagelhout JJ. *Nurse Anesthesia.* 7th ed. St. Louis, MO: Elsevier Saunders; 2023: Chapter 29.

12. Which is a normal functional residual capacity?

    (A) 500 mL
    (B) 1,200 mL
    (C) 2,300 mL
    (D) 1,100 mL

    Rationale: (A) is tidal volume, (B) residual volume and (D) is expiratory reserve volume. Functional residual capacity is a combination of maximal volume that can be expired below tidal volume and the volume remaining after maximal exhalation.
    References: Butterworth JF IV, Mackey DC, Wasnick JD, eds. *Morgan & Mikhail's Clinical Anesthesiology.* 7th ed. New York, NY: McGraw Hill; 2022: Chapter 23.
    Elisha S, Heiner JS, Nagelhout JJ. *Nurse Anesthesia.* 7th ed. St. Louis, MO: Elsevier Saunders; 2023: Chapter 29.

13. What are the three most used pharmacological agents for treating ischemic heart disease?

    (A) Nitrates, alpha-blockers, and ACE-inhibitors
    (B) Nitrates, beta-blockers, and calcium channel blockers
    (C) Beta-blockers, calcium channel blockers, and ACE-inhibitors
    (D) Calcium channel blockers, nitrates, and ARBs

    Rationale: Nitrates, beta-blockers, and calcium channel blockers are the most used pharmacological agents for treating ischemic heart disease.
    References: Butterworth JF IV, Mackey DC, Wasnick JD, eds. *Morgan & Mikhail's Clinical Anesthesiology.* 7th ed. New York, NY: McGraw Hill; 2022: Chapter 21.
    Hines RL, Marschall KE. *Stoelting's Anesthesia and Co-existing Disease.* 7th ed. Philadelphia, PA: Elsevier Saunders; 2018: Chapter 1.

14. Which narcotic does not cause histamine release?

    (A) Fentanyl
    (B) Morphine
    (C) Hydromorphone
    (D) Meperidine

Rationale: Lowered systemic vascular resistance results from bolus doses of morphine, hydromorphone, and meperidine. Fentanyl administration may result in vagus-mediated bradycardia.
Reference: Butterworth JF IV, Mackey DC, Wasnick JD, eds. *Morgan & Mikhail's Clinical Anesthesiology.* 7th ed. New York, NY: McGraw Hill; 2022: Chapter 10.

15. Which of the following occurs following administration of morphine?

    (A) Increased hypoxic drive
    (B) Decreased apneic threshold
    (C) Decreased hypoxic drive
    (D) Decreased $PaCO_2$

    Rationale: When administering narcotics, the hypoxic drive decreases as the $PaCO_2$ increases along with the apneic threshold.

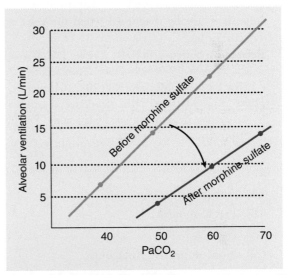

FIG. 1-1. Opioids depress ventilation. This is graphically displayed by a shift of the carbon dioxide (CO_2) curve downward and to the right. (Reproduced with permission from Butterworth JF IV, Mackey DC, Wasnick JD, eds. *Morgan & Mikhail's Clinical Anesthesiology.* 7th ed. New York, NY: McGraw Hill; 2022.)

Reference: Butterworth JF IV, Mackey DC, Wasnick JD, eds. *Morgan & Mikhail's Clinical Anesthesiology.* 7th ed. New York, NY: McGraw Hill; 2022: Chapter 10.

16. The patient is shivering in the postanesthesia care unit. Which intravenous medication will you use?

    (A) Meperidine 10 to 25 mg
    (B) Fentanyl 25 µg
    (C) Morphine 5 mg
    (D) Hyromorphone 5 mg

Rationale: Compared to other narcotics, meperidine 10 to 25 mg IV decreases shivering in postoperative patients.

Reference: Butterworth JF IV, Mackey DC, Wasnick JD, eds. *Morgan & Mikhail's Clinical Anesthesiology.* 7th ed. New York, NY: McGraw Hill; 2022: Chapter 10.

17. A patient with mitral valve stenosis is asymptomatic with occasional mild symptoms upon exertion. Which mitral valve area is associated with these symptoms?

    (A) 0.2 to 0.5 cm^2
    (B) 0.5 to 1.0 cm^2
    (C) 1.5 to 2.0 cm^2
    (D) 2.0 to 2.5 cm

    Rationale: Patients with valve areas between 1.5 and 2.0 cm^2 are usually asymptomatic or have only mild symptoms with exertion. Critical mitral stenosis is associated with valve are 0.5 to 1.0 cm^2 or less. Mitral stenosis is usually diagnosed when the valve area is 1.5 cm^2 or less.

    References: Butterworth JF IV, Mackey DC, Wasnick JD, eds. *Morgan & Mikhail's Clinical Anesthesiology.* 7th ed. New York, NY: McGraw Hill; 2022: Chapter 21.
    Hines RL, Marschall KE. *Stoelting's Anesthesia and Co-existing Disease.* 7th ed. Philadelphia, PA: Elsevier Saunders; 2018: Chapter 2.

18. Which term describes full drug activation of a receptor?

    (A) Antagonist
    (B) Partial agonist
    (C) Agonist
    (D) Noncompetitive Antagonist

    Rationale: Drugs that are agonists fully activate a receptor. Partial agonists activate parts of a receptor. Antagonists bind, but do not activate receptors. Noncompetitive antagonists irreversibly bind to a receptor.

    References: Elisha S, Heiner JS, Nagelhout JJ. *Nurse Anesthesia.* 7th ed. St. Louis, MO: Elsevier Saunders; 2023: Chapter 5.
    Pardo MC, Miller RD. *Miller's Basics of Anesthesia.* 8th ed. Philadelphia, PA: Elsevier; 2023: Chapter 4.

19. A 60-year-old female with mitral valve stenosis has the following post-induction vital signs: HR-125, B/P-70/45 followed by sudden supraventricular tachycardia (SVT). What will you do first?

    (A) Cardioversion
    (B) Ephedrine

    (C) Phenylephrine
    (D) Vasopressin

    Rationale: Marked hemodynamic deterioration in a patient with mitral stenosis from sudden SVT is cause for immediate cardioversion.

    References: Butterworth JF IV, Mackey DC, Wasnick JD, eds. *Morgan & Mikhail's Clinical Anesthesiology.* 7th ed. New York, NY: McGraw Hill; 2022: Chapter 21.
    Hines RL, Marschall KE. *Stoelting's Anesthesia and Co-existing Disease.* 7th ed. Philadelphia, PA: Elsevier Saunders; 2018: Chapter 2.

20. Which adrenergic agonist has the greatest effect on heart rate?

    (A) Norepinephrine
    (B) Dobutamine
    (C) Ephedrine
    (D) Isoproterenol

    Rationale: Heart rate is affected least by phenylephrine and norepinephrine (decreased); and ephedrine (increased). Administering isoproterenol increases heart rate the greatest.

    Reference: Butterworth JF IV, Mackey DC, Wasnick JD, eds. *Morgan & Mikhail's Clinical Anesthesiology.* 7th ed. New York, NY: McGraw Hill; 2022: Chapter 14.

21. What is the onset of analgesia following administration of epidural morphine 5 mg?

    (A) 30 to 60 minutes
    (B) 15 to 30 minutes
    (C) 5 to 15 minutes
    (D) 60 minutes

    Rationale: The onset of epidural morphine is 30 to 60 minutes. The duration of analgesia is 12 to 24 hours. Larger doses of epidural morphine are needed for analgesia. However, delayed respiratory depression may result.

    Reference: Butterworth JF IV, Mackey DC, Wasnick JD, eds. *Morgan & Mikhail's Clinical Anesthesiology.* 7th ed. New York, NY: McGraw Hill; 2022: Chapter 41.

22. Which of the following local anesthetics and dosages are used for cesarean section with spinal anesthesia?

    (A) Lidocaine (100 mg)
    (B) Tetracaine (14 mg)
    (C) Bupivacaine (12 mg)
    (D) Mepivacaine (16 mg)

Rationale: The dose of spinal lidocaine for cesarean section is 50 to 60 mg; bupivacaine (10-15 mg); and tetracaine (7-10 mg). Mepivacaine is not administered for spinal anesthesia for cesarean section.

Reference: Butterworth JF IV, Mackey DC, Wasnick JD, eds. *Morgan & Mikhail's Clinical Anesthesiology.* 7th ed. New York, NY: McGraw Hill; 2022: Chapter 41.

23. Which anticholinergic is classified as a quaternary amine?

    (A) Scopolamine

    (B) Atropine

    (C) Neostigmine

    (D) Glycopyrrolate

Rationale: Atropine and scopolamine are classified as tertiary amines. Neostigmine contains a quaternary ammonium.

Reference: Butterworth JF IV, Mackey DC, Wasnick JD, eds. *Morgan & Mikhail's Clinical Anesthesiology.* 7th ed. New York, NY: McGraw Hill; 2022: Chapter 13.

24. Which anticholinergic cannot cross the blood–brain barrier?

    (A) Glycopyrrolate

    (B) Atropine

    (C) Scopolamine

    (D) Scopolamine and atropine

Rationale: Tertiary amines atropine and scopolamine easily cross the blood–brain barrier.

Quaternary amines (glycopyrrolate) are unable to cross the blood–brain barrier.

Reference: Butterworth JF IV, Mackey DC, Wasnick JD, eds. *Morgan & Mikhail's Clinical Anesthesiology.* 7th ed. New York, NY: McGraw Hill; 2022: Chapter 13.

25. Which variable increases minimal alveolar concentration (MAC)?

    (A) Hypernatremia

    (B) Hyperthermia

    (C) Acute intoxication

    (D) Ketamine

Rationale: Hyperthermia, acute intoxication, and ketamine decrease MAC. Hypernatremia increases MAC.

Reference: Butterworth JF IV, Mackey DC, Wasnick JD, eds. *Morgan & Mikhail's Clinical Anesthesiology.* 7th ed. New York, NY: McGraw Hill; 2022: Chapter 8.

TABLE 1-2. Factors affecting MAC.[1]

Variable	Effect on MAC	Comments
Temperature		
Hypothermia	↓	↑ if >42°C
Hyperthermia	↓	
Age		
Young	↑	
Older adult	↓	
Alcohol		
Acute intoxication	↓	
Chronic abuse	↑	
Anemia		
Hematocrit <10%	↓	
PaO_2		
<40 mmHg	↓	
$PaCO_2$		Caused by <pH in CSF
>95 mmHg	↓	
Thyroid		
Hyperthyroid	No change	
Hypothyroid	No change	
Blood pressure		
Mean arterial pressure <40 mmHg	↓	
Electrolytes		
Hypercalcemia	↓	Caused by altered CSF
Hypernatremia	↑	Caused by altered CSF
Hyponatremia	↓	
Pregnancy	↓	MAC decreased by one-third at 8 weeks' gestation; normal by 72-hour postpartum
Drugs		Except cocaine
Local anesthetics	↓	Except cocaine
Opioids	↓	
Ketamine	↓	
Barbiturates	↓	
Benzodiazepines	↓	
Verapamil	↓	
Lithium	↓	
Sympatholytics	↓	
Methyldopa	↓	
Clonidine	↓	
Dexmedetomidine	↓	
Sympathomimetics	↑	
Amphetamine		
Chronic	↓	
Acute		
Cocaine		
Ephedrine		

[1]These conclusions are based on human and animal studies.
CSF, cerebrospinal fluid; MAC, minimum alveolar concentration.
(Reproduced with permission from Butterworth JF IV, Mackey DC, Wasnick JD, eds. *Morgan & Mikhail's Clinical Anesthesiology.* 7th ed. New York, NY: McGraw Hill; 2022.)

26. Which factors will exacerbate mitral regurgitation?

    (A) Tachycardia and acute increases in afterload
    (B) Tachycardia and acute decreases in afterload
    (C) Bradycardia and acute increases in afterload
    (D) Bradycardia and acute decreases in afterload

    Rationale: Although the anesthetic management will be tailored according to the severity of the mitral regurgitation, factors such as slow heart rate and acute increases in afterload should be avoided to prevent exacerbation of disease. A normal to slightly fast heart rate as well as afterload reduction will improve forward flow.

    References: Butterworth JF IV, Mackey DC, Wasnick JD, eds. *Morgan & Mikhail's Clinical Anesthesiology.* 7th ed. New York, NY: McGraw Hill; 2022: Chapter 21.

    Hines RL, Marschall KE. *Stoelting's Anesthesia and Co-existing Disease.* 7th ed. Philadelphia, PA: Elsevier Saunders; 2018: Chapter 2.

27. Which volumes are included in vital capacity?

    (A) Tidal volume and residual volume
    (B) Residual volume and expiratory reserve volume
    (C) Expiratory reserve volume and inspiratory capacity volume
    (D) Inspiratory capacity volume and residual volume

    Rationale: Expiratory reserve volume and inspiratory capacity volume comprise vital capacity.

    References: Butterworth JF IV, Mackey DC, Wasnick JD, eds. *Morgan & Mikhail's Clinical Anesthesiology.* 7th ed. New York, NY: McGraw Hill; 2022: Chapter 23.

    Elisha S, Heiner JS, Nagelhout JJ. *Nurse Anesthesia.* 7th ed. St. Louis, MO: Elsevier Saunders; 2023:Chapter 29.

28. Your patient's hemodynamic profile is as follows: HR = 100 beats/min, cardiac output (CO) = 5.0 L/min, end-diastolic volume (EDV) = 100 mL. **Calculate the ejection fraction and write answer in the box below:**

50		%

    Rationale:

    STEP 1: $EF = \dfrac{EDV - ESV}{EDV} = \dfrac{SV}{EDV}$

    STEP 2: Must realize that SV is not given but can be calculated from: $CO = HR \times SV$

STEP 3:

$$EF = \frac{CO/HR}{EDV} = \frac{5{,}000\,mL/100}{100} = \frac{50}{100} = \frac{1}{2} = 0.50$$

STEP 4: Convert to % by multiplying $\times\, 100 = 50\%$

References: Butterworth JF IV, Mackey DC, Wasnick JD, eds. *Morgan & Mikhail's Clinical Anesthesiology.* 7th ed. New York, NY: McGraw Hill; 2022: Chapter 20.

Elisha S, Heiner JS, Nagelhout JJ. *Nurse Anesthesia.* 7th ed. St. Louis, MO: Elsevier Saunders; 2023: Chapter 25.

29. What classic triad of symptoms is associated with aortic stenosis with a valve area <1 cm^2?

    (A) Hypotension, dyspnea on exertion, and pulmonary congestion
    (B) Hoarseness, chest pain, and pulmonary emboli
    (C) Chest pains, arrhythmias, and embolic events
    (D) Dyspnea on exertion, angina, and exertional syncope

    Rationale: Patients with advanced aortic stenosis have a classic triad of symptoms: dyspnea on exertion (usually associated with congestive heart failure), angina, and exertional syncope. (A) is associated with mitral regurgitation. (B) is associated with mitral stenosis. (C) is associated with mitral valve prolapse.

    References: Butterworth JF IV, Mackey DC, Wasnick JD, eds. *Morgan & Mikhail's Clinical Anesthesiology.* 7th ed. New York, NY: McGraw Hill; 2022: Chapter 21.

    Elisha S, Heiner JS, Nagelhout JJ. *Nurse Anesthesia.* 7th ed. St. Louis, MO: Elsevier Saunders; 2023: Chapter 25.

30. How does the elimination half-time of remifentanyl differ from alfentanil?

    (A) Elimination half-time is longer for remifentanyl.
    (B) Elimination half-time is shorter for alfentanil.
    (C) Elimination half-time is similar for alfentanil and remifentanyl.
    (D) Elimination half-time is shorter for remifentanyl.

    Rationale: Ester hydrolysis results in shorter elimination half-life for remifentanil as compared to all other opioids.

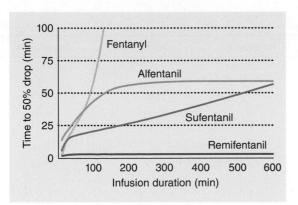

FIG. 1-2. In contrast to other opioids, the time necessary to achieve a 50% decrease in the plasma concentration of remifentanil (its half-time) is very short and is not influenced by the duration of the infusion (it is not context sensitive). (Reproduced with permission from Egan TD. The pharmacokinetics of the new short-acting opioid remifentanil [GI87084B] in healthy adult male volunteers. *Anesthesiology.* 1993;79(5):881-892.)

Reference: Butterworth JF IV, Mackey DC, Wasnick JD, eds. *Morgan & Mikhail's Clinical Anesthesiology.* 7th ed. New York, NY: McGraw Hill; 2022: Chapter 10.

31. One goal during a general anesthetic is to decrease the neuroendocrine stress response to surgical stimulation. Which medication will be helpful?

    (A) Vecuronium
    (B) Midazolam
    (C) Lidocaine
    (D) Fentanyl

    Rationale: Narcotics in large doses help decrease release of catecholamines, cortisol, and antidiuretichormone. Muscle relaxants, benzodiazepines, and local anesthetics do not produce similar effects.
    Reference: Butterworth JF IV, Mackey DC, Wasnick JD, eds. *Morgan & Mikhail's Clinical Anesthesiology.* 7th ed. New York, NY: McGraw Hill; 2022: Chapter 10.

32. You administered meperidine IV. Immediately following administration, the patient developed profound hypotension, hyperpyrexia, and respiratory arrest. What drug interaction do you suspect?

    (A) Interaction with monoamine oxidase inhibitors (MAOs)
    (B) Interaction with erythromycin
    (C) Interaction with sodium pentathol
    (D) Interaction with etomidate

    Rationale: Patients receiving MAO inhibitors should not receive meperidine. In addition to hypotension, hypertension, hyperpyrexia, and respiratory arrest, coma

may result. Interaction of alfentanil and ethrythomycin may lead to respiratory depression and prolonged somnolence. Meperidine and other narcotics combined with central nervous system depressants foster synergism that affects the respiratory and cardiac systems.
Reference: Butterworth JF IV, Mackey DC, Wasnick JD, eds. *Morgan & Mikhail's Clinical Anesthesiology.* 7th ed. New York, NY: McGraw Hill; 2022: Chapter 10.

33. What is the normal aortic valve area?

    (A) 0.5 to 1.0 cm^2
    (B) 1.0 to 1.5 cm^2
    (C) 1.5 to 2.5 cm^2
    (D) 2.5 to 3.5 cm^2

    Rationale: The normal aortic valve has an area of 2.5 to 3.5 cm^2.
    References: Elisha S, Heiner JS, Nagelhout JJ. *Nurse Anesthesia.* 7th ed. St. Louis, MO: Elsevier Saunders; 2023: Chapter 25.
    Hines RL, Marschall KE. *Stoelting's Anesthesia and Co-existing Disease.* 7th ed. Philadelphia, PA: Elsevier Saunders; 2018: Chapter 2.

34. For which severity of aortic stenosis is spinal anesthesia contraindicated?

    (A) 0.5 to 1.0 cm^2
    (B) 1 to 1.5 cm^2
    (C) 1.5 to 2.5 cm^2
    (D) 2.5 to 3.5 cm^2

    Rationale: An aortic valve area of 0.7 cm^2 is associated with sudden death. In general, neuraxial anesthesia is used cautiously with spinal anesthesia being relatively contraindicated due to the sympathectomy-induced drop in SVR.
    References: Butterworth JF IV, Mackey DC, Wasnick JD, eds. *Morgan & Mikhail's Clinical Anesthesiology.* 7th ed. New York, NY: McGraw Hill; 2022: Chapter 21.
    Elisha S, Heiner JS, Nagelhout JJ. *Nurse Anesthesia.* 7th ed. St. Louis, MO: Elsevier Saunders; 2023: Chapter 25.

35. Which agent results in an increased heart rate during inhalational anesthesia?

    (A) Desflurane 0.75 MAC
    (B) Sevoflurane >1.5 MAC
    (C) Desflurane 0.5 MAC
    (D) Sevoflurane <1 MAC

TABLE 1-3. Clinical pharmacology of inhalational anesthetics.

	Nitrous Oxide	Halothane	Isoflurane	Desflurane	Sevoflurane
Cardiovascular					
Blood pressure	N/C	↓↓	↓↓	↓↓	↓
Heart rate	N/C	↓	↑	N/C or ↑	N/C
Systemic vascular resistance	N/C	N/C	↓↓	↓↓	↓
Cardiac output[1]	N/C	↓	N/C	N/C or ↓	↓
Respiratory					
Tidal volume	↓	↓↓	↓↓	↓	↓
Respiratory rate	↑	↑↑	↑	↑	↑
PaCO$_2$					
Resting	N/C	↑	↑	↑↑	↑
Challenge	↑	↑	↑	↑↑	↑
Cerebral					
Blood flow	↑	↑↑	↑	↑	↑
Intracranial pressure	↑	↑↑	↑	↑	↑
Cerebral metabolic rate	↑	↓	↓↓	↓↓	↓↓
Seizures	↓	↓	↓	↓	↓
Neuromuscular					
Nondepolarizing blockade[2]	↑	↑↑	↑↑↑	↑↑↑	↑↑
Renal					
Renal blood flow	↓↓	↓↓	↓↓	↓	↓
Glomerular filtration rate	↓↓	↓↓	↓↓	↓	↓
Urinary output	↓↓	↓↓	↓↓	↓	↓
Hepatic					
Blood flow	↓	↓↓	↓	↓	↓
Metabolism[3]	0.004%	15-20%	0.2%	<0.1%	5%

[1]Controlled ventilation.
[2]Depolarizing blockage is probably also prolonged by these agents, but this is usually not clinically significant.
[3]Percentage of absorbed anesthetic undergoing metabolism. N/C, no change.
(Reproduced with permission from Butterworth JF IV, Mackey DC, Wasnick JD, eds. *Morgan & Mikhail's Clinical Anesthesiology*. 7th ed. New York, NY: McGraw Hill; 2022.)

Rationale: Heart rate increases linearly with dose. There is a minimal increase in heart rate with desflurane when using less than 1 MAC. The heart rate increases with sevoflurane at 1.5 MAC or greater.
References: Butterworth JF IV, Mackey DC, Wasnick JD, eds. *Morgan & Mikhail's Clinical Anesthesiology*. 7th ed. New York, NY: McGraw Hill; 2022: Chapter 8.
Pardo MC, Miller RD. *Miller's Basics of Anesthesia*. 8th ed. Philadelphia, PA: Elsevier; 2023: Chapter 7.

36. The anesthetic plan includes an inhalational induction. Which inhalational agent is the least desirable for a patient with chronic bronchitis and a 50-pack year history of smoking?

    (A) Desflurane
    (B) Sevoflurane
    (C) Halothane
    (D) Nitrous oxide

Rationale: Irritation of the airway is common with desflurane and isoflurane. These inhalational agents are pungent. Less pungency exists with nitrous oxide, sevoflurane, halothane, and therefore less airway irritation.
References: Butterworth JF IV, Mackey DC, Wasnick JD, eds. *Morgan & Mikhail's Clinical Anesthesiology*. 7th ed. New York, NY: McGraw Hill; 2022: Chapter 5.
Pardo MC, Miller RD. *Miller's Basics of Anesthesia*. 8th ed. Philadelphia, PA: Elsevier; 2023: Chapter 7.

37. Which local anesthetic is metabolized by *0*-toluidine?

    (A) Nesicaine
    (B) Cocaine
    (C) Prilocaine
    (D) Mepivacaine

Rationale: Prilocaine is the only amide local anesthetic not metabolized by P-450 microsomal enzymes. Ester local anesthetics nesicaine is metabolized by pseudocholinesterase whereas N-methylation and ester hydrolysis is responsible for cocaine metabolism. Mepivacaine is metabolized by P-450 microsomal enzymes.

Reference: Butterworth JF IV, Mackey DC, Wasnick JD, eds. *Morgan & Mikhail's Clinical Anesthesiology.* 7th ed. New York, NY: McGraw Hill; 2022: Chapter 16.

38. Which local anesthetic is linked to methemoglobinemia?

    (A) Prilocaine
    (B) EMLA
    (C) Lidocaine
    (D) Cocaine

    Rationale: Methemoglobinemia is caused by prilocaine's metabolic pathway that includes *o*-toluidine. EMLA cream is associated with skin blanching, erythema, and edema. Cauda equine syndrome has been associated with lidocaine. Cardiac symptoms include profound arrhythmias and hypertension.

    Reference: Butterworth JF IV, Mackey DC, Wasnick JD, eds. *Morgan & Mikhail's Clinical Anesthesiology.* 7th ed. New York, NY: McGraw Hill; 2022: Chapter 16.

39. Which risk factor contributes to myocardial ischemia in a patient with aortic regurgitation?

    (A) Heart rate 40 to 50 beats/min
    (B) Heart rate 50 to 70 beats/min
    (C) Heart rate 80 to 100 beats/min
    (D) Heart rate 110 to 120 beats/min

    Rationale: One anesthetic goal of managing a patient with aortic regurgitation is to maintain the heart rate toward the upper limits of normal (i.e., 80-100 beats/min, i.e., [**C**]). A heart rate that is too slow or an increase in systemic vascular resistance will increase the regurgitant volume ([A] and [B]). Tachycardia, on the other hand, will contribute to myocardial ischemia in a patient with aortic regurgitation.

    References: Butterworth JF IV, Mackey DC, Wasnick JD, eds. *Morgan & Mikhail's Clinical Anesthesiology.* 7th ed. New York, NY: McGraw Hill; 2022: Chapter 21.

    Elisha S, Heiner JS, Nagelhout JJ. *Nurse Anesthesia.* 7th ed. St. Louis, MO: Elsevier Saunders; 2023: Chapter 25.

40. Prior to general anesthesia the patient reports taking daily imipramine. What is your most serious concern for this patient?

    (A) Dry mouth
    (B) Sedation
    (C) Orthostatic hypotension
    (D) Sympathomimetic activity

    Rationale: Dry mouth, sedation, orthostatic hypotension, prolonged QT interval, dry mouth, blurred vision, and urinary retention are sides effects linked to tricyclic antidepressants-TCAs (imipramine). The most serious concern for patients taking TCAs is sympathomimetic activity resulting in hypertensive crisis and cardiac arrhythmias.

    References: Butterworth JF IV, Mackey DC, Wasnick JD, eds. *Morgan & Mikhail's Clinical Anesthesiology.* 7th ed. New York, NY: McGraw Hill; 2022: Chapter 28.

    Elisha S, Heiner JS, Nagelhout JJ. *Nurse Anesthesia.* 7th ed. St. Louis, MO: Elsevier Saunders; 2023: Chapters 20 & 26.

41. Where is the primary location of hepatic microsomal enzymes?

    (A) Hepatic smooth endoplasmic reticulum
    (B) Kidneys
    (C) Gastrointestinal system
    (D) Small intestine

    Rationale: The primary location of hepatic microsomal enzyme activity is the hepatic smooth endoplasmic reticulum. Microsomal enzymes are also located in the kidneys and gastrointestinal system to a lesser extent. Most reactions in the small intenstine involve P-450 enzymes.

    References: Butterworth JF IV, Mackey DC, Wasnick JD, eds. *Morgan & Mikhail's Clinical Anesthesiology.* 7th ed. New York, NY: McGraw Hill; 2022: Chapter 5.

    Flood P, Rathmell JP, Urbam RD, eds. *Stoelting's Pharmacology & Physiology in Anesthetic Practice.* 6th ed. Philadelphia, PA: Wolters Kluwer; 2022: Chapter 5.

42. In which valvular disease is the pulmonary capillary wedge pressure (PCWP) an overestimation of the left ventricular end-diastolic pressure (LVEDP)?

    (A) Mitral stenosis
    (B) Mitral regurgitation
    (C) Aortic stenosis
    (D) Aortic regurgitation

    Rationale: Because of the abnormal transvalvular gradient in mitral stenosis, the PCWP overestimates the LVEDP.

    References: Butterworth JF IV, Mackey DC, Wasnick JD, eds. *Morgan & Mikhail's Clinical Anesthesiology.* 7th ed. New York, NY: McGraw Hill; 2022: Chapter 5.

    Elisha S, Heiner JS, Nagelhout JJ. *Nurse Anesthesia.* 7th ed. St. Louis, MO: Elsevier Saunders; 2023: Chapter 25.

43. Which of the following medications block alpha- and beta-receptors?

(A) Phentolamine
(B) Isoproterenol
(C) Propanolol
(D) Labetolol

Rationale: Alpha-1, beta-1, and beta-2 receptors are blocked by labetolol. A competitive block is produced by phentolamine (alpha-1 and alpha-2 receptors). Isoproterenol is a selective beta-blocker whereas propanolol is a nonselective beta-1 and beta-2 receptor blockers.

Reference: Butterworth JF IV, Mackey DC, Wasnick JD, eds. *Morgan & Mikhail's Clinical Anesthesiology.* 7th ed. New York, NY: McGraw Hill; 2022: Chapter 14.

44. The patient arrives in the operating room following a motor vehicle accident. Forty percent of the body is burned. When is it permissible to use succinylcholine?

(A) There is no time parameter.
(B) Succinylcholine is used within 48 hours of injury.
(C) Succinylcholine is used after 48 hours of injury.
(D) No succinylcholine is used for patients with burns.

Rationale: Succinylcholine may be used for burn patients within 48 hours of injury. Significant elevation of potassium occurs when succinylcholine is administered after 48 hours.

Reference: Butterworth JF IV, Mackey DC, Wasnick JD, eds. *Morgan & Mikhail's Clinical Anesthesiology.* 7th ed. New York, NY: McGraw Hill; 2022: Chapter 39.

45. What variables are needed to calculate systemic vascular resistance (SVR)?

(A) Body surface area, cardiac output, and central venous pressure
(B) Mean arterial pressure, heart rate, and pulmonary capillary wedge pressure
(C) Mean arterial pressure, cardiac output, and pulmonary capillary wedge pressure
(D) Mean arterial pressure, cardiac output, and central venous pressure

Rationale: $SVR = 80 \times [MAP - CVP]/CO$.

References: Butterworth JF IV, Mackey DC, Wasnick JD, eds. *Morgan & Mikhail's Clinical Anesthesiology.* 7th ed. New York, NY: McGraw Hill; 2022: Chapter 20.

Elisha S, Heiner JS, Nagelhout JJ. *Nurse Anesthesia.* 7th ed. St. Louis, MO: Elsevier Saunders; 2023: Chapter 30.

46. The patient is scheduled for a tympanoplasty. Which inhalational agent will you avoid?

(A) Sevoflurane
(B) Nitrous oxide
(C) Desflurane
(D) Isoflurane

Rationale: When using nitrous oxide, air-filled cavities expand. The blood-gas partition coefficient of nitrous oxide is 0.46. The rapid movement of gas into air-filled cavities is 34 times greater than nitrogen. In this case, the middle ear is subject to increased pressures. The other inhalational agents are not preferential for air-filled cavities.

References: Butterworth JF IV, Mackey DC, Wasnick JD, eds. *Morgan & Mikhail's Clinical Anesthesiology.* 7th ed. New York, NY: McGraw Hill; 2022: Chapter 5.
Pardo MC, Miller RD. *Miller's Basics of Anesthesia.* 8th ed. Philadelphia, PA: Elsevier; 2023: Chapter 7.

47. Which agent increases the cerebral metabolic rate for oxygen ($CMRO_2$)?

(A) Halothane
(B) Isoflurane
(C) Sevoflurane
(D) Nitrous oxide

Rationale: Cerebral vasodilatation and increased cerebral blood flow is linked to nitrous oxide administration without volatile anesthetics. Isoflurane, sevoflurane, desflurane, and halothane decrease $CMRO_2$.

Reference: Butterworth JF IV, Mackey DC, Wasnick JD, eds. *Morgan & Mikhail's Clinical Anesthesiology.* 7th ed. New York, NY: McGraw Hill; 2022: Chapter 8.

48. Which hemodynamic event will decrease coronary perfusion pressure the most?

(A) Decreased systolic blood pressure
(B) Decrease in left ventricular end-diastolic pressure (LVEDP)
(C) Increase in pulmonary capillary wedge pressure (PCWP)
(D) Increase in diastolic blood pressure

Rationale: Coronary perfusion pressure = arterial diastolic pressure minus the LVEDP. Any decreases in aortic pressure or increases in ventricular end-diastolic pressure will reduce coronary perfusion pressure. Since PCWP is an indirect measure of LVEDP, an increase in PCWP will decrease coronary perfusion pressure.

References: Butterworth JF IV, Mackey DC, Wasnick JD, eds. *Morgan & Mikhail's Clinical Anesthesiology.* 7th ed. New York, NY: McGraw Hill; 2022: Chapter 20.

Elisha S, Heiner JS, Nagelhout JJ. *Nurse Anesthesia.* 7th ed. St. Louis, MO: Elsevier Saunders; 2023: Chapter 25.

49. Which antibiotic is not classified as a beta-lactam?

(A) Penicillin

(B) Gentamicin

(C) Erythromycin

(D) Ciprofloxin

Rationale: Gentamicin is an aminoglycoside, erythromycin a macrolide, and ciprofloxin is classified as a fluoroquinolone.

Reference: Flood P, Rathmell JP, Urbam RD, eds. *Stoelting's Pharmacology & Physiology in Anesthetic Practice.* 6th ed. Philadelphia, PA: Wolters Kluwer; 2022: Chapter 28.

50. To avoid hypotension and possible cardiac arrest what is the best method for administering IV vancomycin?

(A) >60 minutes

(B) <30 minutes

(C) >20 minutes

(D) <10 minutes

Rationale: Rapidly infused vancomycin (<30 minutes) results in life-threatening hypotension.

Patient's experience head to toe erythema often termed "red man" syndrome.

References: Flood P, Rathmell JP, Urbam RD, eds. *Stoelting's Pharmacology & Physiology in Anesthetic Practice.* 6th ed. Philadelphia, PA: Wolters Kluwer; 2022: Chapter 28.

51. What is the most common cause of myocardial remodeling?

(A) Congenital heart disease

(B) Myocardial ischemic injury

(C) Chronic lung disease

(D) Cardiomyopathy

Rationale: Ischemic injury is the most common cause of myocardial remodeling and encompasses both hypertrophy and dilation of the left ventricle.

References: Butterworth JF IV, Mackey DC, Wasnick JD, eds. *Morgan & Mikhail's Clinical Anesthesiology.* 7th ed. New York, NY: McGraw Hill; 2022: Chapter 20.

Hines RL, Marschall KE. *Stoelting's Anesthesia and Co-existing Disease.* 7th ed. Philadelphia, PA: Elsevier Saunders; 2018: Chapter 6.

52. A 55-year-old male with congestive heart failure, status post-cardiac transplantation is now undergoing elective surgery for hernia repair. Thirty minutes into the case, his heart rate drops to 28. What medication will you give for bradycardia?

(A) Atropine

(B) Ephedrine

(C) Isoproterenol

(D) Dexmedetomidine

Rationale: When the denervated heart post-cardiac transplantation is bradycardic, a direct-acting beta-adrenergic agonist such as isoproterenol or epinephrine must be given to achieve an increase in heart rate.

References: Elisha S, Heiner JS, Nagelhout JJ. *Nurse Anesthesia.* 7th ed. St. Louis, MO: Elsevier Saunders; 2023: Chapter 26.

Hines RL, Marschall KE. *Stoelting's Anesthesia and Co-existing Disease.* 7th ed. Philadelphia, PA: Elsevier Saunders; 2018: Chapter 6.

53. The patient with renal disease is scheduled for an exploratory laparotomy. What muscle relaxant is the best choice for this patient?

(A) Vecuronium

(B) Pancuronium

(C) Rocuronium

(D) Cisatracurium

Rationale: Ester hydrolysis and Hofmann elimination make cisatracurium the best choice for muscle relaxation for patients with renal disease. Rocuronium and vecuronium elimination is mainly hepatic. However, 20% of vecuronium is eliminated renally. Prolonged neuromuscular relaxation is linked to rocuronium. Both drugs may be used for patients with renal disease. Pancuronium depends on primary renal elimination.

TABLE 1-4. Drugs with a potential for significant accumulation in patients with renal impairment.

- **Muscle relaxants**
  - Pancuronium
- **Anticholinergics**
  - Atropine
  - Glycopyrrolate
- **Metoclopramide**
- **H$_2$-receptor antagonists**
  - Cimetidine
  - Ranitidine
- **Digitalis**
- **Diuretics**
- **Calcium channel antagonists**
  - Diltiazem
  - Nifedipine
- **β-Adrenergic blockers**
  - Atenolol
  - Nadolol
  - Pindolol
  - Propranolol
- **Antihypertensives**
  - Captopril
  - Clonidine
  - Enalapril
  - Hydralazine
  - Lisinopril
  - Nitroprusside (thiocyanate)
- **Antiarrhythmics**
  - Bretylium
  - Disopyramide
  - Encainide (genetically determined)
  - Procainamide
  - Tocainide
- **Bronchodilators**
  - Terbutaline
- **Psychiatric**
  - Lithium
- **Antibiotics**
  - Aminoglycosides
  - Cephalosporins
  - Penicillins
  - Tetracycline
  - Vancomycin
- **Anticonvulsants**
  - Carbamazepine
  - Ethosuximide
  - Primidone

(Reproduced with permission from Butterworth JF IV, Mackey DC, Wasnick JD, eds. *Morgan & Mikhail's Clinical Anesthesiology.* 5th ed. New York, NY: McGraw Hill; 2013.)

References: Butterworth JF IV, Mackey DC, Wasnick JD, eds. *Morgan & Mikhail's Clinical Anesthesiology.* 7th ed. New York, NY: McGraw Hill; 2022: Chapter 30.

Hines RL, Marschall KE. *Stoelting's Anesthesia and Co-existing Disease.* 7th ed. Philadelphia, PA: Elsevier Saunders; 2018: Chapter 17.

54. The patient's glomerular filtration rate is 20 mL/min. What condition most likely exists?

  (A) Acute glomerulonephritis
  (B) Uremia
  (C) Renal calculi
  (D) Acute kidney failure

Rationale: When a patient's GFR falls below 25 mL/min uremia exists. Chronic glomerulonephritis, diabetic nephropathy, hypertensive nephrosclerosis, and polycystic kidney disease characterize uremia.

References: Butterworth JF IV, Mackey DC, Wasnick JD, eds. *Morgan & Mikhail's Clinical Anesthesiology.* 7th ed. New York, NY: McGraw Hill; 2022: Chapter 30.

Hines RL, Marschall KE. *Stoelting's Anesthesia and Co-existing Disease.* 7th ed. Philadelphia, PA: Elsevier Saunders; 2018: Chapter 17.

55. What arterial line waveform might you observe in a patient with severe aortic regurgitation?

  (A) Pulsus paradoxus
  (B) Pulsus alternans
  (C) Pulsus bisferiens
  (D) Anacrotic pulse

Rationale: Pulsus bisferiens may be present in patients with moderate to severe aortic insufficiency because of rapid ejection of a large stroke volume.

References: Butterworth JF IV, Mackey DC, Wasnick JD, eds. *Morgan & Mikhail's Clinical Anesthesiology.* 7th ed. New York, NY: McGraw Hill; 2022: Chapter 24.

Elisha S, Heiner JS, Nagelhout JJ. *Nurse Anesthesia.* 7th ed. St. Louis, MO: Elsevier Saunders; 2023: Chapter 25.

56. Which characteristic describes a typical patient with diastolic heart failure?

  (A) Left ventricular ejection fraction less than 40%
  (B) Dilated left ventricular cavity size
  (C) Persistent atrial fibrillation
  (D) Fourth heart sound

Rationale: Fourth heart sound is a characteristic finding in diastolic heart failure. The other characteristics are typical for systolic heart failure.

References: Elisha S, Heiner JS, Nagelhout JJ. *Nurse Anesthesia.* 7th ed. St. Louis, MO: Elsevier Saunders; 2023: Chapter 24.

Hines RL, Marschall KE. *Stoelting's Anesthesia and Co-existing Disease.* 7th ed. Philadelphia, PA: Elsevier Saunders; 2018: Chapter 6.

57. How does the mechanism of action of methylxanthines affect patients with asthma?

  (A) Blocks degranulation of mast cells
  (B) Bronchodilates via beta-2 receptors
  (C) Bronchodilates via beta-1 receptors
  (D) Inhibits phosphodiesterase

Rationale: Commonly used methylxanthines, such as theopylline and aminophylline, bronchodilate asthmatic patients by inhibiting phosphodiesterase. In addition, catecholamine release, histamine blockade, and stimulation of the diaphragm promote stability in asthmatic conditions.

TABLE 1-5.   A comparison of commonly used bronchodilators.[1]

Agent	Adrenergic Activity	
	β_1	β_2
Albuterol (Ventolin)	$+^1$	+++
Bitolterol (Tornalate)	+	++++
Epinephrine	++++	++
Fenoterol (Berotec)	+	+++
Formoterol (Foradil)	+	++++
Isoetharine (Bronkosol)	++	+++
Isoproterenol (Isuprel)	++++	—
Metaproterenol (Alupent)	+	+
Pirbuterol (Maxair)	+	++++
Salmeterol (Serevent)	+	++++
Terbutaline (Brethaire)	+	+++

[1]+ Indicates level of activity.
(Reproduced with permission from Butterworth JF IV, Mackey DC, Wasnick JD, eds. *Morgan & Mikhail's Clinical Anesthesiology*. 5th ed. New York, NY: McGraw Hill; 2013.)

Reference: Butterworth JF IV, Mackey DC, Wasnick JD, eds. *Morgan & Mikhail's Clinical Anesthesiology*. 7th ed. New York, NY: McGraw Hill; 2022: Chapter 24.

58. A 42-year-old female with multiple sclerosis is scheduled for major surgery with general anesthesia. She has been taking corticosteroid therapy. Which approximate equivalent dose achieves the anti-inflammatory potency of prednisone 50 mg?

(A) 8 mg dexamethasone

(B) 100 mg methylprednisone

(C) 25 mg prednisolone

(D) 300 mg cortisone

Rationale:

(A) is correct: 50 mg prednisone = 8 mg dexamethasone (4:25 potency ratio, i.e., 1/6 the dose).

(B) is incorrect: 50 mg prednisone = 40 mg methylprednisone (4:5 potency ratio, i.e., 4/5 of dose).

(C) is incorrect: 50 mg prednisone = 50 mg prednisolone (1:1 potency ratio, equivalent doses).

(D) is incorrect: 50 mg prednisone = 250 mg cortisone (4:0.8 potency ratio, i.e., 5× the dose).

References: Flood P, Rathmell JP, Urbam RD, eds. *Stoelting's Pharmacology & Physiology in Anesthetic Practice*. 6th ed. Philadelphia, PA: Wolters Kluwer; 2022: Chapter 23.
Elisha S, Heiner JS, Nagelhout JJ. *Nurse Anesthesia*. 7th ed. St. Louis, MO: Elsevier Saunders; 2023: Chapter 37.

59. A patient with rheumatoid arthritis has been receiving long-term corticosteroid therapy and infliximab. Which statement best describes the major anesthetic implication for this drug regimen?

(A) Avoiding anesthetic drugs that are excreted via kidneys

(B) Administering po dose of infliximab via NGT intraoperatively

(C) Paying meticulous attention to sterile techniques

(D) Monitoring intraoperative labs for hypoglycemia

Rationale: Both long-term steroid therapy and infliximab predispose patients to infection. (A) is incorrect because there is not such contraindication with steroids and TNF-antagonists. (B) is incorrect because there are only IV formulations of infliximab. (D) is incorrect because long-term steroid effects are associated with hyperglycemia, not hypoglycemia.

References: Flood P, Rathmell JP, Urbam RD, eds. *Stoelting's Pharmacology & Physiology in Anesthetic Practice*. 6th ed. Philadelphia, PA: Wolters Kluwer; 2022: Chapter 23.
Elisha S, Heiner JS, Nagelhout JJ. *Nurse Anesthesia*. 7th ed. St. Louis, MO: Elsevier Saunders; 2023: Chapter 36.

60. A patient with a prosthetic heart valve presents for a scheduled total abdominal hysterectomy with a heparin infusion. How far in advance of surgery will you recommend this heparin be discontinued?

(A) 2 to 4 hours

(B) 4 to 6 hours

(C) 24 hours

(D) 48 hours

Rationale: Heparin should be discontinued 4 to 6 hours prior to surgery and then re-started postoperatively when the risk of bleeding has diminished.

References: Butterworth JF IV, Mackey DC, Wasnick JD, eds. *Morgan & Mikhail's Clinical Anesthesiology*. 7th ed. New York, NY: McGraw Hill; 2022: Chapter 21.
Hines RL, Marschall KE. *Stoelting's Anesthesia and Co-existing Disease*. 7th ed. Philadelphia, PA: Elsevier Saunders; 2018: Chapter 2.

61. What is the predicted FEV_1/FVC ratio for a patient whose history includes a 55-pack year history of smoking with wheezing on auscultation?

(A) FEV_1/FVC ratio of >0.7

(B) FEV_1/FVC ratio equal to 0.08

(C) FEV$_1$/FVC ratio equal to >0.9

(D) FEV$_1$/FVC ratio of <0.7

Rationale: The combination of greater than 55-pack year history, wheezing on auscultation, and patient self-reported wheezing almost assures that obstruction (FEV$_1$/FVC ratio of <0.7).

Reference: Elisha S, Heiner JS, Nagelhout JJ. *Nurse Anesthesia.* 7th ed. St. Louis, MO: Elsevier Saunders; 2023: Chapter 29.

62. Where do local anesthetics exert their primary mechanism of action?

(A) Sodium channel alpha subunit

(B) Calcium channel

(C) Vanilloid 1 channel

(D) Potassium channel

Rationale: While local anesthetics may bind to calcium, potassium, and vanilloid 1, the primary mechanism of action is exerted at the alpha subunit of the sodium channel.

Reference: Butterworth JF IV, Mackey DC, Wasnick JD, eds. *Morgan & Mikhail's Clinical Anesthesiology.* 7th ed. New York, NY: McGraw Hill; 2022: Chapter 16.

63. Which neuromuscular blocker is considered an acetylcholine (ACh) receptor agonist?

(A) Vecuronium

(B) Rocuronium

(C) Cisatracurium

(D) Succinylcholine

Rationale: Depolarizing muscle relaxants (Succinylcholine) mimic acetylcholine. Nondepolarizing muscle relaxants (vecuroniium, rocuronium, and cisatracurium) are competitive antagonists binding ACh receptors.

Reference: Butterworth JF IV, Mackey DC, Wasnick JD, eds. *Morgan & Mikhail's Clinical Anesthesiology.* 7th ed. New York, NY: McGraw Hill; 2022: Chapter 11.

64. When administering neuromuscular blockers to patients with myasthenia gravis, what do you expect?

(A) Up-regulation

(B) Profound response to succincylcholine

(C) Down-regulation

(D) Decreased sensitivity to vecuronium

Rationale: Up-regulation occurs when more receptors are depolarized and then results in a profound response to depolarizing muscle relaxants. Down-regulation occurs when there are less acetycholine receptors as in myasthenia gravis. Sensitivity to nondepolarizers is increased. There is a resistance to depolarizers.

Reference: Butterworth JF IV, Mackey DC, Wasnick JD, eds. *Morgan & Mikhail's Clinical Anesthesiology.* 7th ed. New York, NY: McGraw Hill; 2022: Chapter 11.

65. Which fibers are most sensitive to local anesthetics?

(A) A-alpha fibers

(B) Small unmyelinated fibers C fibers

(C) A-gamma

(D) C fibers

Rationale: A-alpha fibers are less sensitive to local anesthetics as compared to A-alpha gamma fibers.

TABLE 1-6. Nerve fiber classification.[1]

Fiber Type	Modality Served	Diameter (mm)	Conduction (m/s)	Myelinated?
Aα	Motor efferent	12-20	70-120	Yes
Aα	Proprioception	12-20	70-120	Yes
Aβ	Touch, pressure	5-12	30-70	Yes
Aγ	Motor efferent (muscle spindle)	3-6	15-30	Yes
Aδ	Pain	2-5	12-30	Yes
	Temperature			
	Touch			
B	Preganglionic autonomic fibers	<3	3-14	Some
C	Pain	0.4-1.2	0.5-2	No
Dorsal root	Temperature			
C	Postganglionic sympathetic fibers	0.3-1.3	0.7-2.3	No
Sympathetic				

[1]An alternative numerical system is sometimes used to classify sensory fibers.

(Reproduced with permission from Butterworth JF IV, Mackey DC, Wasnick JD, eds. *Morgan & Mikhail's Clinical Anesthesiology.* 7th ed. New York, NY: McGraw Hill; 2022.)

C fibers including small unmyelinated C fibers resist local anesthetic action.

Reference: Butterworth JF IV, Mackey DC, Wasnick JD, eds. *Morgan & Mikhail's Clinical Anesthesiology.* 7th ed. New York, NY: McGraw Hill; 2022: Chapter 16.

66. Which ratio of the forced expiratory volume in the first second of exhalation (FEV_1) to the total forced vital capacity (FVC) would signify the greatest degree of obstruction?

(A) FEV_1/FVC ratio of 80%

(B) FEV_1/FVC ratio of 40%

(C) FEV_1/FVC ratio of 20%

(D) FEV_1/FVC ratio of 60%

Rationale: The normal ratio of the forced expiratory volume in the first second of exhalation to the total forced vital capacity is greater than or equal to 80%.

References: Butterworth JF IV, Mackey DC, Wasnick JD, eds. *Morgan & Mikhail's Clinical Anesthesiology.* 7th ed. New York, NY: McGraw Hill; 2022: Chapter 23.

Elisha S, Heiner JS, Nagelhout JJ. *Nurse Anesthesia.* 7th ed. St. Louis, MO: Elsevier Saunders; 2023: Chapter 29.

67. What compensatory mechanism is commonly seen with aortic regurgitation?

(A) Eccentric hypertrophy

(B) Dilated annulus of aortic valve

(C) Concentric hypertrophy

(D) Elevated brain natriuretic peptide

Rationale: A volume-overloaded ventricle will cause the sarcomeres to replicate in series resulting in eccentric hypertrophy. Eccentric hypertrophy is commonly seen in aortic regurgitation.

References: Butterworth JF IV, Mackey DC, Wasnick JD, eds. *Morgan & Mikhail's Clinical Anesthesiology.* 7th ed. New York, NY: McGraw Hill; 2022: Chapter 20.

Elisha S, Heiner JS, Nagelhout JJ. *Nurse Anesthesia.* 7th ed. St. Louis, MO: Elsevier Saunders; 2023: Chapter 25.

68. Which pharmacological agent is contraindicated in the patient with Wolff-Parkinson-White (WPW) syndrome exhibiting atrial fibrillation?

(A) Atropine

(B) Diltiazem

(C) Verapamil

(D) Metoprolol

Rationale: Verapamil is contraindicated in this population because of the risk of accelerating a ventricular response. Atropine can be used cautiously, though not contraindicated. Glycopyrrolate would be a more suitable alternative to atropine.

References: Butterworth JF IV, Mackey DC, Wasnick JD, eds. *Morgan & Mikhail's Clinical Anesthesiology.* 7th ed. New York, NY: McGraw Hill; 2022: Chapter 20.

Elisha S, Heiner JS, Nagelhout JJ. *Nurse Anesthesia.* 7th ed. St. Louis, MO: Elsevier Saunders; 2023: Chapter 13.

69. Your patient has mitral valve prolapse. What is the most common arrhythmia associated with this disease?

(A) Paroxysmal supraventricular tachycardia

(B) Atrial fibrillation

(C) Premature ventricular contraction

(D) Junctional tachycardia

Rationale: Paroxysmal SVT is the most encountered sustained arrhythmia in patients with mitral valve prolapse.

References: Butterworth JF IV, Mackey DC, Wasnick JD, eds. *Morgan & Mikhail's Clinical Anesthesiology.* 7th ed. New York, NY: McGraw Hill; 2022: Chapter 21.

Elisha S, Heiner JS, Nagelhout JJ. *Nurse Anesthesia.* 7th ed. St. Louis, MO: Elsevier Saunders; 2023: Chapter 25.

70. From where do the cardiac sympathetic fibers originate?

(A) T_1–T_4

(B) T_2–T_4

(C) T_3–T_6

(D) T_4–T_8

Rationale: The cardiac sympathetic fibers, also known as the cardioaccelerator fibers, originate from the cells in the intermediolateral columns of the higher thoracic segments of the spinal cord and synapse at the first through fifth thoracic paravertebral ganglia, or T_1-T_4.

References: Butterworth JF IV, Mackey DC, Wasnick JD, eds. *Morgan & Mikhail's Clinical Anesthesiology.* 7th ed. New York, NY: McGraw Hill; 2022: Chapter 20.

Elisha S, Heiner JS, Nagelhout JJ. *Nurse Anesthesia.* 7th ed. St. Louis, MO: Elsevier Saunders; 2023: Chapter 25.

71. Which statement about coronary blood flow is incorrect?

(A) At rest, approximately 4 to 5% of the cardiac output passes through the coronary vessels.

(B) The left ventricle is perfused almost entirely during diastole.

(C) The right ventricle is perfused during systole and diastole.

(D) Increases in the aortic pressure can reduce coronary perfusion pressure.

Rationale: All are correct except for (D). Coronary perfusion pressure is determined by the difference between aortic pressure and left ventricular end-diastolic pressure (LVEDP). Any decrease in aortic pressure or increase in LVEDP will reduce coronary perfusion pressure.

References: Butterworth JF IV, Mackey DC, Wasnick JD, eds. *Morgan & Mikhail's Clinical Anesthesiology.* 7th ed. New York, NY: McGraw Hill; 2022: Chapter 20.

Elisha S, Heiner JS, Nagelhout JJ. *Nurse Anesthesia.* 7th ed. St. Louis, MO: Elsevier Saunders; 2023: Chapter 25.

72. What is indicated by a V/Q ratio that is equal to infinity?

(A) Dead space

(B) Shunting

(C) Normal V/Q ratio

(D) Inadequate ventilation

Rationale: V/Q is a where V is ventilation and Q is perfusion relationship. If perfusion is 0, then the V/Q ratio is infinity.

References: Butterworth JF IV, Mackey DC, Wasnick JD, eds. *Morgan & Mikhail's Clinical Anesthesiology.* 7th ed. New York, NY: McGraw Hill; 2022: Chapter 23.

Elisha S, Heiner JS, Nagelhout JJ. *Nurse Anesthesia.* 7th ed. St. Louis, MO: Elsevier Saunders; 2023: Chapter 29.

73. As compared to other anticholinergics, what are scopolamine's sedative effects?

(A) Less than atropine

(B) Greater than glycopyrrolate

(C) Same as atropine

(D) Same as atropine and glycopyrrolate

Rationale: The sedative effect of anticholinergics is greatest with scopolamine. Gycopyrrolate possesses no sedative effects. Sedation is minimal with atropine.

Reference: Butterworth JF IV, Mackey DC, Wasnick JD, eds. *Morgan & Mikhail's Clinical Anesthesiology.* 7th ed. New York, NY: McGraw Hill; 2022: Chapter 13.

74. Who studied the relationship between volume and temperature when pressure remains constant?

(A) Boyle

(B) Charles

(C) Gay-Lussac

(D) Dalton

Rationale: Boyle examined the relationship of pressure and volume with constant temperature. Gay-Lussac examined pressure and temperature when volume is constant. Dalton's Law says that the sum of individual gas pressures is equal to the total pressure.

Reference: Elisha S, Heiner JS, Nagelhout JJ. *Nurse Anesthesia.* 7th ed. St. Louis, MO: Elsevier Saunders; 2023: Chapter 15.

75. Which factor most negatively affects myocardial oxygen consumption?

(A) Cardiac volume work

(B) Electrical activity

(C) Heart rate

(D) Wall stress

Rationale: There are many factors that increase myocardial oxygen demand: heart rate, pressure work, contractility, wall stress, volume work, and electrical activity. Pressure work and heart rate increase myocardial oxygen consumption the most. Of the options above, heart rate is the most important factor that negatively affects myocardial oxygen consumption.

References: Butterworth JF IV, Mackey DC, Wasnick JD, eds. *Morgan & Mikhail's Clinical Anesthesiology.* 7th ed. New York, NY: McGraw Hill; 2022: Chapter 20.

Elisha S, Heiner JS, Nagelhout JJ. *Nurse Anesthesia.* 7th ed. St. Louis, MO: Elsevier Saunders; 2023: Chapter 25.

76. What is the functional residual capacity for an adult patient in the supine position following induction of general anesthesia?

(A) 500 mL

(B) 800 mL

(C) 1,300 mL

(D) 2,300 mL

Rationale: The supine position reduces the functional residual capacity by 800 to 1,000 mL, and induction of general anesthesia further reduces the functional residual capacity by another 500 mL.

References: Butterworth JF IV, Mackey DC, Wasnick JD, eds. *Morgan & Mikhail's Clinical Anesthesiology.* 7th ed. New York, NY: McGraw Hill; 2022: Chapter 23.

Elisha S, Heiner JS, Nagelhout JJ. *Nurse Anesthesia.* 7th ed. St. Louis, MO: Elsevier Saunders; 2023: Chapter 29.

77. What is the normal coronary blood flow at rest?

   (A) 175 to 200 mL/min
   (B) 200 to 225 mL/min
   (C) 225 to 250 mL/min
   (D) 250 to 275 mL/min

   Rationale: At rest, approximate 4 to 5% of the cardiac output, or 225 to 250 mL/min of blood passes the coronary vessels at rest.
   References: Butterworth JF IV, Mackey DC, Wasnick JD, eds. *Morgan & Mikhail's Clinical Anesthesiology.* 7th ed. New York, NY: McGraw Hill; 2022: Chapter 20.
   Elisha S, Heiner JS, Nagelhout JJ. *Nurse Anesthesia.* 7th ed. St. Louis, MO: Elsevier Saunders; 2023: Chapter 25.

78. If a 64-kg woman receives a standard initial dose of dantrolene during malignant hyperthermia crisis, how many grams of mannitol have been administered?

   (A) 12
   (B) 16
   (C) 20
   (D) 24

   Rationale: Standard initial dose is 2.5 mg/kg, or 160 mg in this case. Each vial contains 20 mg of dantrolene; 8 vials would be needed. Each vial contains 3 g of mannitol. 8 vials × 3 g each = 24 g of mannitol.
   References: Butterworth JF IV, Mackey DC, Wasnick JD, eds. *Morgan & Mikhail's Clinical Anesthesiology.* 7th ed. New York, NY: McGraw Hill; 2022: Chapter 52.
   Longnecker DE, Mackey SC, Newman MF, Sandberg WS, Zapol WM, eds. *Anesthesiology.* 3rd ed. McGraw Hill; 2018: Chapter 87.

79. Which statement about protamine is incorrect?

   (A) A hypotensive reaction can be treated with incremental doses of phenylephrine.
   (B) Administering protamine over 10 to 15 minutes will decrease risk of hypotension reaction.
   (C) The normal dose is 10 mg of protamine for every 100 units of heparin.
   (D) Supplementary doses of 50 to 100 mg can be administered to reverse residual anticoagulation.

   Rationale: All are correct, except C. The typical dose is 1 to 1.3 mg of protamine per 100 units of heparin.
   References: Butterworth JF IV, Mackey DC, Wasnick JD, eds. *Morgan & Mikhail's Clinical Anesthesiology.* 7th ed. New York, NY: McGraw Hill; 2022: Chapter 20.

Elisha S, Heiner JS, Nagelhout JJ. *Nurse Anesthesia.* 7th ed. St. Louis, MO: Elsevier Saunders; 2023: Chapter 25.

80. What pathology can increase alveolar dead space?

   (A) Mucous plug
   (B) Pulmonary embolism
   (C) Hyperventilation
   (D) Hypoventilation

   Rationale: Alveolar dead space is defined as ventilation without perfusion.
   References: Butterworth JF IV, Mackey DC, Wasnick JD, eds. *Morgan & Mikhail's Clinical Anesthesiology.* 7th ed. New York, NY: McGraw Hill; 2022: Chapter 23.
   Elisha S, Heiner JS, Nagelhout JJ. *Nurse Anesthesia.* 7th ed. St. Louis, MO: Elsevier Saunders; 2023: Chapter 29.

81. How is residual volume defined?

   (A) Maximum volume of air expired from resting end-expiratory level
   (B) Maximum volume of air inspired from the resting end inspiratory level
   (C) Normal breath
   (D) Volume remaining after maximal exhalation

   Rationale: Residual volume is the air that remains in the lungs after a maximal exhalation which is about 1,200 mL in an average adult.
   References: Butterworth JF IV, Mackey DC, Wasnick JD, eds. *Morgan & Mikhail's Clinical Anesthesiology.* 7th ed. New York, NY: McGraw Hill; 2022: Chapter 23.
   Elisha S, Heiner JS, Nagelhout JJ. *Nurse Anesthesia.* 7th ed. St. Louis, MO: Elsevier Saunders; 2023: Chapter 29.

82. Which patient does not pose an increased risk for an allergic reaction to protamine sulfate?

   (A) A patient who has a history of two previous cardiac catheterizations
   (B) A patient who is currently undergoing aortic valve replacement
   (C) A diabetic patient on maintenance of NPH insulin therapy
   (D) A patient who is maintained on a weekly hemodialysis regimen

Rationale: There is an increased incidence of reactions to protamine in patients sensitized to protamine from previous cardiac catheterization, hemodialysis, cardiac surgery, or exposure to neutral protamine Hagedorn (NPH) insulin. A patient who is undergoing their aortic valve replacement for the first time is not at increased risk.

References: Butterworth JF IV, Mackey DC, Wasnick JD, eds. *Morgan & Mikhail's Clinical Anesthesiology.* 7th ed. New York, NY: McGraw Hill; 2022: Chapter 22.

Barash PG, Cullen BF, Stoelting RK, et al, eds. *Clinical Anesthesia.* 8th ed. Lippincott Williams & Wilkins; 2017: Chapter 41.

83. Compared to neostigmine, what is the onset of action of pyridostigmine?

    (A) Longer than neostigmine
    (B) Same as neostigmine
    (C) Slower than neostigmine
    (D) Clinically inconsequential

    Rationale: The onset of action of pyridostigmine (10-15 minutes) is slower than neostigmine (5 minutes).

    Reference: Butterworth JF IV, Mackey DC, Wasnick JD, eds. *Morgan & Mikhail's Clinical Anesthesiology.* 7th ed. New York, NY: McGraw Hill; 2022: Chapter 12.

84. Which condition potentiates neuromuscular blockade?

    (A) Hypomagnesemia
    (B) Hypercalcemia
    (C) Hyperkalemia
    (D) Hypothermia

    Rationale: Factors potentiating neuromuscular blockade include hypothermia, respiratory acidosis, hypermagnesemia, hypocalcemia, and hypokalemia. In addition, volatile anesthetics, dantrolene, verapamil, furosemide, lidocaine, and antibiotics (aminoglycosides, polymiyxin B, neomycin, tetracycline, clindamycin) potentiate neuromuscular blockade.

    Reference: Butterworth JF IV, Mackey DC, Wasnick JD, eds. *Morgan & Mikhail's Clinical Anesthesiology.* 7th ed. New York, NY: McGraw Hill; 2022: Chapter 12.

85. What is the result of acetylcholine acting on the muscarinic receptor (M2) in the sinoatrial node?

    (A) Positive dromotropic effects
    (B) Negative dromotropic effects
    (C) Positive chronotropic effects
    (D) Positive inotropic effects

    Rationale: Acetylcholine acting on the cardiac muscarinic receptors (M2) will produce negative chronotropic, negative dromotropic, and negative inotropic effects.

    References: Butterworth JF IV, Mackey DC, Wasnick JD, eds. *Morgan & Mikhail's Clinical Anesthesiology.* 7th ed. New York, NY: McGraw Hill; 2022: Chapter 20.

    Elisha S, Heiner JS, Nagelhout JJ. *Nurse Anesthesia.* 7th ed. St. Louis, MO: Elsevier Saunders; 2023: Chapter 25.

86. Which paradoxical cardiac wall motion, when diagnosed with transesophageal echocardiography (TEE) is indicative of myocardial infarction?

    (A) Dyskinesia
    (B) Hypokinesia
    (C) Akinesia
    (D) Hyperkinesia

    Rationale: Dyskinesia, paradoxical movement, is the hallmark of myocardial infarction. Akinesia is absence of motion (not paradoxical motion) but can be associated with myocardial infarction. Hypokinesia describes less vigorous contractions than normal. Hyperkinesia is not an associated term with TEE abnormal wall motion.

    References: Butterworth JF IV, Mackey DC, Wasnick JD, eds. *Morgan & Mikhail's Clinical Anesthesiology.* 7th ed. New York, NY: McGraw Hill; 2022: Chapter 20.

    Elisha S, Heiner JS, Nagelhout JJ. *Nurse Anesthesia.* 7th ed. St. Louis, MO: Elsevier Saunders; 2023: Chapter 17.

87. You plan a standard induction for an 80-kg patient scheduled for cholecystecomy. What induction dose of cisatracurium will you use?

    (A) 16 mg
    (B) 8 mg
    (C) 1.6 mg
    (D) 0.8 mg

    Rationale: The intubating dose of cisatracurium is 0.2 mg/kg.

    Reference: Butterworth JF IV, Mackey DC, Wasnick JD, eds. *Morgan & Mikhail's Clinical Anesthesiology.* 7th ed. New York, NY: McGraw Hill; 2022: Chapter 11.

TABLE 1-7. Additional considerations of muscle relaxants in special populations.

Pediatric	Succinylcholine: should not be used routinely Nondepolarizing agents: faster onset Vecuronium: long-acting in neonates
Older adult	Decreased clearance: prolonged duration, except with cisatracurium
Obese	Dosage 20% more than lean body weight; onset unchanged Prolonged duration, except with cisatracurium
Liver disease	Increased volume of distribution Pancuronium and vecuronium: prolonged elimination due to hepatic metabolism and biliary excretion Cisatracurium: unchanged Pseudocholinesterase decreased; prolonged action may be seen with succinylcholine in severe disease
Kidney failure	Vecuronium: prolonged Rocuronium: relatively unchanged Cisatracurium: safest alternative
Critically ill	Myopathy, polyneuropathy, nicotinic acetylcholine receptor upregulation

(Reproduced with permission from Butterworth JF IV, Mackey DC, Wasnick JD, eds. *Morgan & Mikhail's Clinical Anesthesiology*. 7th ed. New York, NY: McGraw Hill; 2022.)

88. Following topical administration of a local anesthetic you note erythema, skin blanching, and edema. Which local anesthetic did you apply?

    (A) Chloroprocaine
    (B) Tetracaine
    (C) Ropivacaine
    (D) EMLA

    Rationale: Chloroprocaine and ropivacaine are not administered topically. Tetracaine is topically administered to the eye.
    Reference: Butterworth JF IV, Mackey DC, Wasnick JD, eds. *Morgan & Mikhail's Clinical Anesthesiology*. 7th ed. New York, NY: McGraw Hill; 2022: Chapter 16.

89. Which rate of systemic absorption of local anesthetics is true?

    (A) Intravenous > tracheal > intercostals > paracervical > epidural > brachial plexus > sciatic > subcutaneous
    (B) Tracheal > intercostals > intravenous > paracervical > epidural > brachial plexus > sciatic > subcutaneous
    (C) Intravenous < tracheal < intercostals < paracervical < epidural < brachial plexus < sciatic < subcutaneous
    (D) Tracheal < intercostals < intravenous < paracervical < epidural < brachial plexus < sciatic < subcutaneous

    Rationale: One factor that determines systemic absorption of local anesthetics is the site of the injection. The intravenous route has the greatest absorption of local anesthetic.
    Reference: Butterworth JF IV, Mackey DC, Wasnick JD, eds. *Morgan & Mikhail's Clinical Anesthesiology*. 7th ed. New York, NY: McGraw Hill; 2022: Chapter 16.

90. What do you expect when adding epinephrine to local anesthetic?

    (A) Vasodilation at the site of injection
    (B) Increased absorption
    (C) Decreased duration of action
    (D) Vasoconstriction at the site of injection

    Rationale: Adding epinephrine to local anesthetic solutions causes vasoconstriction at the site of injection. There is less absorption of the local anesthetic. An increased duration of action results.
    Reference: Butterworth JF IV, Mackey DC, Wasnick JD, eds. *Morgan & Mikhail's Clinical Anesthesiology*. 7th ed. New York, NY: McGraw Hill; 2022: Chapter 16.

91. During surgery for a bowel obstruction, you note persistent tachycardia and hypertension. What neuromuscular blocker was most likely used?

    (A) Rocuronium
    (B) Cisatracurium
    (C) Atracurium
    (D) Pancuronium

    Rationale: Vagal blockade and sympathetic stimulation result in tachycardiac and hypertension when using pancuronium. Nonsignificant cardiac effects are associated with cisatracurium, atracurium, and rocuronium.

Reference: Butterworth JF IV, Mackey DC, Wasnick JD, eds. *Morgan & Mikhail's Clinical Anesthesiology.* 7th ed. New York, NY: McGraw Hill; 2022: Chapter 11.

92. Which factor is a relative contraindication to pulmonary artery (PA) catheterization?

    (A) Left bundle branch block
    (B) Right bundle branch block
    (C) A patient in septic shock
    (D) A patient undergoing thoracic aortic aneurysm repair

    Rationale: Left bundle branch block is a relative contraindication to PA catheterization because of the concern for complete heart block. (C) and (D) are cases where PA catheterization should be strongly considered to measure cardiac index, preload, volume status, and mixed venous blood oxygenation.
    References: Butterworth JF IV, Mackey DC, Wasnick JD, eds. *Morgan & Mikhail's Clinical Anesthesiology.* 7th ed. New York, NY: McGraw Hill; 2022: Chapter 5.
    Barash PG, Cullen BF, Stoelting RK, et al, eds. *Clinical Anesthesia.* 8th ed. Lippincott Williams & Wilkins; 2017: Chapter 16.

93. Which statement about the central venous waveform *a* wave is correct?

    (A) It is produced by the passive filling of the right atrium.
    (B) It is produced by right atrial contraction.
    (C) It is produced by the closure of the tricuspid valve.
    (D) It is produced by the venous return against a closed tricuspid valve.

    Rationale: The *a* wave is produced by atrial contraction.
    References: Butterworth JF IV, Mackey DC, Wasnick JD, eds. *Morgan & Mikhail's Clinical Anesthesiology.* 7th ed. New York, NY: McGraw Hill; 2022: Chapter 5.
    Elisha S, Heiner JS, Nagelhout JJ. *Nurse Anesthesia.* 7th ed. St. Louis, MO: Elsevier Saunders; 2023: Chapter 17.

94. Which statement is false regarding nitric oxide (NO)?

    (A) NO regulates pulmonary vascular resistance.
    (B) NO inhibits platelet activation.
    (C) NO regulates systemic vascular resistance.
    (D) NO is an exogenous neurotransmitter.

    Rationale: Nitric oxide (NO), an endogenous neurotransmitter, affects multiple body systems. NO regulates pulmonary and systemic vascular resistance and inhibits platelet aggregation. Multiple actions including immune function and nervous system effects are notable.
    Reference: Butterworth JF IV, Mackey DC, Wasnick JD, eds. *Morgan & Mikhail's Clinical Anesthesiology.* 7th ed. New York, NY: McGraw Hill; 2022: Chapter 15.

95. The patient is taking gabapentin. In which patient would you decrease the dose?

    (A) Hepatic compromised patients
    (B) Cardiac compromised patients
    (C) Renal compromised patients
    (D) Respiratory compromised patients

    Rationale: Gabapentin is excreted unchanged in the kidneys. Dose requirements are lower for patients with renal disease. Gabapentin is neither metabolized in the liver nor bound to plasma proteins.
    Reference: Elisha S, Heiner JS, Nagelhout JJ. *Nurse Anesthesia.* 7th ed. St. Louis, MO: Elsevier Saunders; 2023: Chapter 56.

96. Which statement about monitoring the CVP waveform in a patient with atrial fibrillation is correct?

    (A) There are large *v* waves.
    (B) The *v* waves are absent.
    (C) There are giant, "cannon" *a* waves.
    (D) The *a* waves are absent.

    Rationale: The *a* waves are absent in a patient with atrial fibrillation. Commonly, only the *v* waves are present.
    References: Butterworth JF IV, Mackey DC, Wasnick JD, eds. *Morgan & Mikhail's Clinical Anesthesiology.* 7th ed. New York, NY: McGraw Hill; 2022: Chapter 5.
    Elisha S, Heiner JS, Nagelhout JJ. *Nurse Anesthesia.* 7th ed. St. Louis, MO: Elsevier Saunders; 2023: Chapter 17.

97. Which pathologic state will not cause giant, "cannon" *a* waves on the CVP waveform?

    (A) Tricuspid stenosis
    (B) Tricuspid regurgitation
    (C) Mitral stenosis
    (D) Ventricular hypertrophy

    Rationale: All conditions will cause cannon *a* waves except tricuspid regurgitation which will cause large *v* waves.

References: Butterworth JF IV, Mackey DC, Wasnick JD, eds. *Morgan & Mikhail's Clinical Anesthesiology.* 7th ed. New York, NY: McGraw Hill; 2022: Chapter 5.

Elisha S, Heiner JS, Nagelhout JJ. *Nurse Anesthesia.* 7th ed. St. Louis, MO: Elsevier Saunders; 2023: Chapter 17.

98. The patient received streptokinase. When is surgery permitted?

    (A) 3 days following administration
    (B) 5 days following administration
    (C) 7 days following administration
    (D) 10 days following administration

    Rationale: Patients receiving thrombolytic therapy should not be scheduled for surgery within 10 days of administration.

    Reference: Pardo MC, Miller RD. *Miller's Basics of Anesthesia.* 8th ed. Philadelphia, PA: Elsevier; 2023: Chapter 23.

99. Where does acetazolamide exert its action?

    (A) Proximal convoluted tubule
    (B) Ascending Loop of Henle
    (C) Distal Convoluted Tubule
    (D) Collecting ducts

    Rationale: Carbonic anhydrase inhibitors including acetazolamide exert their action in the proximal convoluted tubule. Loop diuretics act in the ascending Loop of Henle; thiazide diuretics at the distal convoluted tubules; and potassium sparing diuretics at the collecting ducts.

    References: Butterworth JF IV, Mackey DC, Wasnick JD, eds. *Morgan & Mikhail's Clinical Anesthesiology.* 7th ed. New York, NY: McGraw Hill; 2022: Chapter 46.

    Hemmings HC Jr, Egan TD, eds. *Pharmacology and Physiology for Anesthesia: Foundations and Clinical Application.* 2nd ed. Philadelphia, PA: Elsevier Saunders; 2019: Chapter 34.

100. Which hemodynamic profile is consistent with pulmonary embolism?

	CVP	PCWP
(A)	High	High
(B)	High	Normal
(C)	High	Low
(D)	Normal	High

    Rationale: A patient with pulmonary embolism will demonstrate an elevated central venous pressure and a normal pulmonary capillary wedge pressure.

References: Butterworth JF IV, Mackey DC, Wasnick JD, eds. *Morgan & Mikhail's Clinical Anesthesiology.* 7th ed. New York, NY: McGraw Hill; 2022: Chapter 24.

Elisha S, Heiner JS, Nagelhout JJ. *Nurse Anesthesia.* 7th ed. St. Louis, MO: Elsevier Saunders; 2023: Chapter 17.

101. Which antibiotic would you avoid in patients with myasthenia gravis?

    (A) Chloramphenicol
    (B) Amphotercin B
    (C) Ciprofloxin
    (D) Gentamicin

    Rationale: Aminoglycosides that includes gentamicin result in skeletal muscle weakness. Skeletal muscle weakness due to myasthenia gravis is aggravated by the aminoglycosides as compared to other antibiotic groups. Nondepolarizing neuromuscular blockers effects are prolonged.

    Reference: Flood P, Rathmell JP, Urbam RD, eds. *Stoelting's Pharmacology & Physiology in Anesthetic Practice.* 6th ed. Philadelphia, PA: Wolters Kluwer; 2022: Chapter 28.

102. Which chemotherapeutic agent is strongly associated with pulmonary fibrosis?

    (A) 5-FU
    (B) Cyclophosphamide
    (C) Doxorubicin
    (D) Bleomycin

    Rationale: Bleomycin is strongly associated with pulmonary fibrosis, pulmonary hypertension, and pulmonary toxicity. 5-FU is commonly associated with cerebellar ataxia, cardiac toxicity, gastritis, and myelosuppression. Cyclophosphamide side effects include encephalopathy, hemorrhagic cystitis, myelosuppression, cardiac symptoms, and pulmonary fibrosis. Doxorubicin is strongly associated with cardiotoxicity.

    Reference: Hines RL, Marschall KE. *Stoelting's Anesthesia and Co-existing Disease.* 7th ed. Philadelphia, PA: Elsevier Saunders; 2018: Chapter 23.

103. Which hemodynamic profile reflects chronic left ventricular failure?

	CVP	PCWP
(A)	High	High
(B)	High	Normal
(C)	High	Low
(D)	Normal	High

Rationale: A patient with chronic left ventricular failure will demonstrate an elevated central venous pressure (CVP) and an elevated pulmonary capillary wedge pressure (PCWP). In acute left ventricular failure, the CVP will be normal and the PCWP will be elevated.

References: Butterworth JF IV, Mackey DC, Wasnick JD, eds. *Morgan & Mikhail's Clinical Anesthesiology.* 7th ed. New York, NY: McGraw Hill; 2022: Chapter 5.

Elisha S, Heiner JS, Nagelhout JJ. *Nurse Anesthesia.* 7th ed. St. Louis, MO: Elsevier Saunders; 2023: Chapter 17.

104. In which West zone must the tip of the pulmonary artery catheter lie for the pulmonary artery wedge pressure (PAWP) measurement to be accurate?

    (A) I
    (B) II
    (C) III
    (D) IV

Rationale: The goal for placement of a PA catheter is West zone III because the bulk of pulmonary blood flow lies within this lung region. Zone III allows for direct physiologic communication between the right heart and pulmonary pressures with the left heart pressures.

References: Elisha S, Heiner JS, Nagelhout JJ. *Nurse Anesthesia.* 7th ed. St. Louis, MO: Elsevier Saunders; 2023: Chapter 17.

Gropper MA, Cohen NH, Eriksson LI, et al, eds. *Miller's Anesthesia.* 9th ed. Philadelphia, PA: Churchill Livingstone Elsevier, 2020: Chapter 40.

105. How do codeine and morphine differ?

    (A) Codeine undergoes O-demethylation.
    (B) Codeine is less antitussive than morphine.
    (C) Codeine undergoes 2-glucuronide conjugation.
    (D) Codeine's equipotent dose is 1.5 mg.

Rationale: Codeine is an effective antitussive but is less potent than morphine. Morphine undergoes 2-glucuronide conjugation resulting in morphine-6-glucuronide. Codeine's equipotent dose to morphine is 75 mg.

References: Elisha S, Heiner JS, Nagelhout JJ. *Nurse Anesthesia.* 7th ed. St. Louis, MO: Elsevier Saunders; 2023: Chapter 5.

Brunton LL, Hilal-Dandan R, Knollmann BC, eds. *Goodman & Gilman's: The Pharmacological Basis of Therapeutics.* 13th ed. McGraw Hill; 2017: Chapter 18.

106. What is the characteristic pulmonary artery catheter (PAC) pressure waveform that tells you the catheter has entered the pulmonary artery?

    (A) A sharp, upstroke/down stroke waveform with the highest point reaching the 10 mmHg point
    (B) A brisk upstroke followed by a steep down stroke returning to mean central venous pressure levels
    (C) A brisk upstroke followed by a notched, sloping down stroke with acute rise in diastolic pressure
    (D) An undulating waveform that occurs near the 10 mmHg point

Rationale: The acute rise in diastolic pressure is characteristic of PAP waveform compared to the lower diastolic pressure reading of the right ventricle. *A* describes the RA waveform; *B* describes the RV, and *D* describes the PAOP.

References: Butterworth JF IV, Mackey DC, Wasnick JD, eds. *Morgan & Mikhail's Clinical Anesthesiology.* 7th ed. New York, NY: McGraw Hill; 2022: Chapter 5.

Elisha S, Heiner JS, Nagelhout JJ. *Nurse Anesthesia.* 7th ed. St. Louis, MO: Elsevier Saunders; 2023: Chapter 17.

107. Which statement about correlation of the CVP waveform and the EKG waveform is incorrect?

    (A) The *a* wave follows the P wave on the ECG.
    (B) The *c* wave immediately follows the start of the QRS complex on ECG.
    (C) The *v* wave appears shortly after the start of the T wave on the ECG.
    (D) The *y* descent occurs during the QRS complex on the ECG.

Rationale: All are correct except (D). The *y* descent of the CVP waveform corresponds to the opening of the tricuspid valve during diastole and therefore is observed immediately following the *v* wave on CVP and shortly after the T wave on the ECG.

References: Butterworth JF IV, Mackey DC, Wasnick JD, eds. *Morgan & Mikhail's Clinical Anesthesiology.* 7th ed. New York, NY: McGraw Hill; 2022: Chapter 5.

Elisha S, Heiner JS, Nagelhout JJ. *Nurse Anesthesia.* 7th ed. St. Louis, MO: Elsevier Saunders; 2023: Chapter 17.

108. During induction of anesthesia you note the inability to ventilate the patient. The chest wall appears rigid. Which medication did you administer?

(A) Sufentanil

(B) Versed

(C) Etomidate

(D) Methohexital

Rationale: The fentanyl family is known to produce chest wall rigidity (fentanyl, sufenta, alfenta, and remifentanil). All narcotics may produce chest wall rigidity in high doses.

Reference: Butterworth JF IV, Mackey DC, Wasnick JD, eds. *Morgan & Mikhail's Clinical Anesthesiology.* 7th ed. New York, NY: McGraw Hill; 2022: Chapter 10.

109. Which of the following is false regarding the mechanism of action of opioids?

(A) Coupling to G proteins

(B) Binding to Mu receptors

(C) Inhibition of voltage gated sodium channels

(D) Inhibition of adenylyl cyclase

Rationale: The mechanisms of action of opioids include coupling to G proteins, binding to agonists and inhibition of adenylyl cyclase. Inhibition of calcium, not sodium channels, is inhibited by opioids.

Reference: Butterworth JF IV, Mackey DC, Wasnick JD, eds. *Morgan & Mikhail's Clinical Anesthesiology.* 7th ed. New York, NY: McGraw Hill; 2022: Chapter 10.

110. How do COX-1 and COX-2 enzymes differ?

(A) COX-1 responds to inflammation.

(B) COX-1 inhibition increases thrombosis.

(C) COX-2 inhibition increases heart attack risk.

(D) COX-1 sites attract large molecules.

Rationale: Large molecules are preferential to COX-2 receptors. COX-2 inhibition may result in thrombosis, stroke, and myocardial infarction. COX-1 inhibition decreases thrombosis. Inflammatory response prompts production of COX-2.

Reference: Butterworth JF IV, Mackey DC, Wasnick JD, eds. *Morgan & Mikhail's Clinical Anesthesiology.* 7th ed. New York, NY: McGraw Hill; 2022: Chapter 10.

111. If amiodarone is not available, what antiarrhythmic will you use to treat unsuccessful defibrillation?

(A) Lidocaine

(B) Diltiazem

(C) Dobutamine

(D) Magnesium

Rationale: Lidocaine is used as a second-line therapy for PVCs and V-Tach that is unresponsive to defibrillation. Diltiazem improves atrial fibrillation or flutter. Dobutamine is indicated for the treatment of systolic heart failure while magnesium is given for torsades de pointes with prolonged QT interval.

Reference: Butterworth JF IV, Mackey DC, Wasnick JD, eds. *Morgan & Mikhail's Clinical Anesthesiology.* 7th ed. New York, NY: McGraw Hill; 2022: Chapter 55.

112. What is the mechanism of action of aspirin?

(A) Irreversible inhibition of COX-2

(B) Low binding to plasma proteins

(C) Plasma esterase hydrolysis

(D) Irreversible inhibition of COX-1

Rationale: Aspirin prevents thrombosis and is useful in treatment for myocardial infarction by irreversibly inhibiting COX-1. COX inhibitors are highly bound to plasma proteins and undergo hepatic biotransformation.

Reference: Butterworth JF IV, Mackey DC, Wasnick JD, eds. *Morgan & Mikhail's Clinical Anesthesiology.* 7th ed. New York, NY: McGraw Hill; 2022: Chapter 10.

113. Which central line site has the shortest distance to the junction of the vena cava and the right atrium?

(A) Left internal jugular

(B) Right internal jugular

(C) Subclavian vein

(D) Right median basilic vein

Rationale: The subclavian vein provides the shortest distance to the junction of the vena cava and the right atrium (approximately 10 cm) compared to other anatomic sites such as the internal jugular veins (15-20 cm); the femoral vein (40 cm); and the right basilica vein (40 cm).

References: Butterworth JF IV, Mackey DC, Wasnick JD, eds. *Morgan & Mikhail's Clinical Anesthesiology.* 7th ed. New York, NY: McGraw Hill; 2022: Chapter 5.

Elisha S, Heiner JS, Nagelhout JJ. *Nurse Anesthesia.* 7th ed. St. Louis, MO: Elsevier Saunders; 2023: Chapter 17.

114. What is the hallmark sign of a catheter-induced pulmonary artery rupture?

(A) Hypotension

(B) Hypoxemia

(C) Hemoptysis

(D) Arrhythmias

Rationale: Hemoptysis is a common sign of PA rupture. Hypotension/hypoxemia would occur because of PA hemorrhage, but it is nonspecific to PA rupture. Arrhythmias are unrelated to the PA rupture.

References: Butterworth JF IV, Mackey DC, Wasnick JD, eds. *Morgan & Mikhail's Clinical Anesthesiology.* 7th ed. New York, NY: McGraw Hill; 2022: Chapter 5.

Gropper MA, Cohen NH, Eriksson LI, et al, eds. *Miller's Anesthesia.* 9th ed. Philadelphia, PA: Churchill Livingstone Elsevier; 2020: Chapter 40.

115. Which law of physics explains why an increase in left ventricular wall thickness will reduce ventricular wall tension?

(A) LaPlace's law

(B) Ohm's law

(C) Poiseuille's law

(D) Fick's law

Rationale: LaPlace's law states that circumferential stress equals intraventricular pressure times ventricular radius divided by the two times the thickness of the ventricular wall. Therefore, the larger the ventricular wall radius, the greater the wall tension. Conversely, an increase in ventricular wall thickness will reduce ventricular wall tension.

References: Butterworth JF IV, Mackey DC, Wasnick JD, eds. *Morgan & Mikhail's Clinical Anesthesiology.* 7th ed. New York, NY: McGraw Hill; 2022: Chapter 20.

Elisha S, Heiner JS, Nagelhout JJ. *Nurse Anesthesia.* 7th ed. St. Louis, MO: Elsevier Saunders; 2023: Chapter 25.

116. Which cardiovascular reflex does not result in an efferent vagal response?

(A) Baroreceptor reflex

(B) Bainbridge reflex

(C) Valsalva maneuver

(D) Oculocardiac reflex

Rationale: Each reflex results in an efferent vagal response and subsequent decreased heart rate except the Bainbridge reflex (also known as the atrial stretch reflex). This reflex is caused by an increased venous return due to hypervolemia causing a stimulation of atrial stretch receptors. The stimulation of atrial stretch receptors results in an increased heart rate.

References: Butterworth JF IV, Mackey DC, Wasnick JD, eds. *Morgan & Mikhail's Clinical Anesthesiology.* 7th ed. New York, NY: McGraw Hill; 2022: Chapter 20.

Elisha S, Heiner JS, Nagelhout JJ. *Nurse Anesthesia.* 7th ed. St. Louis, MO: Elsevier Saunders; 2023: Chapter 25.

117. Which herbal remedy does not delay awakening from anesthesia?

(A) Valerian

(B) Kava kava

(C) St. John's wort

(D) Garlic

Rationale: Valerian, kava kava, and St. John's wort interact with anesthetic drugs including benzodiazepines. The interaction may result in delayed emergence from anesthesia. Garlic potentiates the action of warfarin that may result in bleeding.

References: Elisha S, Heiner J, Nagelhout J. *Nurse Anesthesia.* 7th ed. St. Louis, MO: Elsevier Saunders; 2023: Chapter 20.

Flood P, Rathmell JP, Urbam RD, eds. *Stoelting's Pharmacology & Physiology in Anesthetic Practice.* 6th ed. Philadelphia, PA: Wolters Kluwer; 2022: Chapter 34.

118. While floating a pulmonary artery catheter via the right internal jugular, the patient monitor shows a run of ventricular tachycardia. Which insertion depth is most likely to induce this arrhythmia?

(A) 15 cm

(B) 22 cm

(C) 28 cm

(D) 12 cm

Rationale: A PA catheter inserted through the right internal jugular vein will reach the right ventricle somewhere between 25 and 35 cm, depending on the size of the patient. Transient ectopy from irritation of the right ventricle by the balloon and catheter tip is common.

References: Butterworth JF IV, Mackey DC, Wasnick JD, eds. *Morgan & Mikhail's Clinical Anesthesiology.* 7th ed. New York, NY: McGraw Hill; 2022: Chapter 5.

Elisha S, Heiner JS, Nagelhout JJ. *Nurse Anesthesia.* 7th ed. St. Louis, MO: Elsevier Saunders; 2023: Chapter 17.

119. At what dose is the onset of action of rocuronium like that of succinylcholine for rapid sequence intubation?

(A) 0.9 to 1.2 mg/kg

(B) 1.5 to 2.0 mg/kg

(C) 2 to 2.5 mg/kg

(D) >2.5 mg/kg

Rationale: The standard intubating dose of rocuronium is 0.8 mg/kg. Larger intubating doses (0.9-1.2 mg/kg) facilitate the onset of action to that approximating succinylcholine (0.5 minutes). The normal onset of action of rocuronium is 1.5 minute. The larger dose of rocuronium makes it a viable choice for rapid sequence induction.

Reference: Butterworth JF IV, Mackey DC, Wasnick JD, eds. *Morgan & Mikhail's Clinical Anesthesiology*. 7th ed. New York, NY: McGraw Hill; 2022: Chapter 11.

120. What is the primary neurotransmitter of the parasympathetic nervous system?

(A) Norepinephrine

(B) Acetylcholine

(C) Acetylcoenzyme A

(D) Muscarine

Rationale: Parasympathetic nervous system (cholinergic) effects are due to acetylcholine. Adrenergic effects are due to the transmitter norepinephrine. Acetylcoenzyme A is significant in the synthesis and hydrolysis of acetylcholine. Muscarinic receptors represent one of two major divisions of the cholinergic receptors.

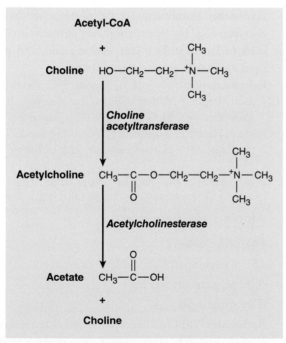

FIG. 1-3. The synthesis and hydrolysis of acetylcholine. (Reproduced with permission from Butterworth JF IV, Mackey DC, Wasnick JD, eds. *Morgan & Mikhail's Clinical Anesthesiology*. 7th ed. New York, NY: McGraw Hill; 2022.)

Reference: Butterworth JF IV, Mackey DC, Wasnick JD, eds. *Morgan & Mikhail's Clinical Anesthesiology*. 7th ed. New York, NY: McGraw Hill; 2022: Chapter 12.

121. Which is correct about the CVP waveform in a patient with tricuspid regurgitation?

(A) Decreasing CVP pressure implies worsening right ventricular dysfunction.

(B) The *x* descent is usually absent.

(C) Giant, "cannon" *a*-waves are apparent.

(D) The *v*-waves become diminished.

Rationale: In the setting of tricuspid regurgitation, central venous pressure will increase, indicating a worsening right ventricular dysfunction. The *x* descent is absent and prominent *v*-waves are usually present on the waveform.

References: Butterworth JF IV, Mackey DC, Wasnick JD, eds. *Morgan & Mikhail's Clinical Anesthesiology*. 7th ed. New York, NY: McGraw Hill; 2022: Chapter 21.

Elisha S, Heiner JS, Nagelhout JJ. *Nurse Anesthesia*. 7th ed. St. Louis, MO: Elsevier Saunders; 2023: Chapter 25.

122. Which sympathomimetic amine structurally related to amphetamine may cause cardiac arrhythmias, myocardial infarction, and stroke?

(A) Echinacea

(B) Ma Huang

(C) Ginkgo biloba

(D) Genseng

Rationale: Ma Huang (ephedra) is a popular herbal formula. Ephedrine is the active form of ephdra responsible for the sympathomimetic effects. Ginseng may cause tachycardia and hypertension especially if combined with other stimulants. Side effects of Ginkgo biloba include gastrointestinal discomfort, headache, dizziness, bleeding, and seizures. Use of Echinacea may result in hypersensitivity reactions.

References: Elisha S, Heiner JS, Nagelhout JJ. *Nurse Anesthesia*. 7th ed. St. Louis, MO: Elsevier Saunders; 2023: Chapter 20.

Flood P, Rathmell JP, Urbam RD, eds. *Stoelting's Pharmacology & Physiology in Anesthetic Practice*. 6th ed. Philadelphia, PA: Wolters Kluwer; 2022: Chapter 34.

123. How does hydromorphone differ from morphine?

(A) Hydromorphone is more potent.

(B) Hydromorphone has a shorter duration of action.

(C) Hydormorphone is less potent.

(D) Hydromorphone is less lipid soluble.

Rationale: Hydromorphone is four to five times more potent than morphine. Both drugs are lipid soluble, but morphine is less lipid soluble than hydromorphone. The duration of action of hydromorphone is the same as morphine.

References: Brunton LL, Hilal-Dandan R, Knollmann BC, eds. *Goodman & Gilman's: The Pharmacological Basis of Therapeutics.* 13th ed. McGraw Hill; 2017: Chapter 18.

Elisha S, Heiner JS, Nagelhout JJ. *Nurse Anesthesia.* 7th ed. St. Louis, MO: Elsevier Saunders; 2023: Chapter 11.

124. What should be used to reconstitute a standard vial of dantrolene?

   (A) 60 mL normal saline

   (B) 100 mL normal saline

   (C) 60 mL sterile water

   (D) 100 mL sterile water

Rationale: Each vial of dantrolene is reconstituted using 60 mL of sterile water.

References: Butterworth JF IV, Mackey DC, Wasnick JD, eds. *Morgan & Mikhail's Clinical Anesthesiology.* 7th ed. New York, NY: McGraw Hill; 2022: Chapter 52.

Hines RL, Marschall KE. *Stoelting's Anesthesia and Co-existing Disease.* 7th ed. Philadelphia, PA: Elsevier Saunders; 2018: Chapter 27.

125. Preoperatively you learn that the patient is taking warfarin. Which herbal remedy poses the potential for bleeding?

   (A) Ginkgo biloba

   (B) Evening primrose

   (C) Kola nut

   (D) Goldenseal

Rationale: Ginkgo biloba is linked to bleeding and hemorrhage due to antiplatelet activity. Use of Evening primrose may lead to nausea and vomiting. Kola nut interacts with stimulants and may result in irritability and insomnia. There are no known drug interactions with goldenseal, but the herbal remedy is known to cause hypertension and edema.

References: Elisha S, Heiner JS, Nagelhout JJ. *Nurse Anesthesia.* 7th ed. St. Louis, MO: Elsevier Saunders; 2023: Chapter 20.

Flood P, Rathmell JP, Urbam RD, eds. *Stoelting's Pharmacology & Physiology in Anesthetic Practice.* 6th ed. Philadelphia, PA: Wolters Kluwer; 2022: Chapter 34.

126. Which antibiotic should not be administered during pregnancy?

   (A) Penicillin

   (B) Aminoglycosides

   (C) Tetracycline

   (D) Erythromycin

Rationale: Each of the antibiotics is safe to administer during pregnancy except tetracycline. Tetracycline is absorbed in teeth and bones resulting in brown, discolored teeth.

Reference: Flood P, Rathmell JP, Urbam RD, eds. *Stoelting's Pharmacology & Physiology in Anesthetic Practice.* 6th ed. Philadelphia, PA: Wolters Kluwer; 2022: Chapter 28.

127. How is emphysema characterized?

   (A) Narrowing of small airways by inflammation and mucus

   (B) Destruction of parenchyma that leads to loss of surface area, elastic recoil, and structural support to maintain the airway

   (C) Antigen binding to immunoglobulin E on the surface of mast cells causing degranulation

   (D) Reversible enlargement of the airways distal to terminal bronchioles with damage of the alveolar septa

Rationale: Emphysema is an obstructive disorder characterized by destruction of parenchyma that leads to loss of surface area, elastic recoil, and structural support to maintain the airway.

References: Butterworth JF IV, Mackey DC, Wasnick JD, eds. *Morgan & Mikhail's Clinical Anesthesiology.* 7th ed. New York, NY: McGraw Hill; 2022: Chapter 24.

Elisha S, Heiner JS, Nagelhout JJ. *Nurse Anesthesia.* 7th ed. St. Louis, MO: Elsevier Saunders; 2023: Chapter 29.

128. Preoperatively, the patient shares that they were treated with vincristine for Hodgkin's disease. What side effect would you expect?

   (A) Paresthesias

   (B) Coagulopathy

   (C) Magnesium wasting

   (D) Arthralgias

Rationale: Peripheral neuropathy and paresthesias are strongly linked to vincristine. Asparaginase is responsible for coagulopathies and hepatic dysfunction. Magnesium wasting is a side effect of cisplatin while arthralgias are prominent for patients taking palitaxel.

Reference: Hines RL, Marschall KE. *Stoelting's Anesthesia and Co-existing Disease.* 7th ed. Philadelphia, PA: Elsevier Saunders; 2018: Chapter 23.

129. A 70-kg adult patient with mitral valve prolapse is scheduled for an exploratory laparotomy. If the patient has history of anaphylaxis to penicillin, what antibiotic prophylaxis will you administer?

    (A) Cefazolin 1 g IV
    (B) Clindamycin 600 mg IV
    (C) Ampicillin 2 g IV
    (D) Amoxicillin 2 g IV

    Rationale: Antibiotic prophylaxis is recommended for patients with mitral valve prolapse, because of the potential for endocarditis. A penicillin-allergic adult patient can safely receive clindamycin 600 mg IV. The other options are contraindicated for the patient allergic to penicillin, including cephalosporins if the patient has a history of anaphylaxis, angioedema, or urticaria.

    References: Butterworth JF IV, Mackey DC, Wasnick JD, eds. *Morgan & Mikhail's Clinical Anesthesiology.* 7th ed. New York, NY: McGraw Hill; 2022: Chapter 21.
    Elisha S, Heiner JS, Nagelhout JJ. *Nurse Anesthesia.* 7th ed. St. Louis, MO: Elsevier Saunders; 2023: Chapter 25.

130. A 70-year-old female is undergoing a large bowel resection when the following hemodynamic profile is obtained: B/P 100/80, cardiac output 6 L/min, and central venous pressure 3 mmHg. What is the systemic vascular resistance?

    (A) 504 dynes/s/cm^5
    (B) 1,120 dynes/s/cm^5
    (C) 1,160 dynes/s/cm^5
    (D) 2,200 dynes/s/cm^5

    Rationale: The formula for calculating SVR is:

    $$SVR = \frac{[MAP - CVP] \times 80}{CO}$$

    In this question, the MAP can be calculated first by plugging into the formula:

    $$MAP = \frac{(SBP + 2DBP)}{3}$$

    The MAP is 87 mmHg. Next, plug the numbers into the SVR formula to derive the SVR.

    $$SVR = \frac{[87 - 3] \times 80}{6}$$

    The final answer is 1,120 dynes/s/cm^5.

References: Butterworth JF IV, Mackey DC, Wasnick JD, eds. *Morgan & Mikhail's Clinical Anesthesiology.* 7th ed. New York, NY: McGraw Hill; 2022: Chapter 20.
Elisha S, Heiner JS, Nagelhout JJ. *Nurse Anesthesia.* 7th ed. St. Louis, MO: Elsevier Saunders; 2023: Chapter 26.

131. What has been firmly established as the primary environmental risk factor associated with emphysema and bronchitis?

    (A) Homozygous α_1-antitrypsin
    (B) Cigarette smoking
    (C) Antigen binding to immunoglobulin E
    (D) Drug toxicity with bleomycin and nitrofurantoin

    Rationale: Cigarette smoking has been firmly established as the primary environmental risk factor associated with emphysema and bronchitis.

    References: Butterworth JF IV, Mackey DC, Wasnick JD, eds. *Morgan & Mikhail's Clinical Anesthesiology.* 7th ed. New York, NY: McGraw Hill; 2022: Chapter 24.
    Elisha S, Heiner JS, Nagelhout JJ. *Nurse Anesthesia.* 7th ed. St. Louis, MO: Elsevier Saunders; 2023: Chapter 29.

132. What is the most significant precipitating factor leading to obstructive sleep apnea (OSA)?

    (A) History of stroke
    (B) History of type II diabetes
    (C) Obesity
    (D) Hypertension

    Rationale: Obesity is the most significant precipitating factor leading to obstructive sleep apnea (OSA).

    References: Butterworth JF IV, Mackey DC, Wasnick JD, eds. *Morgan & Mikhail's Clinical Anesthesiology.* 7th ed. New York, NY: McGraw Hill; 2022: Chapter 44.
    Elisha S, Heiner JS, Nagelhout JJ. *Nurse Anesthesia.* 7th ed. St. Louis, MO: Elsevier Saunders; 2023: Chapter 29.

133. By what mechanism do local anesthetics depress cardiac contractility?

    (A) By increasing Ca^{2+} influx and release into the myocardial cell
    (B) By decreasing Ca^{2+} influx and release into the myocardial cell
    (C) By enhancing the intracellular levels of cAMP of the myocardial cell
    (D) By enhancing the intracellular levels of cGMP of the myocardial cell

Rationale: Local anesthetics depress cardiac contractility by reducing Ca^{2+} influx and release into the myocardial cell in a dose-dependent fashion.
References: Butterworth JF IV, Mackey DC, Wasnick JD, eds. *Morgan & Mikhail's Clinical Anesthesiology.* 7th ed. New York, NY: McGraw Hill; 2022: Chapter 20.
Elisha S, Heiner JS, Nagelhout JJ. *Nurse Anesthesia.* 7th ed. St. Louis, MO: Elsevier Saunders; 2023: Chapter 25.

134. Which local anesthetic agent depresses cardiac contractility the least?

(A) Bupivacaine
(B) Tetracaine
(C) Ropivacaine
(D) Lidocaine

Rationale: The more potent local anesthetics for nerve block such as bupivicaine, ropivacaine, and tetracaine depress left ventricular contractility more significantly than the less potent local anesthetics such as lidocaine and chlorprocaine.
References: Butterworth JF IV, Mackey DC, Wasnick JD, eds. *Morgan & Mikhail's Clinical Anesthesiology.* 7th ed. New York, NY: McGraw Hill; 2022: Chapter 20.
Elisha S, Heiner JS, Nagelhout JJ. *Nurse Anesthesia.* 7th ed. St. Louis, MO: Elsevier Saunders; 2023: Chapter 10.

135. A patient is scheduled for a general anesthetic. You plan to induce with propofol. What is the best dose for a 70-kg male?

(A) 350 mg
(B) 100 mg
(C) 250 mg
(D) 200 mg

Rationale: The induction dose of propofol is 1 to 2.5 mg/kg. The dose range for the 70-kg patient is 70 to 175 mg/kg.
References: Butterworth JF IV, Mackey DC, Wasnick JD, eds. *Morgan & Mikhail's Clinical Anesthesiology.* 7th ed. New York, NY: McGraw Hill; 2022: Chapter 9.
Pardo MC, Miller RD. *Miller's Basics of Anesthesia.* 8th ed. Philadelphia, PA: Elsevier; 2023: Chapter 8.

136. What clinical sign is not consistent with Cushing syndrome?

(A) Hypoglycemia
(B) Hypertension
(C) Hyperglycemia
(D) Hypokalemia

Rationale: Clinical signs consistent with Cushing syndrome include hyperglycemia, hypertension, hypokalemic metabolic alkalosis, hirsutism, osteoporosis, muscle weakness, mental status disorders, buffalo hump, weight gain, moon face, menstrual changes, and increased likelihood of infection.
References: Butterworth JF IV, Mackey DC, Wasnick JD, eds. *Morgan & Mikhail's Clinical Anesthesiology.* 7th ed. New York, NY: McGraw Hill; 2022: Chapter 34.
Elisha S, Heiner JS, Nagelhout JJ. *Nurse Anesthesia.* 7th ed. St. Louis, MO: Elsevier Saunders; 2023: Chapter 37.

137. What are the electrophysiologic effects of diltiazem on the myocardial cells?

(A) Binding to calcium channels in their resting active state
(B) Binding to T-type calcium channels
(C) Binding to L-type calcium channels
(D) Inhibiting potassium efflux during cardiac repolarization

Rationale: Calcium channel blockers such as diltiazem block Ca^{2+} influx through L-type, but not T-type channels in a dose-dependent fashion.
References: Butterworth JF IV, Mackey DC, Wasnick JD, eds. *Morgan & Mikhail's Clinical Anesthesiology.* 7th ed. New York, NY: McGraw Hill; 2022: Chapter 20.
Elisha S, Heiner JS, Nagelhout JJ. *Nurse Anesthesia.* 7th ed. St. Louis, MO: Elsevier Saunders; 2023: Chapter 10.

138. Which is an appropriate initial intervention to correct intraoperative bronchospasm?

(A) Deepen the level of anesthesia with a volatile agent
(B) Give 10 mg morphine IV
(C) Administer intravenous corticosteroids
(D) Give Labetalol 10 mg IV

Rationale: Morphine can release histamine which could cause bronchoconstriction and labetalol can produce bronchoconstriction related to the beta-2 blocking effects. Administering intravenous corticosteroids will not have an immediate effect. The potent inhalation agents produce bronchial relaxation and have all been successfully used in asthmatic patients.
References: Butterworth JF IV, Mackey DC, Wasnick JD, eds. *Morgan & Mikhail's Clinical Anesthesiology.* 7th ed. New York, NY: McGraw Hill; 2022: Chapter 23.
Elisha S, Heiner JS, Nagelhout JJ. *Nurse Anesthesia.* 7th ed. St. Louis, MO: Elsevier Saunders; 2023: Chapter 29.

139. What is the correct classification of asthma symptoms that limit daily activity and require daily use of a short acting beta agonist?

(A) Mild persistent asthma

(B) Severe persistent asthma

(C) Moderate persistent asthma

(D) Intermittent asthma

Rationale: In intermittent asthma, symptoms occur 0 to 2 days a week, an inhaler is used 0 to 2 days a week and there is no activity limitation. Symptoms occur 2 to 6 days a week in mild persistent asthma. An inhaler is used 3 to 6 days a week and there is minor activity limitation. Severe persistent asthma is characterized by continuous signs and symptoms. An inhaler is used several times a day. There is extremely limited activity. With moderate persistent asthma, there is some activity limitations with daily symptoms. An inhaler is typically used daily.

Reference: Elisha S, Heiner JS, Nagelhout JJ. *Nurse Anesthesia.* 7th ed. St. Louis, MO: Elsevier Saunders; 2023: Chapter 29.

140. What are the two strongest predictors of postoperative pulmonary complications?

(A) Operative site and well-controlled asthma

(B) Operative site and history of dyspnea

(C) Obesity and operative site

(D) History of dyspnea and abnormal chest exam

Rationale: Obesity and well-controlled asthma show good evidence against being a risk factor. Abnormal chest exam is supported by fair evidence for postoperative pulmonary complications. The two strongest predictors of postoperative pulmonary complications are operative site and history of dyspnea, which correlate with the degree of preexisting pulmonary disease.

Reference: Butterworth JF IV, Mackey DC, Wasnick JD, eds. *Morgan & Mikhail's Clinical Anesthesiology.* 7th ed. New York, NY: McGraw Hill; 2022: Chapter 24.

141. Which two interventions lessen air trapping in a COPD patient?

(A) Increase respiratory rate

(B) Decrease respiratory rate

(C) Increase I:E ratio

(D) Increase tidal volume

Rationale: Decreasing respiratory rate and decreasing I:E ratio will give the COPD patient more time to exhale and lessen air trapping.

References: Butterworth JF IV, Mackey DC, Wasnick JD, eds. *Morgan & Mikhail's Clinical Anesthesiology.* 7th ed. New York, NY: McGraw Hill; 2022: Chapter 24.

Elisha S, Heiner JS, Nagelhout JJ. *Nurse Anesthesia.* 7th ed. St. Louis, MO: Elsevier Saunders; 2023: Chapter 29.

142. What is the leading cause of cor pulmonale?

(A) Obesity

(B) Asthma

(C) Sleep apnea

(D) COPD

Rationale: COPD is the leading cause of cor pulmonale superseding sleep apnea, obesity, and asthma.

Reference: Elisha S, Heiner JS, Nagelhout JJ. *Nurse Anesthesia.* 7th ed. St. Louis, MO: Elsevier Saunders; 2023: Chapter 29.

143. Which statement is false concerning anesthetic management of OSA patients?

(A) Patients who use CPAP at home should be encouraged to bring device from home for use in PACU.

(B) The anesthetist should anticipate a difficult intubation.

(C) Increased doses of benzodiazepines and opioids may be needed preoperatively.

(D) The anesthetist should anticipate a reduced FRC.

Rationale: Preoperatively, sedative medications should be used cautiously. As a result of central nervous system sensitization, patients may be hypersensitive to effects of benzodiazepines and opioids.

References: Butterworth JF IV, Mackey DC, Wasnick JD, eds. *Morgan & Mikhail's Clinical Anesthesiology.* 7th ed. New York, NY: McGraw Hill; 2022: Chapter 44.

Elisha S, Heiner JS, Nagelhout JJ. *Nurse Anesthesia.* 7th ed. St. Louis, MO: Elsevier Saunders; 2023: Chapter 29.

144. What type of pulmonary disease demonstrates an FEV_1/FVC ratio that is normal with a reduction in vital capacity?

(A) Asthma

(B) COPD

(C) Emphysema

(D) Pulmonary fibrosis

Rationale: FEV_1/FVC ratio that is normal with a reduction in vital capacity is diagnostic of restrictive pulmonary disease.

References: Butterworth JF IV, Mackey DC, Wasnick JD, eds. *Morgan & Mikhail's Clinical Anesthesiology.* 7th ed. New York, NY: McGraw Hill; 2022: Chapter 24.

Elisha S, Heiner JS, Nagelhout JJ. *Nurse Anesthesia.* 7th ed. St. Louis, MO: Elsevier Saunders; 2023: Chapter 29.

145. What diagnosis of a patient could be made with a pulmonary function test that revealed an FEV_1/FVC ratio that is 0.6 of predicted valve?

    (A) Pulmonary fibrosis

    (B) COPD

    (C) Pulmonary edema

    (D) Aspiration pneumonia

Rationale: FEV_1/FVC ratio that is less than or equal to 0.7 is diagnostic of COPD.

References: Butterworth JF IV, Mackey DC, Wasnick JD, eds. *Morgan & Mikhail's Clinical Anesthesiology.* 7th ed. New York, NY: McGraw Hill; 2022: Chapter 24.

Elisha S, Heiner JS, Nagelhout JJ. *Nurse Anesthesia.* 7th ed. St. Louis, MO: Elsevier Saunders; 2023: Chapter 29.

146. What clinical feature of a pulmonary embolism is false?

    (A) Hypoxemia

    (B) Tachycardia

    (C) Decreased pulmonary vascular resistance

    (D) Hypocapnia

Rationale: There would be an increase in pulmonary vascular resistance. A, B, and D are all clinical features of a pulmonary embolism.

References: Butterworth JF IV, Mackey DC, Wasnick JD, eds. *Morgan & Mikhail's Clinical Anesthesiology.* 7th ed. New York, NY: McGraw Hill; 2022: Chapter 24.

Elisha S, Heiner JS, Nagelhout JJ. *Nurse Anesthesia.* 7th ed. St. Louis, MO: Elsevier Saunders; 2023: Chapter 29.

147. Which I:E ratio is most appropriate in a patient with severe restrictive disease?

    (A) I:E of 1:4

    (B) I:E of 1:2

    (C) I:E of 1:1

    (D) I:E of 1:3

Rationale: An I:E ratio of 1:1 may help to maximize the inspiratory time per tidal volume and minimize the peak and plateau ventilator pressures in patients with severe restrictive disease.

References: Butterworth JF IV, Mackey DC, Wasnick JD, eds. *Morgan & Mikhail's Clinical Anesthesiology.* 7th ed. New York, NY: McGraw Hill; 2022: Chapter 24.

Elisha S, Heiner JS, Nagelhout JJ. *Nurse Anesthesia.* 7th ed. St. Louis, MO: Elsevier Saunders; 2023: Chapter 29.

148. Deficiency in which protease inhibitor is linked to early-onset emphysema?

    (A) Beta-1 antitrypsin

    (B) Alpha-2 antitrypsin

    (C) Alpha-1 antitrypsin

    (D) Beta-2 antitrypsin

Rationale: Alpha-1 antitrypsin is a protease inhibitor that prevents excessive activity of proteolytic enzymes in the lungs.

References: Butterworth JF IV, Mackey DC, Wasnick JD, eds. *Morgan & Mikhail's Clinical Anesthesiology.* 7th ed. New York, NY: McGraw Hill; 2022: Chapter 24.

Elisha S, Heiner JS, Nagelhout JJ. *Nurse Anesthesia.* 7th ed. St. Louis, MO: Elsevier Saunders; 2023: Chapter 29.

149. What is the hallmark sign of aspiration pneumonitis?

    (A) Hypertension

    (B) Pulmonary edema

    (C) Arterial hypoxemia

    (D) Tachycardia

Rationale: (A), (B), and (D) are conditions associated with aspiration pneumonitis. However, arterial hypoxemia is the hallmark clinical feature of aspiration pneumonitis.

References: Butterworth JF IV, Mackey DC, Wasnick JD, eds. *Morgan & Mikhail's Clinical Anesthesiology.* 7th ed. New York, NY: McGraw Hill; 2022: Chapter 24.

Elisha S, Heiner JS, Nagelhout JJ. *Nurse Anesthesia.* 7th ed. St. Louis, MO: Elsevier Saunders; 2023: Chapter 29.

150. Which statements regarding emphysema are true?

    (A) Emphysema is a restrictive lung disease

    (B) Elevated hematocrit

    (C) Copious sputum

    (D) Hyperinflation of the lungs on chest x-ray

Rationale: Emphysema is an obstructive lung disease with a normal hematocrit, minimal sputum and demonstrates hyperinflation of the lungs on chest x-ray.

References: Butterworth JF IV, Mackey DC, Wasnick JD, eds. *Morgan & Mikhail's Clinical Anesthesiology*. 7th ed. New York, NY: McGraw Hill; 2022: Chapter 24.
Elisha S, Heiner JS, Nagelhout JJ. *Nurse Anesthesia*. 7th ed. St. Louis, MO: Elsevier Saunders; 2023: Chapter 29.

151. Which mechanical ventilation modalities would be most appropriate for a patient with COPD?

    (A) Increasing respiratory rate and an I:E ratio of 1:1
    (B) Decreasing respiratory rate and an I:E ratio of 1:1
    (C) Increasing respiratory rate and an I:E ratio of 2:1
    (D) Decreasing respiratory rate and an I:E ratio of 1:3

    Rationale: Decreasing respiratory rate and an I:E ratio of 1:3 allows more time for exhalation.

    References: Butterworth JF IV, Mackey DC, Wasnick JD, eds. *Morgan & Mikhail's Clinical Anesthesiology*. 7th ed. New York, NY: McGraw Hill; 2022: Chapter 24.
    Elisha S, Heiner JS, Nagelhout JJ. *Nurse Anesthesia*. 7th ed. St. Louis, MO: Elsevier Saunders; 2023: Chapter 29.

152. Which four criteria are consistent with the diagnoses of Adult Respiratory Distress Syndrome?

    (A) Acute onset, PaO_2 to FiO_2 ratio < 200 regardless of the level of peep applied, bilateral infiltrates on chest x-ray, and a PA wedge pressure less than or equal to 18 mmHg
    (B) Acute onset, PaO_2 to FiO_2 ratio < 200 regardless of the level of peep applied, normal chest x-ray, and a PA wedge pressure less than or equal to 18 mmHg
    (C) Acute onset, PaO_2 to FiO_2 ratio < 300 regardless of the level of peep applied, bilateral infiltrates on chest x-ray, and a PA wedge pressure less than or equal to 18 mmHg
    (D) Slow onset, PaO_2 to FiO_2 ratio < 200 regardless of the level of peep applied, bilateral infiltrates on chest x-ray, and a PA wedge pressure less than or equal to 18 mmHg

    Rationale: Acute onset, PAO_2 to FiO_2 ratio <200 regardless of the level of peep applied, bilateral infiltrates on chest x-ray, and a PA wedge pressure less than or equal to 18 mmHg is consistent with the diagnoses of adult respiratory distress syndrome.

    Reference: Elisha S, Heiner JS, Nagelhout JJ. *Nurse Anesthesia*. 7th ed. St. Louis, MO: Elsevier Saunders; 2023: Chapter 29.

153. Which criteria are consistent with the diagnoses of pulmonary hypertension?

    (A) A mean pulmonary artery pressure 14 mmHg with a pulmonary capillary occlusion pressure of no more than 15 mmHg
    (B) A mean pulmonary artery pressure at least 25 mmHg with a pulmonary capillary occlusion pressure of no more than 15 mmHg
    (C) A mean pulmonary artery pressure at least 10 mmHg with a pulmonary capillary occlusion pressure of no more than 15 mmHg
    (D) A mean pulmonary artery pressure at least 12 mmHg with a pulmonary capillary occlusion pressure of no more than 15 mmHg

    Rationale: A mean pulmonary artery pressure at least 25 mmHg with a pulmonary capillary occlusion pressure of no more than 15 mmHg is consistent with the diagnoses of pulmonary hypertension.

    References: Butterworth JF IV, Mackey DC, Wasnick JD, eds. *Morgan & Mikhail's Clinical Anesthesiology*. 7th ed. New York, NY: McGraw Hill; 2022: Chapter 24.
    Elisha S, Heiner JS, Nagelhout JJ. *Nurse Anesthesia*. 7th ed. St. Louis, MO: Elsevier Saunders; 2023: Chapter 29.

154. Which of the following statements about chronic bronchitis is true?

    (A) Patients with chronic bronchitis display hyperinflation on the chest x-ray.
    (B) Patients with chronic bronchitis display decreased elastic recoil.
    (C) Patients with chronic bronchitis display a normal hematocrit.
    (D) Patients with chronic bronchitis display an elevated $PaCO_2$.

    Rationale: Choices A to C refer to patients with emphysema.

    References: Butterworth JF IV, Mackey DC, Wasnick JD, eds. *Morgan & Mikhail's Clinical Anesthesiology*. 7th ed. New York, NY: McGraw Hill; 2022: Chapter 24.
    Elisha S, Heiner JS, Nagelhout JJ. *Nurse Anesthesia*. 7th ed. St. Louis, MO: Elsevier Saunders; 2023: Chapter 29.

155. How long should a patient discontinue smoking to decrease secretions and reduce pulmonary complications?

    (A) 1 to 2 weeks
    (B) 2 to 4 weeks
    (C) 3 to 5 days
    (D) 4 to 6 weeks

Rationale: A patient will get the optimal benefit if they discontinue smoking 4 to 6 weeks prior to surgery to decrease secretions and to reduce pulmonary complications.

Reference: Butterworth JF IV, Mackey DC, Wasnick JD, eds. *Morgan & Mikhail's Clinical Anesthesiology.* 7th ed. New York, NY: McGraw Hill; 2022: Chapter 24.

156. What is the acid-base interpretation for a patient with the following ABG, pH 7.29, $PaCO_2$ 52, HCO_3 24?

(A) Uncompensated respiratory alkalosis

(B) Compensated respiratory acidosis

(C) Compensated respiratory alkalosis

(D) Uncompensated respiratory acidosis

Rationale: The HCO_3 24 is normal so there is no compensation; pH 7.29 and $PaCO_2$ 52 indicate respiratory acidosis.

References: Butterworth JF IV, Mackey DC, Wasnick JD, eds. *Morgan & Mikhail's Clinical Anesthesiology.* 7th ed. New York, NY: McGraw Hill; 2022: Chapter 50.

Elisha S, Heiner JS, Nagelhout JJ. *Nurse Anesthesia.* 7th ed. St. Louis, MO: Elsevier Saunders; 2023: Chapter 29.

157. When giving neostigmine, what is the resultant muscarinic effect?

(A) Bradycardia

(B) Tachyarrhythmias

(C) Improved contractility

(D) Increased conduction

Rationale: Cardiovascular muscarinic responses include lowered heart rate and brady arrhythmias. Decreased conduction and contractility are also muscarinic side effects.

TABLE 1-8. Muscarinic side effects of cholinesterase inhibitors.

Organ System	Muscarinic Side Effects
Cardiovascular	Decreased heart rate, bradyarrhythmia
Pulmonary	Bronchospasm, bronchial secretions
Cerebral	Diffuse excitation[1]
Gastrointestinal	Intestinal spasm, increased salivation
Genitourinary	Increased bladder tone
Ophthalmological	Pupillary constriction

[1]Applies only to physostigmine.
(Reproduced with permission from Butterworth JF IV, Mackey DC, Wasnick JD, eds. *Morgan & Mikhail's Clinical Anesthesiology.* 7th ed. New York, NY: McGraw Hill; 2022.)

Reference: Butterworth JF IV, Mackey DC, Wasnick JD, eds. *Morgan & Mikhail's Clinical Anesthesiology.* 7th ed. New York, NY: McGraw Hill; 2022: Chapter 12.

158. Which anticholinesterase crosses the blood–brain barrier?

(A) Edrophonium

(B) Neostigmine

(C) Pyridostigmine

(D) Physotigmine

Rationale: Physostigmine is a tertiary amine with no quarternary ammonium. Edrophonium, neostigmine, and pyridostimine contain quarternary ammonium. Quarternary ammonium limits entry of these anticholinesterases through the blood–brain barrier due to lipid insolubility.

Reference: Butterworth JF IV, Mackey DC, Wasnick JD, eds. *Morgan & Mikhail's Clinical Anesthesiology.* 7th ed. New York, NY: McGraw Hill; 2022: Chapter 12.

159. Your patient's Train-of-Four is ¼. You decide to use neostigmine to reverse neuromuscular blockade. What drug combination and doses will you use?

(A) Neostigmine 0.04 mg/kg and glycopyrrolate 0.2 mg per 1 mg of neostigmine

(B) Neostigmine 0.08 mg/kg and glycopyrrolate 0.2 mg per 1 mg of neostigmine

(C) Neostigmine 0.02 mg/kg and atropine 0.014 mg per 1 mg of neostigmine

(D) Neostigmine 0.01 mg/kg and atropine 0.1 mg per 1 mg of neostigmine

Rationale: The usual dose of neostigmine is 0.04 to 0.08 mg/kg. Glycopyrrolate is given prior to or with the anticholinesterase to minimize the muscarinic effects. There is less tachycardia when administering atropine. Higher doses of neostigmine are given for profound paralysis. Atropine is typically given with edrophonium as the onset of action is similar for both drugs.

Reference: Butterworth JF IV, Mackey DC, Wasnick JD, eds. *Morgan & Mikhail's Clinical Anesthesiology.* 7th ed. New York, NY: McGraw Hill; 2022: Chapter 12.

160. What is the acid-base interpretation for a patient with the following ABG, pH 7.49, PaCO₂ 22, HCO₃ 24?

  (A) Uncompensated respiratory alkalosis

  (B) Compensated respiratory acidosis

  (C) Compensated respiratory alkalosis

  (D) Uncompensated respiratory acidosis

Rationale: The HCO₃ 24 is normal so there is no compensation, pH 7.49, PaCO₂ 22 indicates respiratory alkalosis.

References: Butterworth JF IV, Mackey DC, Wasnick JD, eds. *Morgan & Mikhail's Clinical Anesthesiology.* 7th ed. New York, NY: McGraw Hill; 2022: Chapter 50.

Elisha S, Heiner JS, Nagelhout JJ. *Nurse Anesthesia.* 7th ed. St. Louis, MO: Elsevier Saunders; 2023: Chapter 29.

161. Which cardiovascular effect would you expect when stimulating beta-1 receptors?

  (A) Decreased heart rate

  (B) Decreased conduction

  (C) Increased heart rate

  (D) Decreased contractility

Rationale: Stimulation of myocardial beta-1 receptors results in increased heart rate, conduction, and contractility.

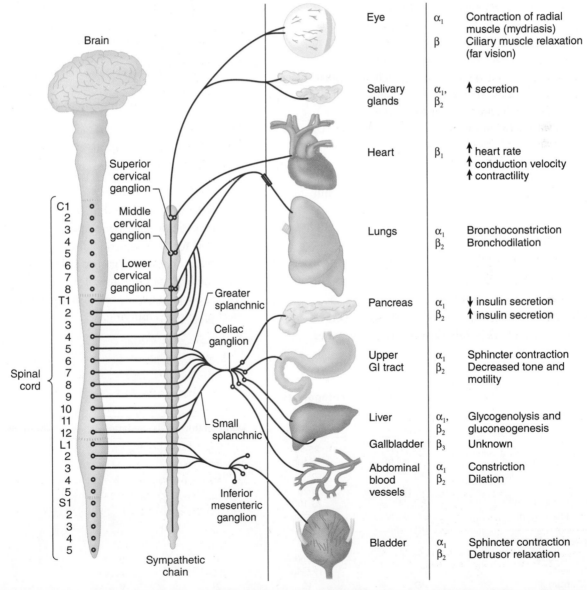

FIG. 1-4. The sympathetic nervous system. Organ innervation, receptor type, and response to stimulation. The origin of the sympathetic chain is the thoracoabdominal (T₁–L₃) spinal cord, in contrast to the craniosacral distribution of the parasympathetic nervous system. Another anatomic difference is the greater distance from the sympathetic ganglion to the visceral structures. GI, gastrointestinal. (Reproduced with permission from Butterworth JF IV, Mackey DC, Wasnick JD, eds. *Morgan & Mikhail's Clinical Anesthesiology.* 7th ed. New York, NY: McGraw Hill; 2022.)

Reference: Butterworth JF IV, Mackey DC, Wasnick JD, eds. *Morgan & Mikhail's Clinical Anesthesiology.* 7th ed. New York, NY: McGraw Hill; 2022: Chapter 14.

162. What statement is true regarding internal cardioverter defibrillators (ICD)?

    (A) ICDs are indicated for left ventricular ejection fractions >35%.
    (B) Placement of ICDs requires general anesthesia.
    (C) ICDs are indicated for intraoperative ventricular fibrillation.
    (D) ICDs are indicated for patients with an ejection fraction <35%.

    Rationale: ICDs are indicated for patients with left ventricular function resulting from a myocardial infarction; ejection fraction <35%; and for those who survive cardiac death. Placement of ICDs may be performed using sedation or general anesthesia. Intraoperative ventricular fibrillation requires defibrillation and pharmacological intervention (amiodarone).
    Reference: Butterworth JF IV, Mackey DC, Wasnick JD, eds. *Morgan & Mikhail's Clinical Anesthesiology.* 7th ed. New York, NY: McGraw Hill; 2022: Chapter 21.

163. How does beta-2 receptor stimulation affect insulin levels?

    (A) Increases insulin
    (B) No change in insulin level
    (C) Decreases insulin
    (D) Alpha-1 decreases insulin

    Rationale: Insulin levels are increased due to beta-2 receptor stimulation. Alpha-1 stimulation decreases insulin secretion.

Reference: Butterworth JF IV, Mackey DC, Wasnick JD, eds. *Morgan & Mikhail's Clinical Anesthesiology.* 7th ed. New York, NY: McGraw Hill; 2022: Chapter 14.

164. What is the acid-base state of a patient with the following ABG, pH 7.35, $PaCO_2$ 50, HCO_3 44?

    (A) Uncompensated respiratory alkalosis
    (B) Compensated respiratory acidosis
    (C) Compensated respiratory alkalosis
    (D) Uncompensated respiratory acidosis

    Rationale: The HCO_3 is elevated so there is compensation; pH 7.35 $PaCO_2$ 50 indicate respiratory acidosis.
    References: Butterworth JF IV, Mackey DC, Wasnick JD, eds. *Morgan & Mikhail's Clinical Anesthesiology.* 7th ed. New York, NY: McGraw Hill; 2022: Chapter 50.
    Elisha S, Heiner JS, Nagelhout JJ. *Nurse Anesthesia.* 7th ed. St. Louis, MO: Elsevier Saunders; 2023: Chapter 29.

165. What is the classification of metoclopramide?

    (A) Antacid
    (B) H_1-receptor antagonist
    (C) Gastrointestinal prokinetic
    (D) H_2-receptor antagonist

    Rationale: Metoclopramide is a prokinetic, speeding gastric emptying, lowering esophageal sphincter tone, and lowering gastric volume. Gastrointestinal prokinetics do not alter gastric pH. Antacids alter the gastric pH. $Histamine_2$ receptor antagonists decrease gastric acid volume. H_1 receptor antagonists have no effect on gastric emptying.

TABLE 1-9. Properties of commonly used H_1-receptor antagonists.[1]

Drug	Route	Dose (mg)	Duration (h)	Sedation	Antiemesis
Diphenhydramine (Benadryl)	PO, IM, IV	25-50	3-6	+++	++
Dimenhydrinate (Dramamine)	PO, IM, IV	50-100	3-6	+++	++
Chlorpheniramine (Chlor-Trimeton)	PO	2-12	4-8	++	0
	IM, IV	5-20			
Hydroxyzine (Atarax, Vistaril)	PO, IM	25-100	4-12	+++	++
Promethazine (Phenergan)	PO, IM, IV	12.5-50	4-12	+++	+++
Cetirizine (Zyrtec)	PO	5-10	24	+	
Cyproheptadine (Periactin)	PO	4	6-8	++	
Fexofenadine (Allegra)	PO	30-60	12	0	
Meclizine (Antivert)	PO	12.5-50	8-24	+	
Loratadine (Claritin)	PO	10	24	0	

[1]0, no effect; ++, moderate activity; +++, marked activity.
IM, intramuscular, IV, intravenous, PO, oral.
(Reproduced with permission from Butterworth JF IV, Mackey DC, Wasnick JD, eds. *Morgan & Mikhail's Clinical Anesthesiology.* 7th ed. New York, NY: McGraw Hill; 2022.)

TABLE 1-10. Pharmacology of aspiration pneumonia prophylaxis.[1]

Drug	Route	Dose	Onset	Duration	Acidity	Volume	LES Tone
Cimetidine (Tagamet)	PO	300-800 mg	1-2 hours	4-8 hours	↓↓↓	↓↓	0
	IV	300 mg					
Ranitidine (Zantac)	PO	150-300 mg	1-2 hours	10-12 hours	↓↓↓	↓↓	0
	IV	50 mg					
Famotidine (Pepcid)	PO	20-40 mg	1-2 hours	10-12 hours	↓↓↓	↓↓	0
	IV	20 mg					
Nizatidine (Axid)	PO	150-300 mg	0.5-1 hours	10-12 hours	↓↓↓	↓↓	0
Nonparticulate antacids (Bicitra, Polycitra)	PO	15-30 mL	5-10 minutes	30-60 minutes	↓↓↓	↑	0
Metoclopramide (Reglan)	IV	10 mg	1-3 minutes	1-2 hours	0	↓↓	↑↑
	PO	10-15 mg		30-60 minutes[2]			

[1]0, no effect; ↓↓, moderate decrease; ↓↓↓, marked decrease; ↑, slight increase; ↑↑, moderate increase.
[2]Oral metoclopramide has a quite variable onset of action and duration of action.
IM, intramuscular, IV, intravenous, LES, lower esophageal sphincter; PO, oral.
(Reproduced with permission from Butterworth JF IV, Mackey DC, Wasnick JD, eds. *Morgan & Mikhail's Clinical Anesthesiology*. 7th ed. New York, NY: McGraw Hill; 2022.)

Reference: Butterworth JF IV, Mackey DC, Wasnick JD, eds. *Morgan & Mikhail's Clinical Anesthesiology*. 7th ed. New York, NY: McGraw Hill; 2022: Chapter 17.

166. Which of the following physiological effects is not associated with serotonin?

(A) Arteriolar and venous vasoconstrictor

(B) Bronchoconstrictor

(C) Increase bleeding time

(D) Decreased peristalsis

Rationale: 5-hydroxytryptamine (5-HT), serotonin, vasoconstricts arterioles, and veins cause platelet aggregation and bronchoconstriction. Serotonin increases gastrointestinal peristalsis.

Reference: Butterworth JF IV, Mackey DC, Wasnick JD, eds. *Morgan & Mikhail's Clinical Anesthesiology*. 7th ed. New York, NY: McGraw Hill; 2022: Chapter 17.

167. Which of the following is a serotonin receptor antagonist?

(A) Droperidol

(B) Decadron

(C) Aprepitant

(D) Dolansetron

Rationale: Droperidol is classified as a butyrophenone; dexmethasone a glucocorticoid; and Aprepitant a neurokinin-1 receptor antagonist. Serotonin receptor antagonists include odansetron, granisetron, and dolasetron.

Reference: Butterworth JF IV, Mackey DC, Wasnick JD, eds. *Morgan & Mikhail's Clinical Anesthesiology*. 7th ed. New York, NY: McGraw Hill; 2022: Chapter 17.

168. Which ABG result is indicative of acute hyperventilation?

(A) pH 7.25, PaCO$_2$ 20, HCO$_3$ 24

(B) pH 7.35, PaCO$_2$ 50, HCO$_3$ 44

(C) pH 7.35, PaCO$_2$ 40, HCO$_3$ 24

(D) pH 7.45, PaCO$_2$ 30, HCO$_3$ 14

Rationale: Uncompensated respiratory alkalosis would be reflected in acute hyperventilation.

References: Butterworth JF IV, Mackey DC, Wasnick JD, eds. *Morgan & Mikhail's Clinical Anesthesiology*. 7th ed. New York, NY: McGraw Hill; 2022: Chapter 50.

Elisha S, Heiner JS, Nagelhout JJ. *Nurse Anesthesia*. 7th ed. St. Louis, MO: Elsevier Saunders; 2023: Chapter 29.

169. What is the physical structure of succinylcholine?

(A) Two joined acetylcholine molecules

(B) Benzylisoquinoline

(C) Steroid ring with two modified Ach molecules

(D) Monoquaternary steroid

Rationale: Atracurium is classified as a benzylisoquinoline. Two modified ACh molecules are separated by a steroid ring in pancuronium. Rocuronium's physical structure consists of a monoquaternary steroid.

Reference: Butterworth JF IV, Mackey DC, Wasnick JD, eds. *Morgan & Mikhail's Clinical Anesthesiology*. 7th ed. New York, NY: McGraw Hill; 2022: Chapter 11.

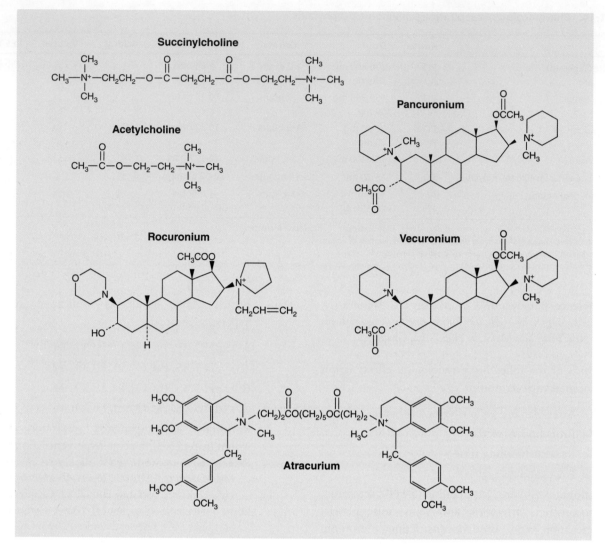

FIG. 1-5. Chemical structures of neuromuscular blocking agents. (Reproduced with permission from Butterworth JF IV, Mackey DC, Wasnick JD, eds. *Morgan & Mikhail's Clinical Anesthesiology.* 7th ed. New York, NY: McGraw Hill; 2022.)

170. Which of the following factors produces 4 to 8 hours of succincylcholine induced neuromuscular blockade?

(A) Homozygous atypical enzyme

(B) Hyperthermia

(C) Heterozygous atypical enzyme

(D) Reduced pseudocholinesterase levels

Rationale: Reduced pseudocholinesterase levels and heterozygous atypical enzyme may results in prolonged succincylcholine block (2-20 minutes and 20-30 minutes) respectively. Hypothermia, pregnancy, renal and liver failure, as well as drugs may prolong succinylcholine neuromuscular blockade. Lengthy prolonged blocks (4-8 hour) are linked to homozygous atypical enzyme. This is commonly associated with the dibucaine resistant allele.

Reference: Butterworth JF IV, Mackey DC, Wasnick JD, eds. *Morgan & Mikhail's Clinical Anesthesiology.* 7th ed. New York, NY: McGraw Hill; 2022: Chapter 11.

171. During a general anesthesia case with mechanical ventilation the ABG results are: pH 7.29, $PaCO_2$ 52 and HCO_3 24. What intervention is appropriate?

(A) Decrease respiratory rate

(B) Decrease tidal volume

(C) Give 150 mEq sodium bicarbonate

(D) Increase respiratory rate

Rationale: The patient is in uncompensated respiratory acidosis likely due to hypoventilation. Increasing ventilation will reduce $PaCO_2$.

References: Butterworth JF IV, Mackey DC, Wasnick JD, eds. *Morgan & Mikhail's Clinical Anesthesiology*. 7th ed. New York, NY: McGraw Hill; 2022: Chapter 50.

Elisha S, Heiner JS, Nagelhout JJ. *Nurse Anesthesia*. 7th ed. St. Louis, MO: Elsevier Saunders; 2023: Chapter 29.

172. What is the primary anesthetic goal for patients with second- and third-degree burns?

(A) Pain management
(B) Restoring circulating volume
(C) Administration of platelets
(D) Administration of colloids

Rationale: Cardiac output declines rapidly for burn patients. Infusion of crystalloids improves survival. In burn patients, kidney failure is associated with the use of hypertonic saline. Patient demise is linked to administration of blood products.

Reference: Butterworth JF IV, Mackey DC, Wasnick JD, eds. *Morgan & Mikhail's Clinical Anesthesiology*. 7th ed. New York, NY: McGraw Hill; 2022: Chapter 39.

173. Hypoxic pulmonary vasoconstriction (HPV) will cause which action in the lungs?

(A) Increased blood flow to nonventilated lung
(B) Decreased blood flow to ventilated lung
(C) Decreased blood flow to nonventilated lung
(D) Increased ventilation to the nonperfused lung

Rationale: Hypoxic pulmonary vasoconstriction (HPV) will cause decreased blood flow to nonventilated lung.

References: Butterworth JF IV, Mackey DC, Wasnick JD, eds. *Morgan & Mikhail's Clinical Anesthesiology*. 7th ed. New York, NY: McGraw Hill; 2022: Chapter 25.

Elisha S, Heiner JS, Nagelhout JJ. *Nurse Anesthesia*. 7th ed. St. Louis, MO: Elsevier Saunders; 2023: Chapter 29.

174. Calculate the oxygen content given the following values: Hb = 14; $PaCO_2 = 60$; $SaO_2 = 90\%$?

(A) 4 mL O_2
(B) 14 mL O_2
(C) 17 mL O_2
(D) 40 mL O_2

Rationale: $CaO_2 = (1.36 \times Hgb \times \%$ arterial Hgb saturation$) + (PaO_2 \times 0.003)$

References: Butterworth JF IV, Mackey DC, Wasnick JD, eds. *Morgan & Mikhail's Clinical Anesthesiology*. 7th ed. New York, NY: McGraw Hill; 2022: Chapter 23.

Elisha S, Heiner JS, Nagelhout JJ. *Nurse Anesthesia*. 7th ed. St. Louis, MO: Elsevier Saunders; 2023: Chapter 29.

175. The Haldane effect is best described by which statement below?

(A) The Haldane effect explains why deoxygenated blood can carry more CO_2.
(B) The Haldane effect explains the influence of pH, PCO_2, and PO_2 on the oxyhemoglobin dissociation curve.
(C) The Haldane effect governs the diffusion of O_2 at the capillary level.
(D) The Haldane effect accounts for the difference in lung volume at inspiration versus expiration.

Rationale: Deoxyhemoglobin more readily accepts the H^+ produced by the dissociation of carbonic acid. This permits more CO_2 to be carried in the form of bicarbonate ions.

Reference: Elisha S, Heiner JS, Nagelhout JJ. *Nurse Anesthesia*. 7th ed. St. Louis, MO: Elsevier Saunders; 2023: Chapter 29.

176. A 22-year-old male emerges from a laparoscopic appendectomy under general anesthesia with and remains intubated. There is no oral airway. During emergence, the patient sits up bucking with teeth clamped down, occluding the endotracheal tube. He forcefully attempts to breathe. Which respiratory phenomenon could occur based on this scenario?

(A) Pulmonary embolism
(B) Pulmonary edema
(C) Aspiration pneumonia
(D) Acute asthma attack

Rationale: During obstruction, forceful inspiratory efforts are ineffective because of the airway obstruction. Ineffective expiration produces an increase in intrathoracic and alveolar pressure. The result of these events is the rapid immense transudation of fluid from the pulmonary interstitium into the alveoli, which consequences pulmonary edema.

Reference: Elisha S, Heiner JS, Nagelhout JJ. *Nurse Anesthesia*. 7th ed. St. Louis, MO: Elsevier Saunders; 2023: Chapter 29.

177. In which lung region are the alveoli most compliant in an upright healthy person?

(A) Apex

(B) Middle

(C) Base

(D) Pleura

Rationale: The smaller alveoli in dependent areas have a lower transpulmonary pressure thus are more compliant and undergo greater expansion during inspiration.

References: Butterworth JF IV, Mackey DC, Wasnick JD, eds. *Morgan & Mikhail's Clinical Anesthesiology.* 7th ed. New York, NY: McGraw Hill; 2022: Chapter 23.

Elisha S, Heiner JS, Nagelhout JJ. *Nurse Anesthesia.* 7th ed. St. Louis, MO: Elsevier Saunders; 2023: Chapter 29.

178. A ventilation:perfusion (V:Q) ratio of zero (0) may be seen in which disorder?

(A) Pulmonary embolism

(B) Low cardiac output

(C) Emphysema

(D) Mucous plug

Rationale: Alveoli that are perfused but not ventilated have a V:Q of 0 which constitutes a intrapulmonary shunt.

References: Butterworth JF IV, Mackey DC, Wasnick JD, eds. *Morgan & Mikhail's Clinical Anesthesiology.* 7th ed. New York, NY: McGraw Hill; 2022: Chapter 23.

Elisha S, Heiner JS, Nagelhout JJ. *Nurse Anesthesia.* 7th ed. St. Louis, MO: Elsevier Saunders; 2023: Chapter 29.

179. In what form is the majority of CO_2 transported in the blood?

(A) Carbonic acid

(B) Bicarbonate

(C) Dissolved

(D) Attached to hemoglobin

Rationale: Carbon dioxide is transported in the blood in three forms: As bicarbonate, dissolved in solution and with proteins. Bicarbonate represents the largest fraction of carbon dioxide in the blood.

References: Butterworth JF IV, Mackey DC, Wasnick JD, eds. *Morgan & Mikhail's Clinical Anesthesiology.* 7th ed. New York, NY: McGraw Hill; 2022: Chapter 23.

Elisha S, Heiner JS, Nagelhout JJ. *Nurse Anesthesia.* 7th ed. St. Louis, MO: Elsevier Saunders; 2023: Chapter 29.

180. Following repeated doses of meperidine, your patient begins to experience tremors, muscle twitches, and seizures. What is the probable cause?

(A) Delta receptor activation

(B) Meperidine's anticholinergic properties

(C) Normeperidine

(D) Kappa agonism

Rationale: Normeperidine is an active metabolite of meperidine. With accumulation of normeperidine, subjects may experience a CNS excitation characterized by tremors, muscle twitches, and seizures.

Reference: Elisha S, Heiner JS, Nagelhout JJ. *Nurse Anesthesia.* 7th ed. St. Louis, MO: Elsevier Saunders; 2023: Chapter 11.

181. Which anticholinergic possesses the least antisialogogue effect?

(A) Atropine

(B) Glycopyrrolate

(C) Scopolamine

(D) Neostigmine

Rationale: Antisialoguge effects are similar for glycopyrrolate and scopolamine. They are less than atropine. Neostigmine is a cholinesterase inhibitor.

TABLE 1-11. Pharmacological characteristics of anticholinergic drugs.[1]

	Atropine	Scopolamine	Glycopyrrolate
Tachycardia	+++	+	++
Bronchodilatation	++	+	++
Sedation	+	+++	0
Antisialagogue effect	++	+++	+++

[1]0, no effect; +, minimal effect; ++, moderate effect; +++, marked effect.
(Reproduced with permission from Butterworth JF IV, Mackey DC, Wasnick JD, eds. *Morgan & Mikhail's Clinical Anesthesiology.* 7th ed. New York, NY: McGraw Hill; 2022.)

Reference: Butterworth JF IV, Mackey DC, Wasnick JD, eds. *Morgan & Mikhail's Clinical Anesthesiology.* 7th ed. New York, NY: McGraw Hill; 2022: Chapter 13.

182. The patient presents for outpatient surgery with a history of asthma. When using glycopyrrolate, what do you expect?

(A) Constriction of bronchial smooth muscle

(B) Increased gastric acid secretion

(C) Decreased body temperature

(D) Relaxation of bronchial smooth muscle

Rationale: Anticholinergics relax bronchial smooth muscle which is significant for asthma patients or those with chronic obstructive pulmonary disease. Decreased gastric acid sections and increased body temperature result from use of anticholinergics.

Reference: Butterworth JF IV, Mackey DC, Wasnick JD, eds. *Morgan & Mikhail's Clinical Anesthesiology.* 7th ed. New York, NY: McGraw Hill; 2022: Chapter 13.

183. How is the action of a single IV bolus dose of Fentanyl terminated?

   (A) Metabolism
   (B) Redistribution
   (C) Distribution
   (D) Elimination

Rationale: The action of a single dose of fentanyl is terminated by redistribution.

Reference: Elisha S, Heiner JS, Nagelhout JJ. *Nurse Anesthesia.* 7th ed. St. Louis, MO: Elsevier Saunders; 2023: Chapter 11.

184. Which type of pneumocytes in the pulmonary epithelium contains surfactant?

   (A) Type I pneumocytes
   (B) Pulmonary alveolar macrophages
   (C) Type II pneumocytes
   (D) Mast cells

Rationale: Type 2 pneumocytes comprise cytoplasmic inclusions which hold surfactant, a substance that reduces surface tension in the alveoli.

References: Butterworth JF IV, Mackey DC, Wasnick JD, eds. *Morgan & Mikhail's Clinical Anesthesiology.* 7th ed. New York, NY: McGraw Hill; 2022: Chapter 23.
Elisha S, Heiner JS, Nagelhout JJ. *Nurse Anesthesia.* 7th ed. St. Louis, MO: Elsevier Saunders; 2023: Chapter 29.

185. Which is the origin of the phrenic nerves?

   (A) T_{10}
   (B) C_2
   (C) C_3–C_5
   (D) T_4–T_6

Rationale: The diaphragm is innervated by the phrenic nerves which arise from C_3–C_5.

References: Butterworth JF IV, Mackey DC, Wasnick JD, eds. *Morgan & Mikhail's Clinical Anesthesiology.* 7th ed. New York, NY: McGraw Hill; 2022: Chapter 23.
Elisha S, Heiner JS, Nagelhout JJ. *Nurse Anesthesia.* 7th ed. St. Louis, MO: Elsevier Saunders; 2023: Chapter 29.

186. What two lung volumes comprise the functional residual capacity?

   (A) Residual volume and tidal volume
   (B) Tidal volume and expiratory reserve volume
   (C) Residual volume and inspiratory reserve volume
   (D) Residual volume and expiratory reserve volume

Rationale: The lung volume at the end of a normal exhalation is called functional residual capacity (FRC). The FRC is a combination of maximal volume that can be expired below tidal volume and the volume remaining after maximal exhalation.

References: Butterworth JF IV, Mackey DC, Wasnick JD, eds. *Morgan & Mikhail's Clinical Anesthesiology.* 7th ed. New York, NY: McGraw Hill; 2022: Chapter 23.
Elisha S, Heiner JS, Nagelhout JJ. *Nurse Anesthesia.* 7th ed. St. Louis, MO: Elsevier Saunders; 2023: Chapter 29.

187. What is vital capacity?

   (A) Volume remaining after maximal exhalation
   (B) Maximal additional volume that can be inspired above tidal volume
   (C) Maximal volume that can be expired below tidal volume
   (D) Maximum volume of gas that can be expired following maximal inspiration

Rationale: Vital capacity is the maximum volume of gas that can be exhaled following maximal inspiration.

References: Butterworth JF IV, Mackey DC, Wasnick JD, eds. *Morgan & Mikhail's Clinical Anesthesiology.* 7th ed. New York, NY: McGraw Hill; 2022: Chapter 23.
Elisha S, Heiner JS, Nagelhout JJ. *Nurse Anesthesia.* 7th ed. St. Louis, MO: Elsevier Saunders; 2023: Chapter 29.

188. Prior to rapid sequence induction of general anesthesia, you plan to administer ranitidine. When is the best time to administer the medication?

   (A) 0.5 to 1 hour preoperatively
   (B) 1 to 1.5 hours preoperatively
   (C) 1 to 2 hours preoperatively
   (D) 1.5 to 2.5 hours preoperatively

Rationale: The onset of action of ranitidine is 1 to 2 hours following IV administration. Decreasing gastric fluid volume and increasing gastric acid pH decreases the risk of aspiration.

Reference: Butterworth JF IV, Mackey DC, Wasnick JD, eds. *Morgan & Mikhail's Clinical Anesthesiology.* 7th ed. New York, NY: McGraw Hill; 2022: Chapter 17.

189. Which H$_2$ receptor antagonist affects the metabolism of warfarin?

   (A) Cimedtidine
   (B) Ranitidine
   (C) Diphenhydramine
   (D) Hydroxyzine

Rationale: Ranitidine metabolism via CP-450 pathways is less than cimetidine. Diphenhydrmiane and hydroxyzine are H$_1$ receptor antagonists.

Reference: Butterworth JF IV, Mackey DC, Wasnick JD, eds. *Morgan & Mikhail's Clinical Anesthesiology.* 7th ed. New York, NY: McGraw Hill; 2022: Chapter 17.

190. Which drug affects the absorption of digoxin?

   (A) Cimetidine
   (B) Bicitra
   (C) Metoclopramide
   (D) Omeprazole

Rationale: Urinary and gastric pH are altered by antacids. Absorption of digoxin, cimetidine, and ranitidine are slowed.

Reference: Butterworth JF IV, Mackey DC, Wasnick JD, eds. *Morgan & Mikhail's Clinical Anesthesiology.* 7th ed. New York, NY: McGraw Hill; 2022: Chapter 1.

191. What is the normal ratio of forced expiratory volume to total forced vital capacity?

   (A) Less than 60%
   (B) Greater than 50%
   (C) Greater than or equal to 80%
   (D) Greater than or equal to 20%

Rationale: The normal ratio of the forced expiratory volume in the first second of exhalation to the total forced vital capacity is greater than or equal to 80%.

References: Butterworth JF IV, Mackey DC, Wasnick JD, eds. *Morgan & Mikhail's Clinical Anesthesiology.* 7th ed. New York, NY: McGraw Hill; 2022: Chapter 23.

Elisha S, Heiner JS, Nagelhout JJ. *Nurse Anesthesia.* 7th ed. St. Louis, MO: Elsevier Saunders; 2023: Chapter 29.

192. In the standard 70-kg patient, what is the functional residual capacity in the supine position?

   (A) 2,300 mL
   (B) 1,300 mL
   (C) 1,200 mL
   (D) 500 mL

Rationale: Normal functional residual capacity is 2,300 mL. The supine position reduces the functional residual capacity by 800 to 1,000 mL.

References: Butterworth JF IV, Mackey DC, Wasnick JD, eds. *Morgan & Mikhail's Clinical Anesthesiology.* 7th ed. New York, NY: McGraw Hill; 2022: Chapter 23.

Elisha S, Heiner JS, Nagelhout JJ. *Nurse Anesthesia.* 7th ed. St. Louis, MO: Elsevier Saunders; 2023: Chapter 29.

193. Which structure classifies local anesthetics?

   (A) Lipophilic group
   (B) Benzene ring
   (C) Hydrophilic group
   (D) Intermediate chain

Rationale: An intermediate chain separates the lipophilic and hydrophilic groups. A benzene ring is noted in the lipophilic group.

TABLE 1-12. Physicochemical properties of local anesthetics.

Generic (Proprietary)	Structure	Relative Lipid Solubility of Unchanged Local Anesthetic	pK_a	Protein Binding (%)
Amides				
Bupivacaine* (Marcaine, Sensorcaine)		8	8.2	96
Etidocaine (Duranest)		16	8.1	94
Lidocaine (Xylocaine)		1	8.2	64
Mepivacaine (Carbocaine)		0.3	7.9	78
Prilocaine (Citanest)		0.4	8.0	53
Ropivacaine (Naropin)		2.5	8.2	94

(continued)

TABLE 1-12. Physicochemical properties of local anesthetics. (continued)

Generic (Proprietary)	Structure	Relative Lipid Solubility of Unchanged Local Anesthetic	pK_a	Protein Binding (%)
Esters				
Chloroprocaine (Nesacaine)		2.3	9.1	NA
Cocaine		NA	8.7	91
Procaine (Novocaine)		0.3	9.1	NA
Tetracaine (Pontocaine)		12	8.6	76

*Carbon atom responsible for optical isomerism.
NA, not available.
(Reproduced with permission from Butterworth JF IV, Mackey DC, Wasnick JD, eds. *Morgan & Mikhail's Clinical Anesthesiology.* 7th ed. New York, NY: McGraw Hill; 2022.)

Reference: Butterworth JF IV, Mackey DC, Wasnick JD, eds. *Morgan & Mikhail's Clinical Anesthesiology.* 7th ed. New York, NY: McGraw Hill; 2022: Chapter 16.

194. Lipid solubility is greatest with which local anesthetic?

(A) Tetracaine
(B) Procaine
(C) Cocaine
(D) Chloroprocaine

Rationale: Lipid solubility is one factor that affects the onset of local anesthetics. Tetracaine possesses the greatest lipid solubility as compared to procaine and chloroprocaine. Cocaine possesses no lipid solubility.
Reference: Butterworth JF IV, Mackey DC, Wasnick JD, eds. *Morgan & Mikhail's Clinical Anesthesiology.* 7th ed. New York, NY: McGraw Hill; 2022: Chapter 16.

195. Which of these factors most influences the duration of action for local anesthetics?

(A) pKa
(B) Ionization
(C) Lipid solubility
(D) Minimum concentration

Rationale: A longer duration of action correlates with high-lipid soluble local anesthetics. Chemical structure modifications influence potency. Onset of action is affected by ionization as well as lipid solubility. Factors influencing duration of action include lipid solubility and potency. Nerve fiber characteristics, nerve stimulation, and electrolyte concentration are factors affecting the minimum concentration of local anesthetic needed to block nerve fibers.

Reference: Butterworth JF IV, Mackey DC, Wasnick JD, eds. *Morgan & Mikhail's Clinical Anesthesiology.* 7th ed. New York, NY: McGraw Hill; 2022: Chapter 16.

196. What factor shifts the hemoglobin dissociation curve to the right?

(A) Normothermia

(B) Hypoventilation

(C) Hyperthermia

(D) Decrease in 2,3,-DPG

Rationale: Acidosis, hyperthermia, and increased 2,3,-DPG shift the oxyhemoglobin dissociation curve to the right. Alkalosis, hypothermia and decreased 2,3,-DPG shift the oxyhemoglobin dissociation curve to the left.

References: Butterworth JF IV, Mackey DC, Wasnick JD, eds. *Morgan & Mikhail's Clinical Anesthesiology.* 7th ed. New York, NY: McGraw Hill; 2022: Chapter 23.

Elisha S, Heiner JS, Nagelhout JJ. *Nurse Anesthesia.* 7th ed. St. Louis, MO: Elsevier Saunders; 2023: Chapter 29.

197. What is the anatomic dead space in a 75-kg healthy adult patient?

(A) 75 mL

(B) 100 mL

(C) 150 mL

(D) 200 mL

Rationale: Anatomic dead space is 2 mL/kg.

References: Butterworth JF IV, Mackey DC, Wasnick JD, eds. *Morgan & Mikhail's Clinical Anesthesiology.* 7th ed. New York, NY: McGraw Hill; 2022: Chapter 23.

Elisha S, Heiner JS, Nagelhout JJ. *Nurse Anesthesia.* 7th ed. St. Louis, MO: Elsevier Saunders; 2023: Chapter 29.

198. What law applies when determining blood flow through an intravenous catheter?

(A) Poiseuille's law

(B) Bernoulli's principle

(C) LaPlace's law

(D) Van der Waal's principle

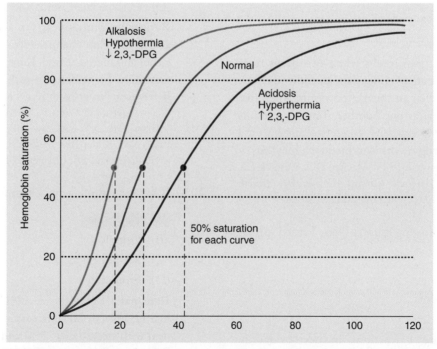

FIG. 1-6. The effects of changes in acid–base status, body temperature, and 2,3-DPG concentration on the hemoglobin–oxygen dissociation curve. (Reproduced with permission from Butterworth JF IV, Mackey DC, Wasnick JD, eds. *Morgan & Mikhail's Clinical Anesthesiology.* 7th ed. New York, NY: McGraw Hill; 2022.)

Rationale: The radius of the intravenous catheter will affect flow as described by Poiseuille. Poiseuille explains the relationship of fluid flow in a tube. In addition, viscosity of the fluid directly influences flow. For example, increased viscosity will decrease blood flow. Bernoulli's principle addresses fluid and gas flow speed through a narrow orifice. The principal shares that with increased flow speed, pressure decreases. The law of LaPlace examines the relationship of radius, pressure, and wall tension. Van der Waal's principle addresses the sum of forces among molecules.

Reference: Butterworth JF IV, Mackey DC, Wasnick JD, eds. *Morgan & Mikhail's Clinical Anesthesiology.* 7th ed. New York, NY: McGraw Hill; 2022: Chapters 4, 5, and 14.

199. During a general anesthetic, fentanyl and versed are administered. The interaction of the drugs produces a greater effect than the sum of the two medications. What is the interaction called?

(A) Addition
(B) Synergism
(C) Tolerance
(D) Tachyphylaxis

Rationale: Synergism results when two drugs react to create a greater effect rather than an additive effect. Addition means that an equal effect results when two drugs are given after one another. Tolerance results from chronic drug exposure. Acute tolerance after a few doses of a drug results is termed tachyphylaxis.

Reference: Butterworth JF IV, Mackey DC, Wasnick JD, eds. *Morgan & Mikhail's Clinical Anesthesiology.* 7th ed. New York, NY: McGraw Hill; 2022: Chapter 9.

200. Which of the following is not a Phase I reaction?

(A) Oxidation
(B) Reduction
(C) Conjugation
(D) Hydrolysis

Rationale: Phase I reactions include oxidation, reduction, and hydrolysis. Conjugation is classified as a Phase II reaction.

References: Butterworth JF IV, Mackey DC, Wasnick JD, eds. *Morgan & Mikhail's Clinical Anesthesiology.* 7th ed. New York, NY: McGraw Hill; 2022: Chapter 7.

Flood P, Rathmell JP, Urbam RD, eds. *Stoelting's Pharmacology & Physiology in Anesthetic Practice.* 6th ed. Philadelphia, PA: Wolters Kluwer; 2022: Chapter 5.

201. Which inhalational agent's metabolism produces Compound A?

(A) Sevoflurane with low flow
(B) Desflurane with low flow
(C) Sevoflurane with high flow
(D) Desflurane with high flow

Rationale: Sevoflurane's metabolites include Compound A. In long anesthetics, using low flows (1 L/m) production of Compound A is more likely than in longer cases using high gas flows.

References: Butterworth JF IV, Mackey DC, Wasnick JD, eds. *Morgan & Mikhail's Clinical Anesthesiology.* 7th ed. New York, NY: McGraw Hill; 2022: Chapter 5.

Pardo MC, Miller RD. *Miller's Basics of Anesthesia.* 8th ed. Philadelphia, PA: Elsevier; 2023: Chapter 7.

202. How is propofol classified?

(A) Alkylphenol
(B) Barbituric acid
(C) Phencyclidine
(D) Carboxylated imidazole

Rationale: Propofol is an alkylphenol. Barbituric acid is the base chemical structure for sodium pentathol and methohexital. Ketamine is a phencyclidine derivative. Etomidate is a carboxylated imidazole.

References: Butterworth JF IV, Mackey DC, Wasnick JD, eds. *Morgan & Mikhail's Clinical Anesthesiology.* 7th ed. New York, NY: McGraw Hill; 2022: Chapter 9.

Pardo MC, Miller RD. *Miller's Basics of Anesthesia.* 8th ed. Philadelphia, PA: Elsevier; 2023: Chapter 8.

203. What induction agent is least protein bound?

(A) Ketamine
(B) Propofol
(C) Methohexital
(D) Etomidate

Rationale: Ketamine is 12% protein bound. The highest protein binding exists with propofol (97%), next with etomidate (77%) and methohexital (73%).

References: Butterworth JF IV, Mackey DC, Wasnick JD, eds. *Morgan & Mikhail's Clinical Anesthesiology.* 7th ed. New York, NY: McGraw Hill; 2022: Chapter 9.

Pardo, MC, Miller RD. *Miller's Basics of Anesthesia.* 8th ed. Philadelphia, PA: Elsevier; 2023: Chapter 8.

204. Clearance of which benzodiazepine is greatest?

(A) Diazepam

(B) Lorazepam

(C) Midazolam

(D) Zaleplon

Rationale: Clearance for midazolam is 6.4 to 11 mL/kg/min. Clearance for lorazepam and diazepam is 0.8 to 01.2 mL/kg/min and 0.2 to 0.5 mL/kg/min respectively. Zaleplon is a nonbenzodiazepine hypnotic.

References: Butterworth JF IV, Mackey DC, Wasnick JD, eds. *Morgan & Mikhail's Clinical Anesthesiology.* 7th ed. New York, NY: McGraw Hill; 2022: Chapter 9.

Pardo MC, Miller RD. *Miller's Basics of Anesthesia.* 8th ed. Philadelphia, PA: Elsevier; 2023: Chapter 8.

205. Following administration of a beta-lactam antibiotic, the patient exhibits urticaria, hypotension, and arrhythmias. What is the most likely cause?

(A) Tachyphylaxis reaction

(B) Anaphylaxis reaction

(C) Atopic reaction

(D) Anaphylactoid reaction

Rationale: Anaphylaxis is commonly associated with antibiotic administration. Beta-lactam drugs including penicillin are primarily responsible for the reaction involving IgE antibodies. The signs and symptoms include pruritus, urticaria, hypotension, wheezing, bronchospasm, abdominal pain, arrhythmias, and possibly angioedema. Individuals who exhibit greater tendencies for allergic reactions are atopic. Acute tolerance after a few doses of a drug results in tachyphylaxis. Tachyphylaxis results in acute tolerance following a few drug doses but does not result in signs and symptoms associated with analphylaxis. Anaphylactoid reactions involve non-IgE antibodies.

References: Elisha S, Heiner JS, Nagelhout JJ. *Nurse Anesthesia.* 7th ed. St. Louis, MO: Elsevier Saunders; 2023: Chapter 46.

Flood P, Rathmell JP, Urbam RD, eds. *Stoelting's Pharmacology & Physiology in Anesthetic Practice.* 6th ed. Philadelphia, PA: Wolters Kluwer; 2022: Chapter 5.

206. Which would be best in the care of a patient in myxedema coma needing emergent surgery?

(A) Propylthiouracil

(B) Liothyronine

(C) Thyroxine

(D) Thyroid stimulating hormone

Rationale: Liothyronine (T_3) can be used for rapid emergent treatment of myxedema coma.

References: Butterworth JF IV, Mackey DC, Wasnick JD, eds. *Morgan & Mikhail's Clinical Anesthesiology.* 7th ed. New York, NY: McGraw Hill; 2022: Chapter 52.

Gropper MA, Cohen NH, Eriksson LI, et al, eds. *Miller's Anesthesia.* 9th ed. Philadelphia, PA: Churchill Livingstone Elsevier; 2020: Chapter 35.

207. Which indicates primary hypothyroidism?

(A) Decreased thyroid stimulating hormone with decreased triiodothyronine and thyroxine

(B) Increased thyroid stimulating hormone with decreased triiodothyronine and thyroxine

(C) Decreased thyroid stimulating hormone with increased triiodothyronine and thyroxine

(D) Increased thyroid stimulating hormone with increased triiodothyronine and thyroxine

Rationale: Increased thyroid stimulating hormone levels with decreased thyroid hormone levels indicate primary hypothyroidism.

References: Butterworth JF IV, Mackey DC, Wasnick JD, eds. *Morgan & Mikhail's Clinical Anesthesiology.* 7th ed. New York, NY: McGraw Hill; 2022: Chapter 52.

Hines RL, Marschall KE. *Stoelting's Anesthesia and Co-existing Disease.* 7th ed. Philadelphia, PA: Elsevier Saunders; 2018: Chapter 19.

208. Which statement is true regarding phenytoin?

(A) Chronic treatment with phenytoin leads to prolonged neuromuscular blockade.

(B) Lower doses of neuromuscular blockers are required.

(C) Elimination of neuromuscular blockers is decreased.

(D) Higher doses of neuromuscular blockers are required.

Rationale: Higher doses of neuromuscular blockers are needed due to increased elimination in patients taking phenytoin.

Reference: Flood P, Rathmell JP, Urbam RD, eds. *Stoelting's Pharmacology & Physiology in Anesthetic Practice.* 6th ed. Philadelphia, PA: Wolters Kluwer; 2022: Chapter 30.

209. Which antiemetic will you avoid for patients with Parkinson's disease?

(A) Dolasetron

(B) Metoclopramide

(C) Odansetron

(D) Diphenhydramine

Rationale: Metoclopramide may precipitate or worsen Parkinson's disease. Dolasetron, odansetron, and diphenhydramine may be given safely to patients with Parkinson's disease.

Reference: Hines RL, Marschall KE. *Stoelting's Anesthesia and Co-existing Disease.* 7th ed. Philadelphia, PA: Elsevier Saunders; 2018: Chapter 28.

210. During surgery for breast cancer, the patient receives isosulfan blue dye. What will you expect?

(A) Increased SaO_2

(B) Tachycardia

(C) Decreased SaO_2

(D) Cardiac arrhythmias

Rationale: A transient decreased oxygenation is common following injection of isosulfan blue dye.

Reference: Hines RL, Marschall KE. *Stoelting's Anesthesia and Co-existing Disease.* 7th ed. Philadelphia, PA: Elsevier Saunders; 2018: Chapter 23.

211. Which analgesic for labor is not associated with significant respiratory depression affecting the mother or fetus?

(A) Morphine

(B) Nalbuphine

(C) Fentanyl

(D) Demerol

Rationale: Nalbuphine is a mixed agonist-antagonist. A respiratory ceiling effect negates unwanted respiratory depression in the mother and fetus. In contrast, morphine, fentanyl, and demerol are associated with significant respiratory depression for the mother and the neonate.

Reference: Butterworth JF IV, Mackey DC, Wasnick JD, eds. *Morgan & Mikhail's Clinical Anesthesiology.* 7th ed. New York, NY: McGraw Hill; 2022: Chapter 41.

212. Why are benzodiazepines avoided during labor and delivery?

(A) Pain on injection

(B) Prolonged neonatal depression

(C) High Apgar scores

(D) Nausea and vomiting

Rationale: Benzodiazepines should be avoided during labor due to prolonged neonatal respiratory depression following delivery. Also, mothers are affected by the amnestic properties of benzodiazepines that may affect memory of childbirth. Low Apgar scores may reflect respiratory depression.

Reference: Butterworth JF IV, Mackey DC, Wasnick JD, eds. *Morgan & Mikhail's Clinical Anesthesiology.* 7th ed. New York, NY: McGraw Hill; 2022: Chapter 41.

213. Which inhalational agent affects the blood pressure the least?

(A) Sevoflurane

(B) Halothane

(C) Isoflurane

(D) Desflurane

Rationale: A dose-dependent decrease in blood pressures occurs with halothane. There is minimal cardiac depression with isoflurane and desflurane. Sevoflurane decreases the arterial blood pressure, but less than isoflurane or desflurane.

Reference: Butterworth JF IV, Mackey DC, Wasnick JD, eds. *Morgan & Mikhail's Clinical Anesthesiology.* 7th ed. New York, NY: McGraw Hill; 2022: Chapter 41.

214. Which analgesic given to renal failure patients results in prolonged respiratory depression?

(A) Remifentanil

(B) Demerol

(C) Sufentanil

(D) Morphine

Rationale: Morphine 3-glucoronide and morphine 6-glucoronide metabolites prolong respiratory depression and narcosis. Remifentanil is metabolized by plasma esterases. Demerol undergoes demethylation producing normeperidine. Seizures are linked to norpeperidine. Fentanyl metabolites are inactive.

Reference: Butterworth JF IV, Mackey DC, Wasnick JD, eds. *Morgan & Mikhail's Clinical Anesthesiology.* 7th ed. New York, NY: McGraw Hill; 2022: Chapter 10.

215. Which COX-2 selective agent is linked to hepatic failure?

(A) Acetominophen

(B) Aspirin

(C) Ketorolac

(D) Celecoxib

Rationale: Acetaminophen results in production of *N*-acetyl-p-benzoquinone imine. Toxic levels cause hepatic failure. Ketorolac is metabolized in the liver with end product excreted unchanged. Inactive metabolites occur following hepatic metabolism of celecoxib. Aspirin is a COX-1 inhibitor.

Reference: Butterworth JF IV, Mackey DC, Wasnick JD, eds. *Morgan & Mikhail's Clinical Anesthesiology.* 7th ed. New York, NY: McGraw Hill; 2022: Chapter 10.

216. Your patient suffers from chronic renal failure. Which nondepolarizer will you avoid?

(A) Vecuronium

(B) Rocuronium

(C) Mivacron

(D) Anectine

Rationale: Prolonged neuromuscular blockade occurs due to partial renal excretion of vecuronium, pancuronium, doxacurium, and pipecuronium for patients in renal failure. Pseudocholinesterase is responsible for mivacron metabolism. The liver is the primary route of elimination for rocuronium. Anectine (succinylcholine) is a depolarizing neuromuscular blocking drug.

Reference: Butterworth JF IV, Mackey DC, Wasnick JD, eds. *Morgan & Mikhail's Clinical Anesthesiology.* 7th ed. New York, NY: McGraw Hill; 2022: Chapter 11.

217. What is the mechanism of action for reversal of succinylcholine?

(A) Metabolism by acetylcholinesterase

(B) Hydrolyzed pseudocholinesterase

(C) Complex formation with steroidal nondepolarizers

(D) Chemical degradation by L-cysteine

Rationale: Succinylcholine is hydrolyzed in the plasma and liver by the enzyme pseudocholinesterase following release from the Ach receptors. Suggamadex forms complexes with steroidal nondepolarizers resulting in reversal. Investigative nondepolarizers undergo chemical degradation.

Reference: Butterworth JF IV, Mackey DC, Wasnick JD, eds. *Morgan & Mikhail's Clinical Anesthesiology.* 7th ed. New York, NY: McGraw Hill; 2022: Chapter 11.

218. The patient undergoing cataract extraction takes echothiophate for glaucoma. If given succinylcholine, what will you expect?

(A) Duration <5 minutes

(B) Duration <10 minutes

(C) Duration >10 minutes

(D) No effect on duration of action

Rationale: Echothiophate eye drops, an organophosphate, decreases pseudocholinesterase activity. This may increase the duration of neuromuscular blockade following administration of succinylcholine. The normal duration of action of succinylcholine is approximately 10 minutes.

Reference: Butterworth JF IV, Mackey DC, Wasnick JD, eds. *Morgan & Mikhail's Clinical Anesthesiology.* 7th ed. New York, NY: McGraw Hill; 2022: Chapter 11.

219. You administered propofol 2 mg/kg, succinylcholine 1.5 mg/kg, and fentanyl 2 µg/kg to a 70-kg patient undergoing emergent appendectomy. Following the 45-minute case you observe no respiratory effort. What is the best choice for this patient?

(A) Administer naloxone

(B) Maintain ventilatory support with sedation

(C) Administer neostigmine

(D) Check the ventilator settings

Rationale: Maintaining ventilator support is the best choice given this patient's lack of respiratory effort. Consider variables affecting prolonged neuromuscular blockade with succinylcholine. Depolarizing neuromuscular blockade is not reversed with neostigmine. The dose of fentanyl is not likely to produce prolonged depressed ventilation.

Reference: Butterworth JF IV, Mackey DC, Wasnick JD, eds. *Morgan & Mikhail's Clinical Anesthesiology.* 7th ed. New York, NY: McGraw Hill; 2022: Chapter 11.

220. Considering hyperkalemia, rhabdomyolysis, and cardiac arrest which neuromuscular blocking agent will you avoid in children?

(A) Rocuronium

(B) Succinylcholine

(C) Atracurium

(D) Cisatracurium

Rationale: Succinylcholine is strongly linked to hyperkalemia, rhabdomyolysis, and cardiac arrest particularly in children with undiagnosed myopathies. A relative contraindication exists for the routine use of succinylcholine in pediatric anesthesia. Nondepolarizing muscular blockers do not possess the same concerns.

Reference: Butterworth JF IV, Mackey DC, Wasnick JD, eds. *Morgan & Mikhail's Clinical Anesthesiology*. 7th ed. New York, NY: McGraw Hill; 2022: Chapter 11.

221. Which medication blocks muscarinic receptors?

(A) Atropine

(B) Rocuronium

(C) Pyridostigmine

(D) Neostigmine

Rationale: Atropine, an anticholinergic, blocks muscarinic receptors. Nondepolarizing neuromuscular blockers, also cholinergic antagonists such as rocurnoium, work at the nicotinic receptors of skeletal muscle. The cholinesterase inhibitors pyridostigmine and neostigmine act at both cholinergic and nicotinic receptors.

Reference: Butterworth JF IV, Mackey DC, Wasnick JD, eds. *Morgan & Mikhail's Clinical Anesthesiology*. 7th ed. New York, NY: McGraw Hill; 2022: Chapter 13.

222. What part of the structure of glycopyrrolate is responsible for binding to acetylcholine receptors?

(A) Organic base

(B) Ester linkage

(C) Aromatic base

(D) Benzene ring

Rationale: While each of the structure of anticholinergic drugs are present, the ester linkage is significant for binding thereby exerting a competitive blockade.

Reference: Butterworth JF IV, Mackey DC, Wasnick JD, eds. *Morgan & Mikhail's Clinical Anesthesiology*. 7th ed. New York, NY: McGraw Hill; 2022: Chapter 13.

223. What manifestation occurs because of anticholinergic overdose?

(A) Tachycardia

(B) Oral secretions

(C) Bradycardia

(D) Cutaneous vasoconstriction

Rationale: Central anticholinergic syndrome results in tachycardia, excessive dry mouth, and cutaneous vasodilation (also known as atropine flush).

Reference: Butterworth JF IV, Mackey DC, Wasnick JD, eds. *Morgan & Mikhail's Clinical Anesthesiology*. 7th ed. New York, NY: McGraw Hill; 2022: Chapter 13.

224. How is EMLA cream formulated?

(A) 1:1 mixture of 0.5% lidocaine and 0.5% prilocaine

(B) 2:1 mixture of 1.5% lidocaine and 2.5% prilocaine

(C) 1:1 mixture of 0.75% benzocaine and 0.5% lidocaine

(D) 2:1 mixture of 0.75% benzocaine and 1.5% lidocaine

Rationale: EMLA's formulation is a 1:1 mixture of prilocaine and lidocaine. The concentration of benzocaine is 20%.

Reference: Butterworth JF IV, Mackey DC, Wasnick JD, eds. *Morgan & Mikhail's Clinical Anesthesiology*. 7th ed. New York, NY: McGraw Hill; 2022: Chapter 16.

225. During an inguinal hernia repair, the surgeon asks how much bupivacaine is allowed for local infiltration. What is the correct maximum dose?

(A) 12 mg/kg

(B) 8 mg/kg

(C) 4.5 mg/kg

(D) 3 mg/kg

Rationale: The maximum dose for chloroprocaine is 12 mg/kg; 8 mg/kg for prilocaine; and 4.5 mg/kg for lidocaine and mepivacaine without epinephrine.

Reference: Butterworth JF IV, Mackey DC, Wasnick JD, eds. *Morgan & Mikhail's Clinical Anesthesiology*. 7th ed. New York, NY: McGraw Hill; 2022: Chapter 16.

226. How does the duration of epidural ropivacaine differ from lidocaine?

(A) The duration of lidocaine is shorter than ropivacaine.

(B) The duration of lidocaine and ropivacaine is similar.

(C) The duration of lidocaine is longer than ropivacaine.

(D) Ropivacaine is similar to amides.

Rationale: The duration of action of lidocaine is shorter than ropivacaine. Ropivacaine is longer acting than other amides including lidocaine, mepivacaine, and prilocaine. The duration is like bupivacaine.

Reference: Butterworth JF IV, Mackey DC, Wasnick JD, eds. *Morgan & Mikhail's Clinical Anesthesiology.* 7th ed. New York, NY: McGraw Hill; 2022: Chapter 16.

227. Which local anesthetic is metabolized by pseudocholinesterase?

    (A) Lidocaine
    (B) Bupivacaine
    (C) Ropivacaine
    (D) Tetracaine

    Rationale: Lidocaine, bupivacaine, and ropivacaine are amide local anesthetics. Amide local anesthetics are metabolized in the liver by P-450 microsomal enzymes.
    Reference: Butterworth JF IV, Mackey DC, Wasnick JD, eds. *Morgan & Mikhail's Clinical Anesthesiology.* 7th ed. New York, NY: McGraw Hill; 2022: Chapter 16.

228. Prolong neurological deficits have been associated with which local anesthetic?

    (A) Epidural chloroprocaine
    (B) EMLA
    (C) Topical chloroprocaine
    (D) Intrathecal lidocaine

    Rationale: Inadvertant dural puncture with chloroprocaine has caused total spinal anesthesia, severe hypotension, severe back pain, and neurological deficits. Sodium bisulfate preservative in chloroprocaine has been implicated as the causative agent. Topical local anesthetics are not linked to neurological deficits. Chloroprocaine is administered via epidural, infiltration, peripheral nerve block, and spinal routes.
    Reference: Butterworth JF IV, Mackey DC, Wasnick JD, eds. *Morgan & Mikhail's Clinical Anesthesiology.* 7th ed. New York, NY: McGraw Hill; 2022: Chapter 16.

229. What part of the body houses the greatest concentration of histamine?

    (A) Parietal cells
    (B) Circulating basophils and mast cells
    (C) Gastric mucosa
    (D) Peripheral tissues

    Rationale: Histamine facilitates the release of hydrochloric acid by parietal cells in the gastric mucosa. While histamine can be found in the central nervous system, peripheral tissues, and the gastric mucosa, the greatest concentration is found in circulating basophils and mast cells.

Reference: Butterworth JF IV, Mackey DC, Wasnick JD, eds. *Morgan & Mikhail's Clinical Anesthesiology.* 7th ed. New York, NY: McGraw Hill; 2022: Chapter 17.

230. Which cardiovascular effect occurs when administering diphenhydramine?

    (A) Hypertension
    (B) Peripheral arterioloar constriction
    (C) Coronary vasoconstriction
    (D) Hypotension

    Rationale: H_1 receptor antagonist diphendydramine dilates coronary arteries and peripheral arterioles. Heart rate is increased, but blood pressure falls.
    Reference: Butterworth JF IV, Mackey DC, Wasnick JD, eds. *Morgan & Mikhail's Clinical Anesthesiology.* 7th ed. New York, NY: McGraw Hill; 2022: Chapter 17.

231. When administering promethazine, how long will the sedative effects last?

    (A) 3 to 6 hours
    (B) 4 to 12 hours
    (C) 8 to 24 hours
    (D) 24 hours

    Rationale: Diphenhydramine and dimenhydrinate's effect last 3 to 6 hours. The duration of action of meclizine is 8 to 24 hours. Loratidine acts for 24 hours.
    Reference: Butterworth JF IV, Mackey DC, Wasnick JD, eds. *Morgan & Mikhail's Clinical Anesthesiology.* 7th ed. New York, NY: McGraw Hill; 2022: Chapter 17.

232. Which of the following medications is potentiated by hydroxyzine?

    (A) Midazolam
    (B) Claritin
    (C) Fexofenadine
    (D) Metoclopramide

    Rationale: H_1 receptor antagonists potentiate central nervous system depressants. No sedative effects are linked to claritin or fexofenadine. Rare sedative effects occur with metoclopramide.
    Reference: Butterworth JF IV, Mackey DC, Wasnick JD, eds. *Morgan & Mikhail's Clinical Anesthesiology.* 7th ed. New York, NY: McGraw Hill; 2022: Chapter 17.

233. You include dexmedetomidine as an adjunct to general anesthesia. Which drug requirements will most likely decrease?

(A) Vecuronium

(B) Propofol

(C) Ephedrine

(D) Methoxamine

Rationale: Decreasing the dose of central nervous system depressants and anesthetic agents is needed to avoid profound hypotension. Ephedrine and methoxamine, sympathomimetic amines, are used to increase blood pressure. No interaction exists between neuromuscular blockers (vecuronium) and dexmedetomidine.

Reference: Butterworth JF IV, Mackey DC, Wasnick JD, eds. *Morgan & Mikhail's Clinical Anesthesiology.* 7th ed. New York, NY: McGraw Hill; 2022: Chapter 17.

234. What is the primary receptor for phenylephrine?

(A) Beta-1

(B) Alpha-1

(C) Beta-2

(D) Alpha-2

Rationale: Receptor selectivity for adrenergic agonist phenylephrine is primarily alpha-1. There is some alpha-2, but no beta-receptor selectivity.

Reference: Butterworth JF IV, Mackey DC, Wasnick JD, eds. *Morgan & Mikhail's Clinical Anesthesiology.* 7th ed. New York, NY: McGraw Hill; 2022: Chapter 14.

235. How do direct and indirect adrenergic agonists differ?

(A) Indirect agonists bind to the receptor.

(B) Ephedrine binds to the receptor.

(C) Direct agonists bind to the receptor.

(D) Neosynephrine increases neurotransmitter activity.

Rationale: Direct acting adrenergic agonists bind to receptors (neosynephrine). Indirect acting adrenergic agonists (ephedrine) increase the release or decrease the reuptake of norepinephrine.

Reference: Butterworth JF IV, Mackey DC, Wasnick JD, eds. *Morgan & Mikhail's Clinical Anesthesiology.* 7th ed. New York, NY: McGraw Hill; 2022: Chapter 14.

236. What is the primary effect of phenylephrine?

(A) Peripheral vasoconstriction

(B) Decreased vascular resistance

(C) Increased heart rate

(D) Increased cardiac output

Rationale: The cardiac effects of phenylephrine are primarily peripheral vasoconstriction, increased vascular resistance, and arterial blood pressure due to alpha-1 selectivity. Reflex bradycardia may result in decreasing cardiac output.

TABLE 1-13. Receptor selectivity of adrenergic agonists.[1]

Drug	α_1	α_2	β_1	β_2	DA$_1$	DA$_2$
Phenylephrine	+++	+	0	0	0	0
Clonidine	+	++	0	0	0	0
Dexmedetomidine	+	+++	0	0	0	0
Epinephrine[2]	++	++	+++	++	0	0
Ephedrine[3]	++	?	++	+	0	0
Fenoldopam	0	0	0	0	+++	0
Norepinephrine[2]	++	++	++	0	0	0
Dopamine[2]	++	++	++	+	+++	+++
Dobutamine	0	0	+++	+	0	0
Terbutaline	0	0	+	+++	0	0

[1]0, no/minimal effect; +, agonist effect (mild, moderate, marked); ?, unknown effect.
[2]The α_1 effects of epinephrine, norepinephrine, and dopamine become more prominent at high doses.
[3]The primary mode of action of ephedrine is indirect stimulation.
DA$_1$ and DA$_2$, dopaminergic receptors.
(Reproduced with permission from Butterworth JF IV, Mackey DC, Wasnick JD, eds. *Morgan & Mikhail's Clinical Anesthesiology.* 7th ed. New York, NY: McGraw Hill; 2022.)

TABLE 1-14. Effects of adrenergic agonists on organ systems.[1]

Drug	Heart Rate	Mean Arterial Pressure	Cardiac Output	Peripheral Vascular Resistance	Bronchodilation	Renal Blood Flow
Phenylephrine	↓	↑↑↑	↓	↑↑↑	0	↓↓↓
Epinephrine	↑↑	↑	↑↑	↑/↓	↑↑	↓↓
Ephedrine	↑↑	↑↑	↑↑	↑	↑↑	↓↓
Fenoldopam	↑↑	↓↓↓	↓/↑	↓↓	0	↑↑↑
Norepinephrine	↓	↑↑↑	↓/↑	↑↑↑	0	↓↓↓
Dopamine	↑/↑↑	↑	↑↑↑	↑	0	↑↑↑
Isoproterenol	↑↑↑	↓	↑↑↑	↓↓	↑↑↑	↓/↑
Dobutamine	↑	↑	↑↑↑	↓	0	↑

[1]0, no/minimal effect; ↑, increase (mild, moderate, marked); ↓, decrease (mild, moderate, marked); ↓/↑, variable effect; ↑/↑↑, mild-to-moderate increase.
(Reproduced with permission from Butterworth JF IV, Mackey DC, Wasnick JD, eds. *Morgan & Mikhail's Clinical Anesthesiology.* 7th ed. New York, NY: McGraw Hill; 2022.)

Reference: Butterworth JF IV, Mackey DC, Wasnick JD, eds. *Morgan & Mikhail's Clinical Anesthesiology.* 7th ed. New York, NY: McGraw Hill; 2022: Chapter 14.

237. Which of the following halogenated agents potentiates the effects of epinephrine the most?

(A) Desflurane
(B) Sevoflurane
(C) Isoflurane
(D) Halothane

Rationale: Halothane sensitizes the myocardium to catecholamines. Myocardial sensitization to catecholamines is minimal with other halogenated agents.
Reference: Butterworth JF IV, Mackey DC, Wasnick JD, eds. *Morgan & Mikhail's Clinical Anesthesiology.* 7th ed. New York, NY: McGraw Hill; 2022: Chapter 14.

238. You plan to administer ephedrine for hypotension following spinal anesthesia. What do you expect?

(A) Decreased heart rate
(B) Decreased cardiac output
(C) Increased heart rate
(D) Short duration of action

Rationale: Administration of ephedrine results in increased heart rate, blood pressure, cardiac output, and cardiac contractility. A longer duration of action is longer compared to other sympathomimetics (neosynephrine).

Reference: Butterworth JF IV, Mackey DC, Wasnick JD, eds. *Morgan & Mikhail's Clinical Anesthesiology.* 7th ed. New York, NY: McGraw Hill; 2022: Chapter 14.

239. How is ephedrine classified?

(A) Indirect beta-1 and beta-2 agonists
(B) Direct beta agonist
(C) Direct alpha agonist
(D) Indirect alpha-1, beta-1, and beta-2 agonists

Rationale: Ephedrine is classified as an indirect-acting adrenergic agonist. Receptivity includes moderate alpha-1, beta-1, and mild beta-2.
Reference: Butterworth JF IV, Mackey DC, Wasnick JD, eds. *Morgan & Mikhail's Clinical Anesthesiology.* 7th ed. New York, NY: McGraw Hill; 2022: Chapter 14.

240. What cardiac effect do you expect following administration of norepinephrine?

(A) Decreased heart rate
(B) Decreased mean arterial pressure
(C) Increased heart rate
(D) Decreased peripheral vascular resistance

Rationale: Norepinephrine results in a decreased heart rate, increased mean arterial pressure, and increased peripheral vascular resistance.
Reference: Butterworth JF IV, Mackey DC, Wasnick JD, eds. *Morgan & Mikhail's Clinical Anesthesiology.* 7th ed. New York, NY: McGraw Hill; 2022: Chapter 14.

241. You are planning to use clonidine during a general anesthetic. Primary receptor selectivity for clonidine includes which of the following?

(A) Alpha-2

(B) Beta-1

(C) Beta-2

(D) Alpha-1

Rationale: Receptor selectivity for clonidine is primarily alpha-2. Mild alpha-1 receptor selectivity exists. There is no beta-receptor selectivity for clonidine.

Reference: Butterworth JF IV, Mackey DC, Wasnick JD, eds. *Morgan & Mikhail's Clinical Anesthesiology.* 7th ed. New York, NY: McGraw Hill; 2022: Chapter 14.

242. Your patient is taking phenelzine. What is your primary concern when administering epinephrine to this patient?

(A) Profound increase in heart rate

(B) Lowered heart rate

(C) Increased heart rate

(D) Profound decrease in heart rate

Rationale: When administering a catecholamine (epinephrine) to patients taking phenelzine (monoamine oxidase inhibitor) expect a profound cardiac response. Epinephrine is metabolized by monoamine oxidase and catechol-o-transferase.

Reference: Butterworth JF IV, Mackey DC, Wasnick JD, eds. *Morgan & Mikhail's Clinical Anesthesiology.* 7th ed. New York, NY: McGraw Hill; 2022: Chapter 14.

243. You are administering an infusion of dopamine (0.5-3 mcg/kg/min). What do you anticipate?

(A) Beta-1 stimulation

(B) DA_1 stimulation

(C) Alpha-1 stimulation

(D) Beta-2 stimulation

Rationale: Lower doses of dopamine result in primarily dopaminergic receptor (DA_1) stimulation resulting renal vessel dilation. Higher doses (3-10 μg/kg/min) result in beta-1 stimulation effects. Increases in peripheral vascular resistance with a decreased renal blood flow result due to alpha-1 effects include dopamine administered in doses 10 to 20 μg/kg/min.

Reference: Butterworth JF IV, Mackey DC, Wasnick JD, eds. *Morgan & Mikhail's Clinical Anesthesiology.* 7th ed. New York, NY: McGraw Hill; 2022: Chapter 14.

244. A patient scheduled for an open bowel resection presents with congestive heart failure and well-documented coronary artery disease. You note the patient's heart rate is 98. Which of the following adrenergic agonists would be the best choice for this patient?

(A) Dobutamine

(B) Esmolol

(C) Phentolamine

(D) Norepinephrine

Rationale: Dobutamine improves cardiac output and assists in balancing myocardial oxygen consumption particularly in tachycardic patients or those with increased peripheral vascular resistance. While peripheral vasoconstriction and an increased blood pressure occur when using norepinephrine, an increased afterload and reflex bradycardia result. Cardiac output is not improved. Phentolamine is an alpha-blocker. Esmolol is a short-acting beta-blocker.

Reference: Butterworth JF IV, Mackey DC, Wasnick JD, eds. *Morgan & Mikhail's Clinical Anesthesiology.* 7th ed. New York, NY: McGraw Hill; 2022: Chapter 14.

245. A patient presents for removal of a pheochromocytoma. Preoperatively, which medication is most useful?

(A) Phenoxybenzamine

(B) Labetolol

(C) Esmolol

(D) Norepinephrine

Rationale: Lowering the blood pressure prior to surgery is a goal for patients presenting with a pheochromocytoma. Preoperatively, the most frequently used alpha-1 antagonist for patients with a pheochromocytoma is phenoxybenzamine. Phenoxybenzamine is effective in lowering blood pressure due to reversal of vasoconstriction associated with tumor secreting epinephrine and norepinephrine. Esmolol ultrashort duration as well as minimal effect on blood pressure makes it a poor choice for blood pressure control. If the patient presents with tachycardia or ventricular arrhythmias, beta-1 blockers (labetolol) may be useful. Norepinephrine exerts the opposite effect (increased blood pressure).

Reference: Butterworth JF IV, Mackey DC, Wasnick JD, eds. *Morgan & Mikhail's Clinical Anesthesiology.* 7th ed. New York, NY: McGraw Hill; 2022: Chapter 14.

246. During metabolism of nitrates (nitroglycerin and sodium nitroprusside), what substance is released?

(A) Guanylyl cyclase

(B) cGMP

(C) Nitric oxide

(D) Nitrate

Rationale: Metabolism of nitrates results in release of nitric oxide. Nitric oxide activates guanylyl cyclase which synthesizes cyclic guanosine. Nitric oxide is responsible for the vasodilatory effects of nitrates. Production of nitrate may lead to conversion of hemoglobin to methemoglobin.

Reference: Butterworth JF IV, Mackey DC, Wasnick JD, eds. *Morgan & Mikhail's Clinical Anesthesiology*. 7th ed. New York, NY: McGraw Hill; 2022: Chapter 15.

247. You are infusing sodium nitroprusside at 3 μg/kg/min. What condition is likely to result?

(A) Cyanide toxicity

(B) Adsorption of polyvinylchloride

(C) Increased afterload

(D) Cerebral vessel constriction

Rationale: Nitroprusside in doses greater than 500 μg/kg or infusions faster than 2 μg/kg/min is associated with cyanide toxicity. Tubing and glass containers specific for the administration of nitroglycerin are used to avoid adsorption of nitroglycerin to polyvinylchloride. Administration of sodium nitroprusside results in reduced preload and afterload as well as cerebral vessel dilation.

Reference: Butterworth JF IV, Mackey DC, Wasnick JD, eds. *Morgan & Mikhail's Clinical Anesthesiology*. 7th ed. New York, NY: McGraw Hill; 2022: Chapter 15.

248. During esophageal surgery, the endotracheal tube catches fire. What will you do first?

(A) Call for help

(B) Remove the endotracheal tube

(C) Stop the gas flow and remove the endotracheal tube

(D) Remove the surgical drapes

Rationale: Rapidly stopping the gas flow (oxidizers) and removing the endotracheal tube is essential when an airway fire occurs. Removing surgical drapes after turning off gases is needed when a fire involves the patient's body.

Reference: Butterworth JF IV, Mackey DC, Wasnick JD, eds. *Morgan & Mikhail's Clinical Anesthesiology*. 7th ed. New York, NY: McGraw Hill; 2022: Chapter 3.

249. The patient with rheumatoid arthritis complains of long-term throbbing joint pain. Which fibers are activated?

(A) Efferent A and C fibers

(B) Alpha and beta efferent fibers

(C) Afferent A and C fibers

(D) Alpha and beta afferent fibers

Rationale: As compared to peripheral nerve injury, that results in shooting or burning pain, tissue injury or inflammation results in throbbing or aching pain. A and C afferent fibers are activated with tissue injury and inflammation. With nerve injuries, alpha and beta afferent fibers are activated.

References: Butterworth JF IV, Mackey DC, Wasnick JD, eds. *Morgan & Mikhail's Clinical Anesthesiology*. 7th ed. New York, NY: McGraw Hill; 2022: Chapter 47.
Brunton LL, Hilal-Dandan R, Knollmann BC, eds. *Goodman & Gilman's: The Pharmacological Basis of Therapeutics*. 13th ed. McGraw Hill; 2017: Chapter 18.

250. Why is the primary metabolite of tramadol significant?

(A) Greater potency than the parent drug

(B) Shorter elimination half-life than the parent drug

(C) Respiratory depression is not reversible with naloxone

(D) Safety profile when using MAO inhibitors

Rationale: Tramadol's O-demethylated metabolite possesses greater potency than the parent drug. The elimination half-life is 7.5 hours as compared to the parent drug (6 hours). Naloxone is used effectively to reverse respiratory depression but may not entirely reverse analgesia. Tramadol should be avoided for patients taking MAO inhibitors or SSRIs due to the propensity for seizures.

References: Brunton LL, Hilal-Dandan R, Knollmann BC, eds. *Goodman & Gilman's: The Pharmacological Basis of Therapeutics*. 13th ed. New York, NY: McGraw Hill; 2017: Chapter 18.
Hemmings HC Jr, Egan TD, eds. *Pharmacology and Physiology for Anesthesia: Foundations and Clinical Application*. 2nd ed. Philadelphia, PA: Elsevier Saunders; 2019: Chapter 4.

251. Following general anesthesia for right shoulder arthroscopy, the patient complains of pain. The patient's history includes congestive heart failure. Which analgesic will you avoid?

(A) Butorphanol
(B) Morphine
(C) Demerol
(D) Nalbuphine

Rationale: Cardiac effects following administration of butorphanol include increased pulmonary artery pressure and decreased systemic arterial pressure. It is generally avoided in patients with a history of myocardial infarction or congestive heart failure. Comparatively, morphine, Demerol, and nalbuphine administration results in fewer cardiac effects.

Reference: Brunton LL, Hilal-Dandan R, Knollmann BC, eds. *Goodman & Gilman's: The Pharmacological Basis of Therapeutics*. 13th ed. New York, NY: McGraw Hill; 2017: Chapter 18.

252. Which drug would you avoid in an asthmatic patient?

(A) Volatile anesthetics
(B) Nitrous oxide
(C) Morphine
(D) Lidocaine

Rationale: Morphine can release histamine, which could cause bronchoconstriction,

Reference: Elisha S, Heiner JS, Nagelhout JJ. *Nurse Anesthesia*. 7th ed. St. Louis, MO: Elsevier Saunders; 2023: Chapter 29.

253. You decide to give butorphanol 2 mg to the patient postoperatively. What is the equipotent dose of morphine?

(A) 100 mg
(B) 8 mg
(C) 10 mg
(D) 80 mg

Rationale: The equipotent dose of morphine is 10 mg or demerol 80 to 100 mg.

Reference: Brunton LL, Hilal-Dandan R, Knollmann BC, eds. *Goodman & Gilman's: The Pharmacological Basis of Therapeutics*. 13th ed. New York, NY: McGraw Hill; 2017: Chapter 18.

254. Your patient has a history of asthma. Which opioid will you avoid?

(A) Fentanyl
(B) Morphine
(C) Remifentanil
(D) Tramadol

Rationale: Morphine releases histamine and is contraindicated for patients with asthma. Tramadol and fentanyl and derivatives do not release histamine.

References: Butterworth JF IV, Mackey DC, Wasnick JD, eds. *Morgan & Mikhail's Clinical Anesthesiology*. 7th ed. New York, NY: McGraw Hill; 2022: Chapter 10.

Brunton LL, Hilal-Dandan R, Knollmann BC, eds. *Goodman & Gilman's: The Pharmacological Basis of Therapeutics*. 13th ed. McGraw Hill; 2017: Chapter 18.

255. How is remifentanil metabolized?

(A) Hepatic cytochrome P
(B) Hydrolysis by esterase enzymes
(C) Hepatic conjugation
(D) Conjugation with glucuronic acid

Rationale: Most opioids are metabolized in the liver. Metabolic processes include conjugation, cytochrome P, or a combination. Remifentanil is the exception whereby metabolism undergoes hydrolysis in the blood and tissue.

References: Butterworth JF IV, Mackey DC, Wasnick JD, eds. *Morgan & Mikhail's Clinical Anesthesiology*. 7th ed. New York, NY: McGraw Hill; 2022: Chapter 10.

Elisha S, Heiner JS, Nagelhout JJ. *Nurse Anesthesia*. 7th ed. St. Louis, MO: Elsevier Saunders; 2023: Chapter 11.

256. How does digoxin control atrial arrhythmias?

(A) Enhancing vagal tone
(B) Addition of calcium
(C) Decreased intracellular sodium
(D) Decreasing vagal tone

Rationale: Vagal effects result in decreased heart rate, prolonged AV conduction, slowed impulse through the AV node, and a prolonged effective refractory period. Because of the vagal effects it is used to control atrial arrhythmias.

Reference: Elisha S, Heiner JS, Nagelhout JJ. *Nurse Anesthesia*. 7th ed. St. Louis, MO: Elsevier Saunders; 2023: Chapter 13.

257. Your patient is undergoing a cholecystecomy with general anesthesia and an endotracheal tube. The patient takes digoxin for chronic congestive heart failure. What is the first sign of digitalis toxicity under anesthesia?

(A) Bradycardia

(B) Hypotension

(C) Arrhythmias

(D) Hypertension

Rationale: Signs and symptoms associated with digitalis toxicity include headache, CNS dysfunction, diarrhea, nausea and vomiting, fatigue, and arrhythmias. Specifically, when a patient is anesthetized, premature ventricular contractions may be the first sign of digitalis toxicity.

References: Brunton LL, Hilal-Dandan R, Knollmann BC, eds. *Goodman & Gilman's: The Pharmacological Basis of Therapeutics.* 13th ed. McGraw Hill; 2017: Chapter 18.

Elisha S, Heiner JS, Nagelhout JJ. *Nurse Anesthesia.* 7th ed. St. Louis, MO: Elsevier Saunders; 2023: Chapter 13.

258. What medication is indicated for treatment of ventricular fibrillation?

(A) Vasopressin

(B) Verapamil

(C) Ibutilide

(D) Adenosine

Rationale: Vasopressin may be used in place of epinephrine for treatment of ventricular fibrillation. Verapamil is indicated for rate control in atrial flutter, atrial fibrillation, and for stopping paroxysmal supraventricular tachycardia. For cardioversion of atrial fibrillation or atrial flutter, ibutilide is used. Adenosine is used to treat stable supraventricular tachycardia, narrow and wide-complex tachycardias.

Reference: Butterworth JF IV, Mackey DC, Wasnick JD, eds. *Morgan & Mikhail's Clinical Anesthesiology.* 7th ed. New York, NY: McGraw Hill; 2022: Chapter 55.

259. Why is terbutaline preferred for the treatment of asthma over bronkosol?

(A) Bronkosol's beta-1 adrenergic activity is less than terbutaline.

(B) Both bronchodilators are acceptable.

(C) Terbutaline's beta-1 adrenergic activity is less than bronkosol.

(D) Bronkosol's beta-2 activity is greater than terbutaline.

Rationale: The preference for using terbutaline is due to more selective beta-2 activity. Bronkosol's increased beta-1 activity makes it less useful than terbutaline.

Reference: Butterworth JF IV, Mackey DC, Wasnick JD, eds. *Morgan & Mikhail's Clinical Anesthesiology.* 7th ed. New York, NY: McGraw Hill; 2022: Chapter 24.

260. During the preoperative interview, you learn the patient takes daily lithium. How will Lithium affect drugs used for general anesthesia?

(A) Shorten the duration of action of vecuronium

(B) Increase the MAC of Isoflurane

(C) Increase the duration of action of vecuronium

(D) No interaction with lithium exists for drugs used during general anesthesia.

Rationale: Lithium decreases MAC and increases the duration of action of neuromuscular blockers. Neuromuscular monitoring is essential.

References: Butterworth JF IV, Mackey DC, Wasnick JD, eds. *Morgan & Mikhail's Clinical Anesthesiology.* 7th ed. New York, NY: McGraw Hill; 2022: Chapter 24.

Brunton LL, Hilal-Dandan R, Knollmann BC, eds. *Goodman & Gilman's: The Pharmacological Basis of Therapeutics.* 13th ed. McGraw Hill; 2017: Chapter 18.

261. In reviewing the patient's record, you note daily use of lithium and hydrochlorothiazide. What do you expect?

(A) Hypernatremia

(B) Therapeutic lithium levels

(C) Decrease lithium levels

(D) Hyponatremia

Rationale: Patient concomitantly taking lithium and a loop or thiazide diuretic may experience lithium toxicity. Lithium toxicity results from hyponatremia that decreases renal excretion of lithium. Due to the Lithium's narrow therapeutic range (0.8-1.0 mEq/L), preoperative lithium levels should be checked.

References: Brunton LL, Hilal-Dandan R, Knollmann BC, eds. *Goodman & Gilman's: The Pharmacological Basis of Therapeutics.* 13th ed. McGraw Hill; 2017: Chapter 18.

Butterworth JF IV, Mackey DC, Wasnick JD, eds. *Morgan & Mikhail's Clinical Anesthesiology.* 7th ed. New York, NY: McGraw Hill; 2022: Chapter 28.

262. You are called for an emergency exploratory laparoscopy. The patient was involved in a motor vehicle accident and appears intoxicated. What do you expect?

(A) Increased requirements for fentanyl

(B) Decreased requirements for midazolam

(C) Increased requirements for sodium pentathol

(D) Decreased requirements for amphetamines

Rationale: The patient is acutely intoxicated. Acute intoxication results in decreased requirements for opioids, barbiturates, benzodiazepines, and phencyclidine derivatives. By comparison patients with chronic alcoholism require higher requirements for opioids, barbiturates, and benzodiazepines.

TABLE 1-15. Effect of acute and chronic substance abuse on anesthetic requirements.[1]

Substance	Acute	Chronic
Opioids	↓	↑
Barbiturates	↓	↑
Alcohol	↓	↑
Marijuana	↓	0
Benzodiazepines	↓	↑
Amphetamines	↑[2]	↓
Cocaine	↑[2]	0
Phencyclidine	↓	?

[1]↓, decreases; ↑, increases; 0, no effect; ?, unknown.
[2]Associated with marked sympathetic stimulation.
(Reproduced with permission from Butterworth JF IV, Mackey DC, Wasnick JD, eds. *Morgan & Mikhail's Clinical Anesthesiology.* 7th ed. New York, NY: McGraw Hill; 2022.)

References: Brunton LL, Hilal-Dandan R, Knollmann BC, eds. *Goodman & Gilman's: The Pharmacological Basis of Therapeutics.* 13th ed. McGraw Hill; 2017: Chapter 16.
Butterworth JF IV, Mackey DC, Wasnick JD, eds. *Morgan & Mikhail's Clinical Anesthesiology.* 7th ed. New York, NY: McGraw Hill; 2022: Chapter 28.

263. Why do patients who take tranylcypromine need to avoid eating cheese?

(A) Hypotensive crisis due to tyramine

(B) Decreased agitation

(C) Hypertensive crisis due to tyramine

(D) Jaundice

Rationale: Tyramine containing foods, such as cheese and red wine, may result in a hypertensive crisis secondary to generation of norepinephrine for patients taking MAO inhibitors (tranylcypromine). Side effects of MAO inhibitors may include orthostatic hypotension, increased agitation, jaundice, urinary retention, muscle spasms, tremors, and seizures.

References: Brunton LL, Hilal-Dandan R, Knollmann BC, eds. *Goodman & Gilman's: The Pharmacological Basis of Therapeutics.* 13th ed. McGraw Hill; 2017: Chapter 16.
Butterworth JF IV, Mackey DC, Wasnick JD, eds. *Morgan & Mikhail's Clinical Anesthesiology.* 7th ed. New York, NY: McGraw Hill; 2022: Chapter 28.

264. Which narcotic will you avoid in patients taking MAO inhibitors?

(A) Demerol

(B) Fentanyl

(C) Morphine

(D) Sufentanil

Rationale: Administration of demerol to patients taking MAO inhibitors may result in hyperthermia, seizures, coma, and death. All narcotics should be used with caution for patients taking MAO inhibitors.

References: Brunton LL, Hilal-Dandan R, Knollmann BC, eds. *Goodman & Gilman's: The Pharmacological Basis of Therapeutics.* 13th ed. McGraw Hill; 2017: Chapter 16.
Butterworth JF IV, Mackey DC, Wasnick JD, eds. *Morgan & Mikhail's Clinical Anesthesiology.* 7th ed. New York, NY: McGraw Hill; 2022: Chapter 28.
Elisha S, Heiner JS, Nagelhout JJ. *Nurse Anesthesia.* 7th ed. St. Louis, MO: Elsevier Saunders; 2023: Chapter 11.

265. Which of the following medications does not prolong the QT interval?

(A) Fluoxetine

(B) Sertraline

(C) Azithromycin

(D) Gentamicin

Rationale: Classifications of psychiatric drugs known to prolong the QT interval include butyrophenones, phenothiazines, antipsychotics, and SSRIs (fluoxetine, sertraline). Antibiotic classifications associated with prolonging the QT interval include macrolides (azithromycin). Gentamicin, an aminoglycoside, may cause auditory dysfunction.

References: Butterworth JF IV, Mackey DC, Wasnick JD, eds. *Morgan & Mikhail's Clinical Anesthesiology.* 7th ed. New York, NY: McGraw Hill; 2022: Chapter 28.
Elisha S, Heiner JS, Nagelhout JJ. *Nurse Anesthesia.* 7th ed. St. Louis, MO: Elsevier Saunders; 2023: Chapter 26.

266. When treating hypotension for a patient taking doxepin what will you use?

(A) Neosynephrine 10 μg IV

(B) Ephedrine 5 mg IV

(C) Neosynephrine 100 μg IV

(D) Ephedrine 10 mg IV

Rationale: Doxepine, a tricyclic antidepressant, results in an exaggerated response when given indirect-acting vasopressors or sympathetic stimulants. Small doses of direct-acting vasopressors (neosynephrine) are the appropriate treatment for hypotension.

Reference: Butterworth JF IV, Mackey DC, Wasnick JD, eds. *Morgan & Mikhail's Clinical Anesthesiology.* 7th ed. New York, NY: McGraw Hill; 2022: Chapter 28.

267. Your patient is taking amitriptyline. What will you tell your patient about taking this drug?

(A) Continue taking amitriptyline preoperatively.

(B) Stop taking amitryptyline 24 hours before surgery.

(C) Stop taking amitryptyline 1 week before surgery.

(D) Stop taking amitryptyline 2 weeks before surgery.

Rationale: Amitriptyline (Elavil) is a tricyclic antidepressant. Informing the patient to continue taking the medication will avoid possible cholinergic symptoms, cardiac arrhythmias, and extrapyramidal side effects.

References: Brunton LL, Hilal-Dandan R, Knollmann BC, eds. *Goodman & Gilman's: The Pharmacological Basis of Therapeutics.* 13th ed. McGraw Hill; 2017: Chapter 16.

Butterworth JF IV, Mackey DC, Wasnick JD, eds. *Morgan & Mikhail's Clinical Anesthesiology.* 7th ed. New York, NY: McGraw Hill; 2022: Chapter 28.

Elisha S, Heiner JS, Nagelhout JJ. *Nurse Anesthesia.* 7th ed. St. Louis, MO: Elsevier Saunders; 2023: Chapters 20 & 56.

268. Contractions weaken despite use of oxytocin. Prostaglandin is administered. What do you expect?

(A) Constipation

(B) Hypotension

(C) Headache

(D) Bronchodilation

Rationale: Side effects of prostaglandin (hemabate or carboprost) may result in diarrhea, nausea, and vomiting and bronchoconstriction. Hypotension results due to vascular relaxation of smooth muscle.

References: Butterworth JF IV, Mackey DC, Wasnick JD, eds. *Morgan & Mikhail's Clinical Anesthesiology.* 7th ed. New York, NY: McGraw Hill; 2022: Chapter 40.

Elisha S, Heiner JS, Nagelhout JJ. *Nurse Anesthesia.* 7th ed. St. Louis, MO: Elsevier Saunders; 2023: Chapter 51.

269. The patient is scheduled for a cesarean section. You plan to use sevoflurane. How will this choice affect the uterus?

(A) Increase uterine constriction

(B) Decrease uterine bleeding

(C) Increase uterine relaxation

(D) Inhalational agents have no effect on the uterus.

Rationale: Volatile anesthetics relax the uterus. For this reason, decrease the concentration to 0.5 MAC.

Reference: Butterworth JF IV, Mackey DC, Wasnick JD, eds. *Morgan & Mikhail's Clinical Anesthesiology.* 7th ed. New York, NY: McGraw Hill; 2022: Chapter 40.

270. Dantrolene was administered for malignant hyperthermia. What is the most serious complication?

(A) Respiratory insufficiency

(B) Aspiration pneumonia

(C) Hepatic dysfunction

(D) Generalized muscle weakness

Rationale: Generalized muscle weakness may result in respiratory insufficiency and aspiration pneumonia. It is also associated with hepatic dysfunction.

References: Butterworth JF IV, Mackey DC, Wasnick JD, eds. *Morgan & Mikhail's Clinical Anesthesiology.* 7th ed. New York, NY: McGraw Hill; 2022: Chapter 52.

Elisha S, Heiner JS, Nagelhout JJ. *Nurse Anesthesia.* 7th ed. St. Louis, MO: Elsevier Saunders; 2023: Chapter 36.

271. What is the result of an excess of glucocorticoids?

(A) Cushing's syndrome

(B) Addison's disease

(C) Conn syndrome

(D) Pheochromocytoma

Rationale: Excess production or administration of glucocoricoids results in Cushing's syndrome. A deficiency of glucocorticoids results in Addison's disease. Conn syndrome is caused by increased aldosterone (mineralocorticoid) whereas an excess in catecholamines results in a pheochromocytoma.

References: Butterworth JF IV, Mackey DC, Wasnick JD, eds. *Morgan & Mikhail's Clinical Anesthesiology.* 7th ed. New York, NY: McGraw Hill; 2022: Chapter 34.

Elisha S, Heiner JS, Nagelhout JJ. *Nurse Anesthesia.* 7th ed. St. Louis, MO: Elsevier Saunders; 2023: Chapter 37.

272. What is the most effective treatment for moderate to severe Parkinson's disease?

(A) Levodopa

(B) Nonergot derivatives

(C) Levodopa with a decarboxylase inhibitor

(D) Dopamine receptor agonists

Rationale: Levodopa given with a decarboxylase inhibitor increases the central delivery and allows for decreased doses of Levodopa. Dopamine receptor agonists including ergot and nonergot derivatives are useful. Nonergot derivatives are used in early Parkinson's disease treatment.

Reference: Butterworth JF IV, Mackey DC, Wasnick JD, eds. *Morgan & Mikhail's Clinical Anesthesiology.* 7th ed. New York, NY: McGraw Hill; 2022: Chapter 28.

273. The patient is scheduled for a thoracotomy. Upon review of the patient's medical history, you note that lovastatin as part of the medical management. What will you tell the patient preoperatively?

(A) Take the statin as directed prior to surgery.

(B) Stop the statin immediately.

(C) Stop the statin 1 week prior to surgery.

(D) Stop the statin 2 weeks prior to surgery.

Rationale: Anti-lipid lowering medications offer benefits for patients undergoing surgery that include decreasing the length of hospital stay, stroke, MI, renal dysfunction, and death. The anti-inflammatory effects, stabilizing atherosclerotic plaquing, and improved endothelial function offer benefit to high-risk surgical patients. Stopping statins prior to surgery may result in a rebound effect.

References: Elisha S, Heiner JS, Nagelhout JJ. *Nurse Anesthesia.* 7th ed. St. Louis, MO: Elsevier Saunders; 2023: Chapter 20.

Hines RL, Marschall KE. *Stoelting's Anesthesia and Co-existing Disease.* 7th ed. Philadelphia, PA: Elsevier Saunders; 2018: Chapter 1.

Pardo MC, Miller RD. *Miller's Basics of Anesthesia.* 8th ed. Philadelphia, PA: Elsevier; 2023: Chapter 13.

274. What is the percent of total body water in the intracellular compartment?

(A) 25%

(B) 8%

(C) 100%

(D) 67%

Rationale: The total body water in the extracellular compartment is comprised of 25% interstitial and 8% intravascular. The total body water of the intracellular compartment is 67%.

TABLE 1-16. Body fluid compartments (based on an average 70-kg man).

Compartment	Fluid as Percent Body Weight (%)	Total Body Water (%)	Fluid Volume (L)
Intracellular	40	67	28
Extracellular			
Interstitial	15	25	10.5
Intravascular	5	8	3.5
Total	60	100	42

(Reproduced with permission from Butterworth JF IV, Mackey DC, Wasnick JD, eds. *Morgan & Mikhail's Clinical Anesthesiology.* 7th ed. New York, NY: McGraw Hill; 2022.)

References: Butterworth JF IV, Mackey DC, Wasnick JD, eds. *Morgan & Mikhail's Clinical Anesthesiology.* 7th ed. New York, NY: McGraw Hill; 2022: Chapter 49.

Elisha S, Heiner JS, Nagelhout JJ. *Nurse Anesthesia.* 7th ed. St. Louis, MO: Elsevier Saunders; 2023: Chapter 21.

275. What is the major extracellular cation?

(A) Sodium

(B) Potassium

(C) Magnesium

(D) Chloride

Rationale: The major intracellular cation is potassium whereas sodium is the major extracellular cation. Magnesium comprises about 50% of the intracellular compartment as compared to potassium. The anion chloride comprises approximately 60% of the extracellular compartment.

References: Butterworth JF IV, Mackey DC, Wasnick JD, eds. *Morgan & Mikhail's Clinical Anesthesiology.* 7th ed. New York, NY: McGraw Hill; 2022: Chapter 49.

Elisha S, Heiner JS, Nagelhout JJ. *Nurse Anesthesia.* 7th ed. St. Louis, MO: Elsevier Saunders; 2023: Chapter 21.

276. What substance poorly penetrates through the capillary endothelium?

(A) Oxygen

(B) Water

(C) Lipid-soluble substances

(D) Plasma proteins

Rationale: Oxygen, water, lipid-soluble freely as well as low molecular weight substances (sodium, chloride, potassium, and glucose) penetrates the capillary endothelium. High molecular weight substances (plasma proteins) poorly penetrate the endothelial clefts.

References: Butterworth JF IV, Mackey DC, Wasnick JD, eds. *Morgan & Mikhail's Clinical Anesthesiology.* 7th ed. New York, NY: McGraw Hill; 2022: Chapter 49.

Elisha S, Heiner JS, Nagelhout JJ. *Nurse Anesthesia.* 7th ed. St. Louis, MO: Elsevier Saunders; 2023: Chapter 21.

277. At what value do serious complications of hyponatremia manifest?

(A) 150 mEq/L

(B) 145 mEq/L

(C) 130 mEq/L

(D) 120 mEq/L

Rationale: Hypernatremia is sodium >145 mEq/L whereas hyponatremia is sodium <135 mEq/L. Severe hyponatremia (<120 mEq/L) manifests neurologically with cerebral edema, confusion, seizures, coma, and death.

References: Butterworth JF IV, Mackey DC, Wasnick JD, eds. *Morgan & Mikhail's Clinical Anesthesiology.* 7th ed. New York, NY: McGraw Hill; 2022: Chapter 49.

Elisha S, Heiner JS, Nagelhout JJ. *Nurse Anesthesia.* 7th ed. St. Louis, MO: Elsevier Saunders; 2023: Chapter 21.

278. The patient presents for surgery, and you note a potassium level of 6 mEq/L. You choose to administer calcium gluconate. Which drug interaction is most concerning for this patient when administering calcium?

(A) Digoxin

(B) Furosemide

(C) Kayexalate

(D) Sodium bicarbonate

Rationale: Digoxin toxicity is potentiated by calcium. Furosemide, kayexalate, and sodium bicarbonate assist with decreasing potassium.

Reference: Butterworth JF IV, Mackey DC, Wasnick JD, eds. *Morgan & Mikhail's Clinical Anesthesiology.* 7th ed. New York, NY: McGraw Hill; 2022: Chapter 49.

TABLE 1-17. The composition of fluid compartments.

| | Gram-Molecular Weight | Intracellular (mEq/L) | Extracellular | |
			Intravascular (mEq/L)	Interstitial (mEq/L)
Sodium	23.0	10	145	142
Potassium	39.1	140	4	4
Calcium	40.1	<1	3	3
Magnesium	24.3	50	2	2
Chloride	35.5	4	105	110
Bicarbonate	61.0	10	24	28
Phosphorus	31.0[1]	75	2	2
Protein (g/dL)		16	7	2

[1]PO_4^{3-} is 95 g.

(Reproduced with permission from Butterworth JF IV, Mackey DC, Wasnick JD, eds. *Morgan & Mikhail's Clinical Anesthesiology.* 7th ed. New York, NY: McGraw Hill; 2022.)

279. The patient presents with hypercalcemia secondary to a malignancy. What is the most effective means for lower serum calcium?

(A) A loop diuretic followed by rehydration

(B) Bisphosphonate

(C) Rehydration followed by a loop diuretic

(D) Etidronate

Rationale: Rehydrate the patient first. Giving the loop diuretic first will worsen hypovolemia and the hypercalcemia. Biphosphonate and etidronate may be used to lower calcium levels.

References: Butterworth JF IV, Mackey DC, Wasnick JD, eds. *Morgan & Mikhail's Clinical Anesthesiology.* 7th ed. New York, NY: McGraw Hill; 2022: Chapter 49.

Elisha S, Heiner JS, Nagelhout JJ. *Nurse Anesthesia.* 7th ed. St. Louis, MO: Elsevier Saunders; 2023: Chapter 21.

280. What target range is required for therapeutic effects of heparin?

(A) ACT 200 to 400 seconds

(B) aPTT 1.5 to 2.5 times the control value

(C) ACT 100 to 200 seconds

(D) aPTT 2.5 to 3.5 times the control value

Rationale: The aPTT is typically used to determine a therapeutic range for heparin. Activated coagulation time (ACT) is also available with values above 400 to 800 seconds.

Reference: Hemmings HC Jr, Egan TD, eds. *Pharmacology and Physiology for Anesthesia: Foundations and Clinical Application.* 2nd ed. Philadelphia, PA: Elsevier Saunders; 2019: Chapter 37.

281. Which statement is false regarding low molecular weight heparins (LMWHs)?

(A) LMWHs prevent formation of prothrombinase.

(B) Thrombolytic doses do not significantly cross the placenta.

(C) Bioavailability is greater with LMWHs as compared to heparin.

(D) Protamine is the antidote of choice for LMWHs.

Rationale: Protamine reverses the effects of heparin. There is no antidote for LMWHs.

References: Butterworth JF IV, Mackey DC, Wasnick JD, eds. *Morgan & Mikhail's Clinical Anesthesiology.* 7th ed. New York, NY: McGraw Hill; 2022: Chapter 24.

Hemmings HC Jr, Egan TD, eds. *Pharmacology and Physiology for Anesthesia: Foundations and Clinical Application.* 2nd ed. Philadelphia, PA: Elsevier Saunders; 2019: Chapter 37.

282. The patient is taking subcutaneous unfractionated heparin. When is the best time to administer a spinal anesthetic?

(A) 4 to 6 hours after heparin administration

(B) 2 to 4 hours after heparin administration

(C) 12 to 24 hours after heparin administration

(D) 6 to 8 hours after heparin administration

Rationale: For patients taking unfractionated heparin, it is advisable to wait 6 to 8 hours before proceeding with a regional anesthetic technique. For patients taking low molecular weight heparin, wait 12 to 24 hours.

References: Butterworth JF IV, Mackey DC, Wasnick JD, eds. *Morgan & Mikhail's Clinical Anesthesiology.* 7th ed. New York, NY: McGraw Hill; 2022: Chapter 24.

Hemmings H, Egan T. *Pharmacology and Physiology for Anesthesia: Foundations and Clinical Application.* 2nd ed. Philadelphia, PA: Elsevier Saunders; 2019: Chapter 37.

283. What test is used to measure the effect of warfarin on blood coagulation?

(A) aPTT

(B) ACT

(C) AT

(D) INR

Rationale: The aPTT and ACT determine the therapeutic range of heparin. The INR or PT measure the effect of warfarin on blood coagulation. Antithrombin (AT) is the plasma co-factor needed to exert anticoagulation action by heparin.

Reference: Hemmings HC Jr, Egan TD, eds. *Pharmacology and Physiology for Anesthesia: Foundations and Clinical Application.* 2nd ed. Philadelphia, PA: Elsevier Saunders; 2019: Chapter 37.

284. How does renal impairment affect insulin requirements?

(A) Insulin requirements decrease.

(B) No relationship exists between insulin requirements and renal impairment.

(C) Insulin requirements increase.

(D) The kidneys break down insulin to a greater extent.

Rationale: Insulin is broken down in the liver, kidneys, and muscle. For patients with renal disease, the insulin requirements decrease.

References: Butterworth JF IV, Mackey DC, Wasnick JD, eds. *Morgan & Mikhail's Clinical Anesthesiology*. 7th ed. New York, NY: McGraw Hill; 2022: Chapter 34.

Hemmings HC Jr, Egan TD, eds. *Pharmacology and Physiology for Anesthesia: Foundations and Clinical Application*. 2nd ed. Philadelphia, PA: Elsevier Saunders; 2019: Chapter 31.

285. What oral hypoglycemic is relatively contraindicated for patients with renal impairment?

(A) Glyburide

(B) Lipizide

(C) Tolbutamide

(D) Metformin

Rationale: First-generation sulfonylureas (tolbutamide) are used cautiously for patient with renal disease. Second-generation sulfonylureas are better suited for patients with renal disease. Metformin, a biguanide, is relatively contraindicated for patients with renal disease due to unchanged urinary excretion.

References: Butterworth JF IV, Mackey DC, Wasnick JD, eds. *Morgan & Mikhail's Clinical Anesthesiology*. 7th ed. New York, NY: McGraw Hill; 2022: Chapter 34.

Hemmings HC Jr, Egan TD, eds. *Pharmacology and Physiology for Anesthesia: Foundations and Clinical Application*. 2nd ed. Philadelphia, PA: Elsevier Saunders; 2019: Chapter 31.

286. A patient with preexisting hypertension is undergoing an exploratory laparotomy. The blood pressure increases intraoperatively. What will you do first?

(A) Give esmolol

(B) Increase the concentration of isoflurane

(C) Give labetalol

(D) Decrease the concentration of isoflurane

Rationale: Deepening the anesthetic typically precedes pharmacological intervention.

Reference: Butterworth JF IV, Mackey DC, Wasnick JD, eds. *Morgan & Mikhail's Clinical Anesthesiology*. 7th ed. New York, NY: McGraw Hill; 2022: Chapter 21.

287. A patient states they take nitroglycerin for angina. What statement is true regarding nitroglycerin's effect on the heart?

(A) Decreases preload

(B) Increases afterload

(C) Increases preload

(D) Decreases coronary vasodilatation

Rationale: Patients taking nitrates for angina benefit due to decreasing preload and afterload as well as dilating the coronary and systemic circulation.

Reference: Butterworth JF IV, Mackey DC, Wasnick JD, eds. *Morgan & Mikhail's Clinical Anesthesiology*. 7th ed. New York, NY: McGraw Hill; 2022: Chapter 21.

288. What patient history represents the greatest risk for cardiac complications?

(A) Recent angina

(B) Coronary artery disease involving two vessels

(C) History of MI 1 year ago

(D) Coronary artery disease involving three vessels

Rationale: Patients whose history includes extensive coronary artery disease involving three or more vessels or left main; recent history of myocardial infarction or ventricular dysfunction pose the greatest risk for cardiac complications.

Reference: Butterworth JF IV, Mackey DC, Wasnick JD, eds. *Morgan & Mikhail's Clinical Anesthesiology*. 7th ed. New York, NY: McGraw Hill; 2022: Chapter 21.

TABLE 1-18. Comparison of antianginal agents.[1]

| Cardiac Parameter | Nitrates | Calcium Channel Blockers | | | β-Blockers |
		Verapamil	Nifedipine Nicardipine Nimodipine	Diltiazem	
Preload	↓↓	—	—	—	—/↑
Afterload	↓	↓	↓↓	↓	—/↓
Contractility	—	↓↓	—	↓	↓↓↓
SA node automaticity	↑/—	↓↓	↑/—	↓↓	↓↓↓
AV conduction	—	↓↓↓	—	↓↓	↓↓↓
Vasodilatation					
Coronary	↑	↑↑	↑↑↑	↑↑	—/↓
Systemic	↑↑	↑	↑↑	↑	—/↓

[1]↑, increases; —, no change; ↓, decreases.

AV, atrioventricular; SA, sinoatrial.

(Reproduced with permission from Butterworth JF IV, Mackey DC, Wasnick JD, eds. *Morgan & Mikhail's Clinical Anesthesiology*. 7th ed. New York, NY: McGraw Hill; 2022.)

289. What characterizes a second-degree burn?

    (A) Penetrate epidermis and blisters form

    (B) Replace fluids for burns >10% of the total body surface area

    (C) Full thickness

    (D) Requires debridement

Rationale: First-degree burns do not penetrate the epidermis. In comparison, second-degree burns penetrate the epidermis with blister formation. Fluids are replaced for second-degree burns involving more than 20% of the total body surface area. Third-degree burns involve full thickness of the dermis requiring debridement and skin grafting.

Reference: Butterworth JF IV, Mackey DC, Wasnick JD, eds. *Morgan & Mikhail's Clinical Anesthesiology.* 7th ed. New York, NY: McGraw Hill; 2022: Chapter 39.

290. An adult male who weighs 100 kg is burned over 50% of his body. Using the Parkland formula, calculate the fluid requirements for the first 24 hours.

Answer: 20,000 mL

Rationale: The Parkland Formula is used to calculate the fluids needed for resuscitation of burn patients. The calculation includes 4 mL/kg × body weight × percent burned $4 \times 100 \times 50 = 20{,}000$ mL

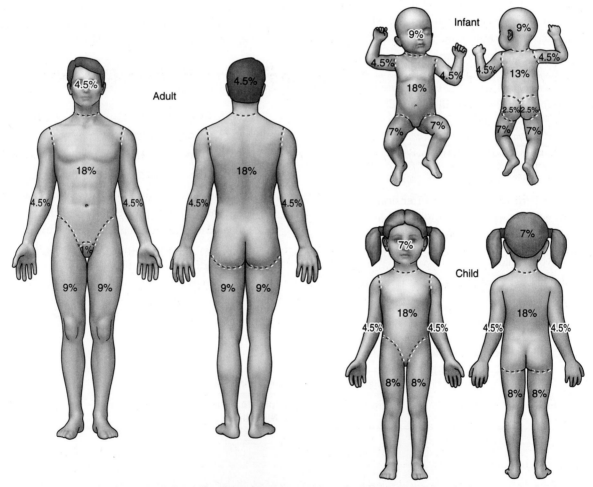

FIG. 1-7. The Rule of Nines, utilized to estimate burned surface area as a percentage of total body surface area (TBSA). (Reproduced with permission from Stone C, Humphries RL, Drigalla D, Stephan M. eds. *CURRENT Diagnosis & Treatment: Pediatric Emergency Medicine.* New York: McGraw Hill; 2014.)

Reference: Butterworth JF IV, Mackey DC, Wasnick JD, eds. *Morgan & Mikhail's Clinical Anesthesiology.* 7th ed. New York, NY: McGraw Hill; 2022: Chapter 39.

291. Which medication decreases the production of aqueous humor in glaucoma patients?

(A) Pilocarpine

(B) Solumedrol

(C) Acetazolamide

(D) Echothiophate

Rationale: Beta-blockers (timolol, betaxolol) and carbonic anhydrase inhibitors (acetazolamide, dorzolamide) aid glaucoma patients by decreasing the production of aqueous humor. Pilocarpine is a cholinergic agonist biotic used for pupillary constriction. Echothiophate, a cholinesterase inhibitor, is useful for patients with glaucoma. The drug causes miosis that improves the outflow of aqueous humor.

Reference: Elisha S, Heiner JS, Nagelhout JJ. *Nurse Anesthesia.* 7th ed. St. Louis, MO: Elsevier Saunders; 2023: Chapter 44.

292. What signs and symptoms are associated with acute opioid intoxication?

(A) Tachypnea and pinpoint pupils

(B) Hypotension and pinpoint pupils

(C) Dilated pupils and hypotension

(D) Dilated pupils and hypertension

Rationale: Acute opioid use is associated with respiratory depression, hypotension, euphoria, bradycardia, pinpoint pupils, and marked decreased consciousness.

References: Butterworth JF IV, Mackey DC, Wasnick JD, eds. *Morgan & Mikhail's Clinical Anesthesiology.* 7th ed. New York, NY: McGraw Hill; 2022: Chapter 28.
Elisha S, Heiner JS, Nagelhout JJ. *Nurse Anesthesia.* 7th ed. St. Louis, MO: Elsevier Saunders; 2023: Chapter 20.

293. How does chronic alcohol ingestion affect anesthetic requirements, including central nervous system hypnotics?

(A) Decreases requirements

(B) Increases requirements

(C) No effect on anesthetic requirements

(D) No effect with central nervous system hypnotics

Rationale: Acute ingestion of alcohol decreases anesthetic requirements whereas chronic ingestion increases the requirements due to tolerance.

TABLE 1-19. Effect of acute and chronic substance abuse on anesthetic requirements.[1]

Substance	Acute	Chronic
Opioids	↓	↑
Barbiturates	↓	↑
Alcohol	↓	↑
Marijuana	↓	0
Benzodiazepines	↓	↑
Amphetamines	↑[2]	↓
Cocaine	↑[2]	0
Phencyclidine	↓	?

[1]↓, decreases; ↑, increases; 0, no effect; ?, unknown.
[2]Associated with marked sympathetic stimulation.
(Reproduced with permission from Butterworth JF IV, Mackey DC, Wasnick JD, eds. *Morgan & Mikhail's Clinical Anesthesiology.* 7th ed. New York, NY: McGraw Hill; 2022.)

References: Butterworth JF IV, Mackey DC, Wasnick JD, eds. *Morgan & Mikhail's Clinical Anesthesiology.* 7th ed. New York, NY: McGraw Hill; 2022: Chapter 28.
Elisha S, Heiner JS, Nagelhout JJ. *Nurse Anesthesia.* 7th ed. St. Louis, MO: Elsevier Saunders; 2023: Chapter 20.

294. Which of the following statements regarding cigarette smoking is true?

(A) Carbon monoxide's affinity for hemoglobin is 100 times greater than oxygen.

(B) Carboxyhemoglobin returns to normal following two nights without smoking.

(C) Smoking cessation within 12 to 48 hours of surgery decreases circulating catecholamines.

(D) Nicotine causes hypotension and tachycardia.

Rationale: Nicotine's effects on the cardiovascular system include tachycardia, hypertension, myocardial oxygen consumption, and decreased delivery of oxygen to the tissue.

Reference: Elisha S, Heiner JS, Nagelhout JJ. *Nurse Anesthesia.* 7th ed. St. Louis, MO: Elsevier Saunders; 2023: Chapter 20.

295. During the preoperative interview, the patient admits to the use of anabolic steroids. What implications for anesthesia are most concerning?

(A) Impaired liver function and myocardial infarction

(B) Cardiomyopathy

(C) Behavioral disturbances

(D) Atherosclerosis

Rationale: Use of anabolic steroids predisposes patients to liver disorders that directly affect selection of medications that require liver metabolism. Risk factors are numerous including psychiatric conditions, cardiac dysfunction including myocardial infarction, stroke, liver cancer, and hypercoagulopathy.

Reference: Elisha S, Heiner JS, Nagelhout JJ. *Nurse Anesthesia.* 7th ed. St. Louis, MO: Elsevier Saunders; 2023: Chapter 20.

296. The patient has a history of porphyria. What drug will you avoid?

(A) Methohexital

(B) Propofol

(C) Vecuronium

(D) Nitrous oxide

Rationale: Metabolism of thiobarbiturates results in production of aminolevulinic acid synthetase. Porphyrin is formed by aminolevulinic acid synthetase. Porphyrin may precipitate an acute porphyric crisis.

References: Butterworth JF IV, Mackey DC, Wasnick JD, eds. *Morgan & Mikhail's Clinical Anesthesiology.* 7th ed. New York, NY: McGraw Hill; 2022: Chapter 28.

Hines RL, Marschall KE. *Stoelting's Anesthesia and Co-existing Disease.* 7th ed. Philadelphia, PA: Elsevier Saunders; 2018: Chapter 15.

297. Which risk factor is not related to latex allergy?

(A) Allergy to passion fruit

(B) Greater than five surgical procedures

(C) Spina stenosis

(D) Chronic exposure to latex

Rationale: Chronic, rather than acute exposure to latex products, represents a significant risk factor for latex allergy. Factors including spina bifida and urologic reconstructive surgery as well as food allergies (mainly fruits) may predispose an individual to latex allergy.

Reference: Elisha S, Heiner JS, Nagelhout JJ. *Nurse Anesthesia.* 7th ed. St. Louis, MO: Elsevier Saunders; 2023: Chapter 20.

298. What statement is true regarding trauma-induced coagulopathy?

(A) Tissue hyperperfusion results in coagulopathy.

(B) Thrombomodulin and activated protein C are released from the endothelium.

(C) Thrombomodulin binds to factor I.

(D) Thrombomodulin binds to protein C.

Rationale: Tissue hypoperfusion results in trauma-induced coagulopathy. Thrombomodulin and activated protein C are released from the endothelium. Thrombomodulin binds to thrombin resulting in impaired clot formation. However, several mechanisms exist.

References: Butterworth JF IV, Mackey DC, Wasnick JD, eds. *Morgan & Mikhail's Clinical Anesthesiology.* 7th ed. New York, NY: McGraw Hill; 2022: Chapter 39.

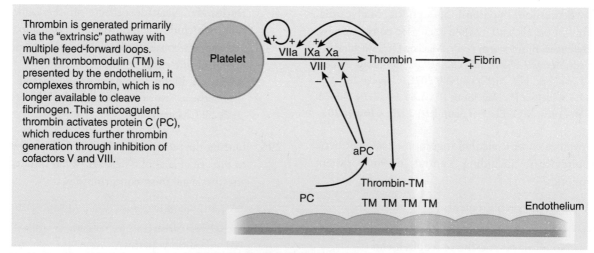

Thrombin is generated primarily via the "extrinsic" pathway with multiple feed-forward loops. When thrombomodulin (TM) is presented by the endothelium, it complexes thrombin, which is no longer available to cleave fibrinogen. This anticoagulent thrombin activates protein C (PC), which reduces further thrombin generation through inhibition of cofactors V and VIII.

FIG. 1-8. Mechanism of trauma-induced coagulopathy. During periods of tissue hypoperfusion, thrombomodulin (TM) released by the endothelium complexes with thrombin. The thrombin–TM complexes prevent cleavage of fibrinogen to fibrin and also activate protein C (PC), reducing further thrombin generation through cofactors V and VIII. (Reproduced with permission from Brohi K, Cohen MJ, Davenport RA. Acute coagulopathy of trauma: mechanism, identification and effect. *Curr Opin Crit Care.* 2007;13(6):680-685.)

Elisha S, Heiner JS, Nagelhout JJ. *Nurse Anesthesia.* 7th ed. St. Louis, MO: Elsevier Saunders; 2023: Chapter 40.

299. Which statement is false regarding epidural hematomas?

(A) It is typically associated with skull fractures.

(B) Patient may present conscious and then lapse into an unconscious state.

(C) When supratentorial hematomas exceed 30 mL volume, surgical decompression is used.

(D) It is typically associated with blunt force injury.

Rationale: Acute subdural hematomas are associated with deceleration or blunt force injury. Mortality is highest with subdural hematomas. Surgical evacuation is employed regardless of the volume.

Reference: Butterworth JF IV, Mackey DC, Wasnick JD, eds. *Morgan & Mikhail's Clinical Anesthesiology.* 7th ed. New York, NY: McGraw Hill; 2022: Chapter 39.

300. What condition results from a deficiency of Complement 1 esterase inhibitor?

(A) Angioedema

(B) Neutropenia

(C) Chronic granulomatous disease

(D) Chediak-Higashi syndrome

Rationale: Angioedema is an autosomal dominant disorder. Complement 1 esterase inhibitor deficiency or dysfunction causes increased vascular permeability, facial and/or laryngeal edema.

Reference: Hines RL, Marschall KE. *Stoelting's Anesthesia and Co-existing Disease.* 7th ed. Philadelphia, PA: Elsevier Saunders; 2018: Chapter 24.

301. What statement is true regarding allergic reactions?

(A) Anaphylaxis is a Type II hypersensitivity reaction.

(B) Type II hypersensitivity include transfusion reactions.

(C) Angioedema is a Type II hypersensitivity reaction.

(D) Anaphylactoid reactions result due to an interaction with IgE.

Rationale: Angioedema is classified as a Type I hypersensitivity reaction. Anaphylactoid reactions are not due to an interaction with IgE.

TABLE 1-20. Hypersensitivity reactions.

Type I (immediate)
  Atopy
  Urticaria—angioedema
  Anaphylaxis
Type II (cytotoxic)
  Hemolytic transfusion reactions
  Autoimmune hemolytic anemia
  Heparin-induced thrombocytopenia
Type III (immune complex)
  Arthus reaction
  Serum sickness
  Acute hypersensitivity pneumonitis
Type IV (delayed, cell-mediated)
  Contact dermatitis
  Tuberculin-type hypersensitivity
  Chronic hypersensitivity pneumonitis

(Reproduced with permission from Butterworth JF IV, Mackey DC, Wasnick JD, eds. *Morgan & Mikhail's Clinical Anesthesiology.* 7th ed. New York, NY: McGraw Hill; 2022.)

References: Butterworth JF IV, Mackey DC, Wasnick JD, eds. *Morgan & Mikhail's Clinical Anesthesiology.* 7th ed. New York, NY: McGraw Hill; 2022: Chapter 54.

Hines RL, Marschall KE. *Stoelting's Anesthesia and Co-existing Disease.* 7th ed. Philadelphia, PA: Elsevier Saunders; 2018: Chapter 24.

302. Which classification of anesthetic agents is most linked to anaphylactic reactions?

(A) Thiobarbiturates

(B) Narcotics

(C) Benzodiazepines

(D) Muscle Relaxants

Rationale: All anesthetic agents may cause anaphylactic reactions. Muscle relaxants (rocuronium, atracurium, succinylcholine) remain the most common. This is primarily due to repeated use of this drug group.

References: Butterworth JF IV, Mackey DC, Wasnick JD, eds. *Morgan & Mikhail's Clinical Anesthesiology.* 7th ed. New York, NY: McGraw Hill; 2022: Chapter 54.

Hines RL, Marschall KE. *Stoelting's Anesthesia and Co-existing Disease.* 7th ed. Philadelphia, PA: Elsevier Saunders; 2018: Chapter 24.

303. What statement about human immunodeficiency virus (HIV) infection and acquired immunodeficiency syndrome (AIDS) is true?

(A) AIDS is caused by a retrovirus.

(B) Seroconversion occurs 2 to 3 months following transmission of the HIV virus.

(C) Seroconversion occurs 4 to 6 weeks following transmission of the HIV virus.

(D) There is no contraindication for the use of spinal anesthesia.

Rationale: Neuraxial anesthesia may be contraindicated for patients with HIV/AIDS when neurologic lesions are present. Neurologic lesions increase intercerebral pressure (ICP).

Reference: Hines RL, Marschall KE. *Stoelting's Anesthesia and Co-existing Disease.* 7th ed. Philadelphia, PA: Elsevier Saunders; 2018: Chapter 24.

304. What signs and symptoms are linked to the pathophysiology of septic shock?

(A) Hypervolemia and wide pulse pressure

(B) Bounding pulse and hypotension

(C) Bradycardia and narrow pulse pressure

(D) Hypotension and narrow pulse pressure

Rationale: Systemic venodilation and fluid shift to the tissues exists in septic shock resulting in hypovolemia and hypotension. Hemodynamic instability is prominent.

References: Butterworth JF IV, Mackey DC, Wasnick JD, eds. *Morgan & Mikhail's Clinical Anesthesiology.* 7th ed. New York, NY: McGraw Hill; 2022: Chapter 57.

Hines RL, Marschall KE. *Stoelting's Anesthesia and Co-existing Disease.* 7th ed. Philadelphia, PA: Elsevier Saunders; 2018: Chapter 22.

305. What is the recommended minimum liter flow to avoid renal injury when using sevoflurane?

(A) 1 L/min

(B) 2 L/min

(C) 3 L/min

(D) 4 L/min

Rationale: To avoid renal injury use a minimum flow of 2 L/min of sevoflurane.

References: Butterworth JF IV, Mackey DC, Wasnick JD, eds. *Morgan & Mikhail's Clinical Anesthesiology.* 7th ed. New York, NY: McGraw Hill; 2022: Chapter 29.

Hines RL, Marschall KE. *Stoelting's Anesthesia and Co-existing Disease.* 7th ed. Philadelphia, PA: Elsevier Saunders; 2018: Chapter 17.

306. What percent of total cardiac output flows through the kidneys?

(A) 10 to 15%

(B) 20 to 25%

(C) 30 to 35%

(D) 40 to 45%

Rationale: 20 to 25% of the cardiac output flows through the kidneys.

References: Butterworth JF IV, Mackey DC, Wasnick JD, eds. *Morgan & Mikhail's Clinical Anesthesiology.* 7th ed. New York, NY: McGraw Hill; 2022: Chapter 29.

Hines RL, Marschall KE. *Stoelting's Anesthesia and Co-existing Disease.* 7th ed. Philadelphia, PA: Elsevier Saunders; 2018: Chapter 17.

307. What is the normal glomerular filtration rate (GFR)?

(A) 440 mL/min

(B) 660 mL/min

(C) 1,200 mL/min

(D) 120 mL/min

Rationale: Renal plasma flow is 660 mL/min; renal blood flow is 1,200 mL/min; and the glomerular filtration rate in men is 120 +/− 25 mL/min. In women, the GFR is 95 +/− 20 mL/min.

References: Butterworth JF IV, Mackey DC, Wasnick JD, eds. *Morgan & Mikhail's Clinical Anesthesiology.* 7th ed. New York, NY: McGraw Hill; 2022: Chapter 29.

Hines RL, Marschall KE. *Stoelting's Anesthesia and Co-existing Disease.* 7th ed. Philadelphia, PA: Elsevier Saunders; 2018: Chapter 17.

308. What drug is associated with acute kidney injury?

(A) Halothane

(B) Demerol

(C) Radiocontrast dye

(D) Morphine

Rationale: Inhalational agents decrease renal vascular resistance but are not linked to acute kidney injury. The exception is Sevoflurane's breakdown product Compound A. The effects of opioids on the kidney are minimal. Radiocontrast agents decrease renal perfusion and cause direct tubular injury and intratubular obstruction. NSAIDs inhibit prostaglandin synthesis and decrease renal perfusion.

TABLE 1-21. Drugs and toxins associated with acute kidney injury.

Type of Injury	Drug or Toxin
Decreased renal perfusion	Nonsteroidal anti-inflammatory drugs (NSAIDs), angiotensin-converting enzyme inhibitors, radiocontrast agents, amphotericin B, cyclosporine, tacrolimus
Direct tubular injury	Aminoglycosides, radiocontrast agents, amphotericin B, methotrexate, cisplatin, foscarnet, pentamidine, heavy metals, myoglobin, hemoglobin, intravenous immunoglobulin, HIV protease inhibitors
Intratubular obstruction	Radiocontrast agents, methotrexate, acyclovir, sulfonamides, ethylene glycol, uric acid, cocaine, lovastatin
Immunological–Inflammatory	Penicillin, cephalosporins, allopurinol, NSAIDs, sulfonamides, diuretics, rifampin, ciprofloxacin, cimetidine, proton pump inhibitors, tetracycline, phenytoin

(Reproduced with permission from Anderson RJ, Barry DW. Clinical and laboratory diagnosis of acute renal failure. *Best Pract Res Clin Anaesthesiol.* 2004;18(1):1-20.)

References: Butterworth JF IV, Mackey DC, Wasnick JD, eds. *Morgan & Mikhail's Clinical Anesthesiology.* 7th ed. New York, NY: McGraw Hill; 2022: Chapter 30.

Hines RL, Marschall KE. *Stoelting's Anesthesia and Co-existing Disease.* 7th ed. Philadelphia, PA: Elsevier Saunders; 2018: Chapter 17.

309. Which narcotic's metabolite is most likely to accumulate in patients with renal dysfunction?

(A) Fentanyl

(B) Demerol

(C) Remifentanil

(D) Morphine

Rationale: Many narcotic metabolites are inactivated in the liver. Demerol and morphine metabolites accumulate in patients with renal disease and increase the likelihood of respiratory depression and/or seizures.

References: Butterworth JF IV, Mackey DC, Wasnick JD, eds. *Morgan & Mikhail's Clinical Anesthesiology.* 7th ed. New York, NY: McGraw Hill; 2022: Chapter 29.

Hines RL, Marschall KE. *Stoelting's Anesthesia and Co-existing Disease.* 7th ed. Philadelphia, PA: Elsevier Saunders; 2018: Chapter 17.

310. What condition is most likely to cause complications during extracorporeal shock wave lithotripsy (ESWL)?

(A) Renal calculi <4 mm

(B) Cardiac arrhythmias

(C) Ecchymosis

(D) Skin blistering

Rationale: ESWL is effect for renal calculi 4 mm to 2 cm. Ecchymosis and skin blistering may occur during or following the procedure. While shock waves are timed with the electrocardiogram, cardiac arrhythmias may result during ESWL.

References: Butterworth JF IV, Mackey DC, Wasnick JD, eds. *Morgan & Mikhail's Clinical Anesthesiology.* 7th ed. New York, NY: McGraw Hill; 2022: Chapter 31.

Hines RL, Marschall KE. *Stoelting's Anesthesia and Co-existing Disease.* 7th ed. Philadelphia, PA: Elsevier Saunders; 2018: Chapter 17.

311. What is the normal hepatic blood flow?

(A) 15 to 20%

(B) 25 to 30%

(C) 20 to 25%

(D) 30 to 35%

Rationale: 25 to 30% of the cardiac output is provided to the liver.

References: Butterworth JF IV, Mackey DC, Wasnick JD, eds. *Morgan & Mikhail's Clinical Anesthesiology.* 7th ed. New York, NY: McGraw Hill; 2022: Chapter 32.

Hines RL, Marschall KE. *Stoelting's Anesthesia and Co-existing Disease.* 7th ed. Philadelphia, PA: Elsevier Saunders; 2018: Chapter 13.

312. Which coagulation factor is not produced in the liver?

(A) Factor V

(B) Factor I

(C) Factor VIII

(D) Factor II

Rationale: Factor VIII and von Willebrand Factor are the only coagulation factors not produced in the liver.

Reference: Butterworth JF IV, Mackey DC, Wasnick JD, eds. *Morgan & Mikhail's Clinical Anesthesiology.* 7th ed. New York, NY: McGraw Hill; 2022: Chapter 32.

313. What factors cause a vitamin K deficiency?

(A) VI, IX, X

(B) VII, IX, X

(C) VIII, IX, X

(D) VII, IX, VI

Rationale: Factors causing a vitamin K deficiency include flawed prothrombin and factors VII, IX, and X.

Reference: Butterworth JF IV, Mackey DC, Wasnick JD, eds. *Morgan & Mikhail's Clinical Anesthesiology*. 7th ed. New York, NY: McGraw Hill; 2022: Chapter 32.

314. What albumin level is associated with chronic liver disease?

(A) 3.5 g/dL

(B) 4.0 g/dL

(C) 4.5 g/dL

(D) 2.5 g/dL

Rationale: Normal albumin levels range from 3.5 to 5.5 g/dL. Values less than 2.5 g/dL indicate chronic liver disease.

Reference: Butterworth JF IV, Mackey DC, Wasnick JD, eds. *Morgan & Mikhail's Clinical Anesthesiology*. 7th ed. New York, NY: McGraw Hill; 2022: Chapter 32.

315. Which of the following is false regarding prothrombin time (PT)?

(A) The normal PT range is 11 to 14 seconds.

(B) PT measures factors V, VII, X, finbrinogen, and prothrombin.

(C) PT assists in the evaluation of chronic and acute liver disease.

(D) PT is decreased in vitamin K deficiency.

Rationale: The PT is increased in vitamin K deficiency, advanced liver disease, DIC, warfarin and heparin therapy, and factor VII deficiency.

TABLE 1-22. Coagulation test abnormalities.

	PT	PTT	TT	Fibrinogen
Advanced liver disease	↑	↑	N or ↑	N or ↓
DIC	↑	↑	↑	↓
Vitamin K deficiency	↑↑	↑	N	N
Warfarin therapy	↑↑	↑	N	N
Heparin therapy	↑	↑↑	↑	N
Hemophilia				
Factor VIII deficiency	N	↑	N	N
Factor IX deficiency	N	↑	N	N
Factor VII deficiency	↑	N	N	N
Factor XIII deficiency	N	N	N	N

DIC, disseminated intravascular coagulation; N, normal; PT, prothrombin time; PTT, partial thromboplastin time; TT, thrombin time.
(Reproduced with permission from Butterworth JF IV, Mackey DC, Wasnick JD, eds. *Morgan & Mikhail's Clinical Anesthesiology*. 7th ed. New York, NY: McGraw Hill; 2022.)

Reference: Butterworth JF IV, Mackey DC, Wasnick JD, eds. *Morgan & Mikhail's Clinical Anesthesiology*. 7th ed. New York, NY: McGraw Hill; 2022: Chapter 33.

316. What is the characteristic of hepatitis B?

(A) Incubation period 20 to 37 days

(B) Fecal-oral transmission

(C) Incubation period 60 to 110 days with progression to chronic liver disease

(D) No progression to chronic liver disease

Rationale: Characteristics of Hepatitis A include fecal-oral transmission with an incubation period of 20 to 37 days. There is no progression to chronic liver disease as compared to Hepatitis B.

References: Butterworth JF IV, Mackey DC, Wasnick JD, eds. *Morgan & Mikhail's Clinical Anesthesiology*. 7th ed. New York, NY: McGraw Hill; 2022: Chapter 32.

Hines RL, Marschall KE. *Stoelting's Anesthesia and Co-existing Disease*. 7th ed. Philadelphia, PA: Elsevier Saunders; 2018: Chapter 13.

317. What are the risk factors for halothane hepatitis?

(A) >40 years, female, and obese

(B) Male gender and obese

(C) Female gender and <40 years

(D) Obese and smoker

Rationale: Females, >40 years, obesity, exposure to multiple anesthetics, and familial predisposition represent risk factors linked to halothane hepatitis.

References: Butterworth JF IV, Mackey DC, Wasnick JD, eds. *Morgan & Mikhail's Clinical Anesthesiology*. 7th ed. New York, NY: McGraw Hill; 2022: Chapter 8.

Elisha S, Heiner JS, Nagelhout JJ. *Nurse Anesthesia*. 7th ed. St. Louis, MO: Elsevier Saunders; 2023: Chapter 33.

318. When evaluating a patient with cirrhosis, what laboratory findings are expected?

(A) Increased bilirubin, decreased albumin, hyponatremia

(B) Increased albumin, hyponatremia

(C) Increased prothrombin time, hyponatremia

(D) Decreased albumin, hypernatremia, decreased bilirubin

Rationale: Laboratory findings consistent with cirrhosis include increased bilirubin, normal or increased AST/ALT, decreased albumin and PT, hyponatremia, thrombocytopenia, and decreased hemoglobin and hematocrit.

TABLE 1-23. Abnormalities in liver tests.[1]

	Parenchymal (Hepatocellular) Dysfunction	Biliary Obstruction or Cholestasis
AST (SGOT)	↑ to ↑↑↑	↑
ALT (SGPT)	↑ to ↑↑↑	↑
Albumin	0 to ↓↓↓	0
Prothrombin time	0 to ↑↑↑	0 to ↑↑[2]
Bilirubin	0 to ↑↑↑	0 to ↑↑↑
Alkaline phosphatase	↑	↑ to ↑↑↑
5'-Nucleotidase	0 to ↑	↑ to ↑↑↑
γ-Glutamyl transpeptidase	↑ to ↑↑↑	↑↑↑

[1]↑, increases; 0, no change; ↓, decreases.
[2]Usually corrects with vitamin K.
ALT, alanine aminotransferase; AST, aspartate aminotransferase; SGOT, serum glutamic-oxaloacetic transaminase; SGPT, serum glutamic pyruvic-transferase. (Reproduced with permission from Wilson JD, Braunwald E, Isselbacher KJ et al. *Harrison's Principles of Internal Medicine.* 12th ed. New York, NY: McGraw Hill; 1991.)

References: Butterworth JF IV, Mackey DC, Wasnick JD, eds. *Morgan & Mikhail's Clinical Anesthesiology.* 7th ed. New York, NY: McGraw Hill; 2022: Chapter 33.
Elisha S, Heiner JS, Nagelhout JJ. *Nurse Anesthesia.* 7th ed. St. Louis, MO: Elsevier Saunders; 2023: Chapter 33.

319. The intoxicated patient arrives for an emergent exploratory laparotomy following a motor vehicle accident. What statement is true regarding this scenario?

(A) Anesthetic requirements are increased.

(B) Alcohol increases MAC.

(C) Alcohol decreases GABA receptor activity.

(D) Alcohol inhibits NMDA receptors.

Rationale: Acute alcohol intoxication decreases MAC thereby decreasing anesthetic requirements. GABA receptor activity is increased resulting in marked effects of central nervous system depressants.
References: Butterworth JF IV, Mackey DC, Wasnick JD, eds. *Morgan & Mikhail's Clinical Anesthesiology.* 7th ed. New York, NY: McGraw Hill; 2022: Chapter 32.
Elisha S, Heiner JS, Nagelhout JJ. *Nurse Anesthesia.* 7th ed. St. Louis, MO: Elsevier Saunders; 2023: Chapter 33.

320. Which statement is true regarding the pneumatic tourniquet?

(A) Hypertension occurs when the tourniquet is released.

(B) Tissue hypoxia occurs within 2 minutes of application.

(C) Metabolic alkalosis occurs after tourniquet release.

(D) Core body temperature increases upon tourniquet release.

Rationale: The pneumatic tourniquet causes hypertension and pain approximately 60 minutes after inflation. Tissue hypoxia occurs shortly after inflating the tourniquet. Once the tourniquet is released products of tissue metabolism cause a brief period of metabolic acidosis and fall in blood pressure and temperature.
Reference: Butterworth JF IV, Mackey DC, Wasnick JD, eds. *Morgan & Mikhail's Clinical Anesthesiology.* 7th ed. New York, NY: McGraw Hill; 2022: Chapter 38.

321. A 65-year-old patient presents for an open reduction and internal fixation following a hip fracture. The patient is short of breath, confused, and you notice petechiae on the chest. What is the most likely cause?

(A) Fat embolism syndrome

(B) Mentation changes due to aging

(C) Deep vein thrombosis

(D) Thromboembolism

Rationale: Classic signs of fat embolism include dypsnea, confusion, and petechiae. The signs occur 1 to 3 days following a long-bone or pelvic fracture.
Reference: Butterworth JF IV, Mackey DC, Wasnick JD, eds. *Morgan & Mikhail's Clinical Anesthesiology.* 7th ed. New York, NY: McGraw Hill; 2022: Chapter 38.

322. Which congenital cardiac malformations may benefit from a modified Blalock-Taussig shunt procedure?

(A) Tetralogy of Fallot

(B) Truncus arteriosus

(C) Bicuspid atresia

(D) Transposition of the great vessels

Rationale: A modified Blalock-Taussig procedure is a shunt between systemic, often subclavian, and pulmonary circulation. This procedure can be useful in tricuspid atresia or palliative in Tetralogy of Fallot.
References: Butterworth JF IV, Mackey DC, Wasnick JD, eds. *Morgan & Mikhail's Clinical Anesthesiology.* 7th ed. New York, NY: McGraw Hill; 2022: Chapter 21.
Jaffe RA, Samuels SI, Schmiesing CA, Golianu B, eds. *Anesthesiologist's Manual of Surgical Procedures.* 5th ed. Philadelphia, PA: Wolters Kluwer Lippincott Williams & Wilkins; 2014: Chapter 12.4.

323. How does the National Asthma Education and Prevention Program Expert Panel Report 3 define asthma?

(A) A chronic inflammatory disorder of the airways

(B) Preventable and treatable disease state characterized by airflow limitation that is not fully reversible

(C) Mechanical obstruction to breathing that occurs during sleep

(D) Right heart failure secondary to pulmonary pathology

Rationale: The National Asthma Education and Prevention Program Expert Panel Report 3 defines asthma as a chronic inflammatory disorder of the airways in which many cells and cellular elements play a role.

References: Butterworth JF IV, Mackey DC, Wasnick JD, eds. *Morgan & Mikhail's Clinical Anesthesiology.* 7th ed. New York, NY: McGraw Hill; 2022: Chapter 23.

Elisha S, Heiner JS, Nagelhout JJ. *Nurse Anesthesia.* 7th ed. St. Louis, MO: Elsevier Saunders; 2023: Chapter 29.

324. How is the clinical diagnosis of chronic bronchitis made?

(A) Presence of a productive cough on most days of 3 consecutive months for a least 2 consecutive years

(B) Presence of an occasional productive cough for 2 consecutive months for at least 1 year

(C) Presence of a productive cough on most days of 3 consecutive weeks for a least 2 consecutive months

(D) Presence of a productive cough on 3 consecutive days for a least 2 consecutive weeks

Rationale: Presence of a productive cough on most days of 3 consecutive months for a least 2 consecutive years is diagnostic of chronic bronchitis.

References: Butterworth JF IV, Mackey DC, Wasnick JD, eds. *Morgan & Mikhail's Clinical Anesthesiology.* 7th ed. New York, NY: McGraw Hill; 2022: Chapter 23.

Elisha S, Heiner JS, Nagelhout JJ. *Nurse Anesthesia.* 7th ed. St. Louis, MO: Elsevier Saunders; 2023: Chapter 29.

325. Which congenital cardiac malformation includes a right-to-left intracardiac shunt?

(A) Tetralogy of Fallot

(B) Atrial septal defect

(C) Ventricular septal defect

(D) Patent ductus arteriosus

Rationale: Tetralogy of Fallot includes a right-to-left shunt. The others result in left-to-right shunting.

References: Butterworth JF IV, Mackey DC, Wasnick JD, eds. *Morgan & Mikhail's Clinical Anesthesiology.* 7th ed. New York, NY: McGraw Hill; 2022: Chapter 21.

Hines RL, Marschall KE. *Stoelting's Anesthesia and Co-existing Disease.* 7th ed. Philadelphia, PA: Elsevier Saunders; 2018: Chapter 3.

326. Which disease does not place the patient at increased risk for developing Cor Pulmonale?

(A) Adenotonsillar hypertrophy

(B) Chronic obstructive pulmonary disease

(C) Obesity

(D) Eaton-Lambert syndrome

Rationale: Cor pulmonale is a right-heart disease of pulmonary origin. (A) and (C) predispose to the development of obstructive sleep apnea which can eventually manifest as right-sided disease and failure. Cor pulmonale is frequently associated with chronic obstructive pulmonary disease.

References: Barash PG, Cullen BF, Stoelting RK, et al, eds. *Clinical Anesthesia.* 8th ed. Lippincott Williams & Wilkins; 2017: Chapter 50.

Butterworth JF IV, Mackey DC, Wasnick JD, eds. *Morgan & Mikhail's Clinical Anesthesiology.* 7th ed. New York, NY: McGraw Hill; 2022: Chapter 34.

Hines RL, Marschall KE. *Stoelting's Anesthesia and Co-existing Disease.* 7th ed. Philadelphia, PA: Elsevier Saunders; 2018: Chapter 6.

327. What is indicated by an apnea/hypopnea index of 42 occurrences per hour?

(A) Normal result

(B) Mild obstructive sleep apnea

(C) Moderate sleep apnea

(D) Severe sleep apnea

Rationale: More than 30 to 40 apnea/hypopnea events per hour indicates severe obstructive disease.

References: Butterworth JF IV, Mackey DC, Wasnick JD, eds. *Morgan & Mikhail's Clinical Anesthesiology.* 7th ed. New York, NY: McGraw Hill; 2022: Chapter 44.

Gropper MA, Cohen NH, Eriksson LI, et al, eds. *Miller's Anesthesia.* 9th ed. Philadelphia, PA: Churchill Livingstone Elsevier; 2020: Chapter 64.

328. What is the most common cause of obstructive sleep apnea?

(A) Ondine's curse

(B) Obesity

(C) Muscular dystrophy

(D) Central apnea

Rationale: Obesity is the most common contributor to development of obstructive sleep apnea.

References: Butterworth JF IV, Mackey DC, Wasnick JD, eds. *Morgan & Mikhail's Clinical Anesthesiology.* 7th ed. New York, NY: McGraw Hill; 2022: Chapter 44.

Elisha S, Heiner JS, Nagelhout JJ. *Nurse Anesthesia.* 7th ed. St. Louis, MO: Elsevier Saunders; 2023: Chapter 29.

329. Which structure is commonly occluded in obstructive hydrocephalus?

(A) Choroid plexus

(B) Foramen of Monro

(C) Aqueduct of Sylvius

(D) Foramen of Magendie

Rationale: Cerebrospinal fluid commonly flows through the aqueduct of Sylvius to the fourth ventricle. Narrowing or obstruction of this path can result in obstructive, or noncommunicating, hydrocephalus.

References: Butterworth JF IV, Mackey DC, Wasnick JD, eds. *Morgan & Mikhail's Clinical Anesthesiology.* 7th ed. New York, NY: McGraw Hill; 2022: Chapter 26.

Hall JE. *Guyton and Hall Textbook of Medical Physiology.* 14th ed. Philadelphia, PA: Saunders Elsevier; 2021: Chapter 61.

330. Which state should be avoided during the anesthetic care of a patient with multiple sclerosis?

(A) Hyperthermia

(B) Hyperoxia

(C) Hypercapnia

(D) Hypertension

Rationale: Hyperthermia should be avoided because increases in temperature may precipitate exacerbations of this condition.

Reference: Butterworth JF IV, Mackey DC, Wasnick JD, eds. *Morgan & Mikhail's Clinical Anesthesiology.* 7th ed. New York, NY: McGraw Hill; 2022: Chapter 28.

331. What causes weakness in myasthenia gravis?

(A) Autoimmune damage to nerve axons

(B) Damage to presynaptic calcium channels

(C) Damage to postsynaptic cholinergic receptors

(D) Autoimmune damage to type I muscle fibers

Rationale: Weakness results from loss of postsynaptic acetylcholine receptors.

References: Butterworth JF IV, Mackey DC, Wasnick JD, eds. *Morgan & Mikhail's Clinical Anesthesiology.* 7th ed. New York, NY: McGraw Hill; 2022: Chapter 35.

Hall JE. *Guyton and Hall Textbook of Medical Physiology.* 14th ed. Philadelphia, PA: Saunders Elsevier; 2021: Chapter 7.

332. What would be the effect on muscle strength if a patient with myasthenia gravis were treated with an anticholinesterase?

(A) No change

(B) Decreased strength

(C) Increased strength

Rationale: Pyridostigmine, an anticholinesterase, is used to improve weakness in patients with this disease.

References: Butterworth JF IV, Mackey DC, Wasnick JD, eds. *Morgan & Mikhail's Clinical Anesthesiology.* 7th ed. New York, NY: McGraw Hill; 2022: Chapter 35.

Longnecker DE, Mackey SC, Newman MF, Sandberg WS, Zapol WM, eds. *Anesthesiology.* 3rd ed. McGraw Hill; 2018: Chapter 54.

333. Is an aneurysm in the brain more likely to occur in a larger vessel or a smaller vessel? Why?

(A) Equally likely in either a large or small vessel because blood pressure is constant

(B) More likely in a larger vessel due to increased diameter

(C) More likely in a smaller vessel due to increased resistance

(D) More likely in a smaller vessel due to decreased flow

Rationale: Brain aneurysms are more common in larger arteries. Application of the law of LaPlace illustrates increasing vessel wall pressure with increasing diameter.

Reference: Butterworth JF IV, Mackey DC, Wasnick JD, eds. *Morgan & Mikhail's Clinical Anesthesiology.* 7th ed. New York, NY: McGraw Hill; 2022: Chapter 27.

334. Which level of spinal cord injury is most associated with autonomic hyperreflexia?

(A) T_5–T_8

(B) T_{10}–L_1

(C) L_1–L_4

(D) L_4–S_1

Rationale: Autonomic hyperreflexia is most associated with spinal cord injuries at or above the mid-thoracic spine.

References: Butterworth JF IV, Mackey DC, Wasnick JD, eds. *Morgan & Mikhail's Clinical Anesthesiology.* 7th ed. New York, NY: McGraw Hill; 2022: Chapter 28.

Elisha S, Heiner JS, Nagelhout JJ. *Nurse Anesthesia.* 7th ed. St. Louis, MO: Elsevier Saunders; 2023: Chapter 40.

335. What is the most important cervical radiographic finding in a patient with rheumatoid arthritis?

(A) Cervical stenosis

(B) Cervical spondylosis

(C) Atlantoaxial subluxation

(D) Lordosis

Rationale: Atlantoaxial subluxation indicates increased risk of spinal cord impingement during airway management.

References: Butterworth JF IV, Mackey DC, Wasnick JD, eds. *Morgan & Mikhail's Clinical Anesthesiology.* 7th ed. New York, NY: McGraw Hill; 2022: Chapter 38.

Hines RL, Marschall KE. *Stoelting's Anesthesia and Co-existing Disease.* 7th ed. Philadelphia, PA: Elsevier Saunders; 2018: Chapter 21.

336. What is the most common form of muscular dystrophy?

(A) Becker

(B) Limb-girdle

(C) Myotonic

(D) Duchenne

Rationale: Duchene occurs most frequently.

References: Butterworth JF IV, Mackey DC, Wasnick JD, eds. *Morgan & Mikhail's Clinical Anesthesiology.* 7th ed. New York, NY: McGraw Hill; 2022: Chapter 35.

Elisha S, Heiner JS, Nagelhout JJ. *Nurse Anesthesia.* 7th ed. St. Louis, MO: Elsevier Saunders; 2023: Chapter 36.

337. Which statement is true regarding Duchenne muscular dystrophy?

(A) The disease is X-linked and occurs more frequently in girls.

(B) The disease occurs equally in boys and girls and is diagnosed in early childhood.

(C) The disease is X-linked and symptoms occur only in boys.

(D) The disease primarily manifests as contractures of the large joints.

Rationale: Duchenne muscular dystrophy is an X-linked disease manifesting clinically in young boys while girls can be carriers who are asymptomatic.

References: Butterworth JF IV, Mackey DC, Wasnick JD, eds. *Morgan & Mikhail's Clinical Anesthesiology.* 7th ed. New York, NY: McGraw Hill; 2022: Chapter 35.

Elisha S, Heiner JS, Nagelhout JJ. *Nurse Anesthesia.* 7th ed. St. Louis, MO: Elsevier Saunders; 2023: Chapter 36.

338. What is the anesthetic implication of a patient taking tricyclic antidepressants who is scheduled to receive general anesthesia?

(A) Meperidine will produce skeletal muscle rigidity and hyperpyrexia.

(B) Tricyclic antidepressants should be discontinued 2 weeks before surgery.

(C) MAC requirements may be increased for inhaled anesthetics.

(D) Ephedrine is preferred agent to treat post-induction hypotension.

Rationale: MAC requirements are increased for patients taking tricyclic antidepressants, possibly related to the enhanced catecholamine activity.

References: Butterworth JF IV, Mackey DC, Wasnick JD, eds. *Morgan & Mikhail's Clinical Anesthesiology.* 7th ed. New York, NY: McGraw Hill; 2022: Chapter 21.

Flood P, Rathmell JP, Urbam RD, eds. *Stoelting's Pharmacology & Physiology in Anesthetic Practice.* 6th ed. Philadelphia, PA: Wolters Kluwer; 2022: Chapter 19.

339. Which characteristic is not shared by malignant hyperthermia and neuroleptic malignant syndrome?

(A) Generalized muscular rigidity

(B) Flaccid paralysis after vecuronium administration

(C) Effectively treated with dantrolene

(D) Hyperthermia

Rationale: The ability of NDMRs to produce flaccid paralysis distinguishes neuroleptic malignant syndrome (NMS) from malignant hyperthermia (MH). MH and NMS share the features such as generalized muscular rigidity and hyperthermia. Further, like MH, supportive measures including dantrolene administration is effective.

References: Butterworth JF IV, Mackey DC, Wasnick JD, eds. *Morgan & Mikhail's Clinical Anesthesiology.* 7th ed. New York, NY: McGraw Hill; 2022: Chapter 52.

Flood P, Rathmell JP, Urbam RD, eds. *Stoelting's Pharmacology & Physiology in Anesthetic Practice.* 6th ed. Philadelphia, PA: Wolters Kluwer; 2022: Chapter 19.

340. A patient is taking an MAO inhibitor. What anesthetic agent can be safely used in this patient?

(A) Phenylephrine

(B) Ketamine

(C) Bupivacaine with epinephrine

(D) Pancuronium

Rationale: Any drug that enhances sympathetic activity, such as ketamine, pancuronium, and epinephrine (including epinephrine in local anesthetics), should be avoided. Phenylephrine, if necessary, can be used in small doses and is preferable to using an indirect-acting agent for treating anesthetic-induced hypotension.

References: Butterworth JF IV, Mackey DC, Wasnick JD, eds. *Morgan & Mikhail's Clinical Anesthesiology.* 7th ed. New York, NY: McGraw Hill; 2022: Chapter 28.

Flood P, Rathmell JP, Urbam RD, eds. *Stoelting's Pharmacology & Physiology in Anesthetic Practice.* 6th ed. Philadelphia, PA: Wolters Kluwer; 2022: Chapter 19.

341. A 25-year-old 50-kg otherwise healthy patient complains of nausea and demonstrates vomiting, refractory to ondansetron and dexamethasone therapy. Which dose of droperidol will achieve a safe therapeutic response?

(A) 1.25 mg IV

(B) 0.625 mg/kg IV

(C) 0.5 mg IV

(D) 12.5 mg IV

Rationale: 1.25 mg IV is associated with greater effectiveness and is the upper limit of therapeutic dosing. 0.625 mg *per* kg (i.e., 31.25 mg) is an overdose. A flat dose of 0.625 mg total would be acceptable. 0.5 mg is a subtherapeutic dose.

References: Butterworth JF IV, Mackey DC, Wasnick JD, eds. *Morgan & Mikhail's Clinical Anesthesiology.* 7th ed. New York, NY: McGraw Hill; 2022: Chapter 19.

Flood P, Rathmell JP, Urbam RD, eds. *Stoelting's Pharmacology & Physiology in Anesthetic Practice.* 6th ed. Philadelphia, PA: Wolters Kluwer; 2022: Chapter 37.

342. Which statement about phenytoin is correct?

(A) Chronic phenytoin therapy requires higher dose requirements of vecuronium.

(B) Chronic phenytoin therapy requires lower dose requirements of vecuronium.

(C) Chronic phenytoin therapy requires higher dose requirements of succinylcholine.

(D) Chronic phenytoin therapy requires lower dose requirements of succinylcholine.

Rationale: Patients taking anticonvulsants demonstrate resistance to nondepolarizing agents and possess higher dosing requirements.

References: Butterworth JF IV, Mackey DC, Wasnick JD, eds. *Morgan & Mikhail's Clinical Anesthesiology.* 7th ed. New York, NY: McGraw Hill; 2022: Chapter 11.

Flood P, Rathmell JP, Urbam RD, eds. *Stoelting's Pharmacology & Physiology in Anesthetic Practice.* 6th ed. Philadelphia, PA: Wolters Kluwer; 2022: Chapter 30.

343. Which statement about gabapentin is false?

(A) Gabapentin is not bound to plasma proteins.

(B) Gabapentin is an effective monotherapy for partial seizures.

(C) Gabapentin is unable to cross blood–brain barrier.

(D) Gabapentin undergoes no metabolism.

Rationale: Gabapentin is a lipid soluble anticonvulsant that can cross the blood–brain barrier (BBB). Gabapentin is not bound to plasma proteins and is an effective monotherapy for partial seizures.

References: Flood P, Rathmell JP, Urbam RD, eds. *Stoelting's Pharmacology & Physiology in Anesthetic Practice.* 6th ed. Philadelphia, PA: Wolters Kluwer; 2022: Chapter 30.

Elisha S, Heiner JS, Nagelhout JJ. *Nurse Anesthesia.* 7th ed. St. Louis, MO: Elsevier Saunders; 2023: Chapter 56.

344. For which pathophysiologic state would gabapentin not be prescribed for management?

(A) Postherpatic neuralgia

(B) Diabetic neuropathy

(C) Acute postoperative pain adjuvant

(D) Status epilepticus

Rationale: Oral gabapentinis used for the management of postherpatic neuralgiadiabetic neuropathy and acute postoperative pain. This agent would not be utilized in the treatment of an acute seizure, such as status epilepticus where an intravenous agent would be more appropriate.

References: Butterworth JF IV, Mackey DC, Wasnick JD, eds. *Morgan & Mikhail's Clinical Anesthesiology*. 7th ed. New York, NY: McGraw Hill; 2022: Chapter 47.

Elisha S, Heiner JS, Nagelhout JJ. *Nurse Anesthesia*. 7th ed. St. Louis, MO: Elsevier Saunders; 2023: Chapter 56.

Flood P, Rathmell JP, Urbam RD, eds. *Stoelting's Pharmacology & Physiology in Anesthetic Practice*. 6th ed. Philadelphia, PA: Wolters Kluwer; 2022: Chapter 30.

345. Which neuromuscular disease is associated with increased resistance to succinylcholine?

(A) Myasthenic syndrome

(B) Myasthenia gravis

(C) Myotonic dystrophy

(D) Muscular dystrophy

Rationale: Patients with myasthenia gravis have fewer acetylcholine receptors and therefore are resistant to succinylcholine. Patients with myasthenic syndrome are sensitive to succinylcholine. In patients with myotonic syndrome, succinylcholine results in prolonged skeletal muscle contraction, indicating a lack of resistance to succinylcholine. Muscular dystrophy patients are very sensitive to succinylcholine.

References: Butterworth JF IV, Mackey DC, Wasnick JD, eds. *Morgan & Mikhail's Clinical Anesthesiology*. 7th ed. New York, NY: McGraw Hill; 2022: Chapter 11.

Hines RL, Marschall KE. *Stoelting's Anesthesia and Co-existing Disease*. 7th ed. Philadelphia, PA: Elsevier Saunders; 2018: Chapter 2.

346. What is the initial dose of dantrolene for a 74-kg man in acute malignant hyperthermia crisis?

(A) 150 mg

(B) 185 mg

(C) 200 mg

(D) 215 mg

Rationale: The first dose of dantrolene should be 2.5 mg/kg.

References: Butterworth JF IV, Mackey DC, Wasnick JD, eds. *Morgan & Mikhail's Clinical Anesthesiology*. 7th ed. New York, NY: McGraw Hill; 2022: Chapter 52.

Hines RL, Marschall KE. *Stoelting's Anesthesia and Co-existing Disease*. 7th ed. Philadelphia, PA: Elsevier Saunders; 2018: Chapter 27.

347. Which of the following is a late sign of malignant hyperthermia?

(A) Increased end-tidal carbon dioxide

(B) Increased heart rate

(C) Increased temperature

(D) Masseter rigidity

Rationale: Hyperthermia is a late manifestation of malignant hyperthermia crisis.

References: Butterworth JF IV, Mackey DC, Wasnick JD, eds. *Morgan & Mikhail's Clinical Anesthesiology*. 7th ed. New York, NY: McGraw Hill; 2022: Chapter 52.

Hines RL, Marschall KE. *Stoelting's Anesthesia and Co-existing Disease*. 7th ed. Philadelphia, PA: Elsevier Saunders; 2018: Chapter 27.

348. Which disease is least likely to be associated with malignant hyperthermia?

(A) King syndrome

(B) Central-core disease

(C) Multi-minicore myopathy

(D) Duchenne muscular dystrophy

Rationale: King, or King-Denborough syndrome, central-core disease, and multi-minicore myopathy are more strongly associated with malignant hyperthermia than Duchenne's.

References: Butterworth JF IV, Mackey DC, Wasnick JD, eds. *Morgan & Mikhail's Clinical Anesthesiology*. 7th ed. New York, NY: McGraw Hill; 2022: Chapter 52.

Hines RL, Marschall KE. *Stoelting's Anesthesia and Co-existing Disease*. 7th ed. Philadelphia, PA: Elsevier Saunders; 2018: Chapter 21.

349. Which would be expected in a patient with Graves' disease?

(A) Increased thyroid stimulating hormone with decreased thyroid hormone

(B) Increased thyroid stimulating hormone with increased thyroid hormone

(C) Decreased thyroid stimulating hormone with decreased thyroid hormone

(D) Decreased thyroid stimulating hormone with increased thyroid hormone

Rationale: Graves' disease is an autoimmune disease where antibodies stimulate the thyroid. Increased thyroid release into circulation decreases pituitary release of thyroid stimulating hormone.

References: Butterworth JF IV, Mackey DC, Wasnick JD, eds. *Morgan & Mikhail's Clinical Anesthesiology*. 7th ed. New York, NY: McGraw Hill; 2022: Chapter 34.

Hall JE. *Guyton and Hall Textbook of Medical Physiology*. 14th ed. Philadelphia, PA: Saunders Elsevier; 2021: Chapter 76.

350. Which diagnosis indicates adrenal insufficiency?

(A) Addison's disease

(B) Conn syndrome

(C) Cushing's disease

(D) Mendelsohn syndrome

Rationale: Addison's disease is glucocorticoid shortage from decreased adrenal function.

References: Butterworth JF IV, Mackey DC, Wasnick JD, eds. *Morgan & Mikhail's Clinical Anesthesiology.* 7th ed. New York, NY: McGraw Hill; 2022: Chapter 34.

Hall JE. *Guyton and Hall Textbook of Medical Physiology.* 14th ed. Philadelphia, PA: Saunders Elsevier; 2021: Chapter 77.

351. Which is secreted from the posterior pituitary?

(A) Antidiuretic hormone

(B) Adrenocorticotropic hormone

(C) Prolactin

(D) Thyroid stimulating hormone

Rationale: Oxytocin and antidiuretic hormone are stored in the posterior pituitary.

References: Butterworth JF IV, Mackey DC, Wasnick JD, eds. *Morgan & Mikhail's Clinical Anesthesiology.* 7th ed. New York, NY: McGraw Hill; 2022: Chapter 27.

Hemmings HC Jr, Egan TD, eds. *Pharmacology and Physiology for Anesthesia: Foundations and Clinical Application.* 2nd ed. Philadelphia, PA: Elsevier Saunders; 2019: Chapter 31.

352. What causes acromegaly?

(A) Hypersecretion of adrenocorticotropic hormone

(B) Hypersecretion of thyroid stimulating hormone

(C) Hypersecretion of growth hormone

(D) Hypersecretion of prolactin

Rationale: Excess growth hormone in adults result in acromegaly.

References: Butterworth JF IV, Mackey DC, Wasnick JD, eds. *Morgan & Mikhail's Clinical Anesthesiology.* 7th ed. New York, NY: McGraw Hill; 2022: Chapter 27.

Hemmings HC Jr, Egan TD, eds. *Pharmacology and Physiology for Anesthesia: Foundations and Clinical Application.* 2nd ed. Philadelphia, PA: Elsevier Saunders; 2019: Chapter 30.

353. What condition results from hypersecretion of growth hormone in a child?

(A) Acromegaly

(B) Dwarfism

(C) Osteomalacia

(D) Gigantism

Rationale: Pituitary hypersecretion of growth hormone in a child results in gigantism.

References: Butterworth JF IV, Mackey DC, Wasnick JD, eds. *Morgan & Mikhail's Clinical Anesthesiology.* 7th ed. New York, NY: McGraw Hill; 2022: Chapter 27.

Hall JE. *Guyton and Hall Textbook of Medical Physiology.* 14th ed. Philadelphia, PA: Saunders Elsevier; 2021: Chapter 75.

354. Which common anesthetic medication should be avoided during the induction of a patient diagnosed with acute intermittent porphyria?

(A) Sufentanil

(B) Propofol

(C) Etomidate

(D) Fentanyl

Rationale: Barbiturates and etomidate should be avoided. Propofol and opioids are commonly regarded as safe for use with this condition.

References: Butterworth JF IV, Mackey DC, Wasnick JD, eds. *Morgan & Mikhail's Clinical Anesthesiology.* 7th ed. New York, NY: McGraw Hill; 2022: Chapter 9.

Hines RL, Marschall KE. *Stoelting's Anesthesia and Co-existing Disease.* 7th ed. Philadelphia, PA: Elsevier Saunders; 2018: Chapter 15.

355. Which correctly describes acute intermittent porphyria?

(A) Accumulation of delta-aminolevulinic acid and porphobilinogen secondary to porphobilinogen deaminase deficiency

(B) Accumulation of protoporphyrin secondary to protoporphyrinogen oxidase deficiency

(C) Accumulation of delta-aminolevulinic acid and protoporphyrin secondary to ferrochelatase deficiency

(D) Accumulation of delta-aminolevulinic acid and coproporphyrinogen secondary to coproporphyrinogen oxidase deficiency

Rationale: Induction of delta-aminolevulinic acid synthetase and overproduction of heme precursors called porphyrins results in various forms of porphyria. Acute intermittent porphyria is specifically related to porphobilinogen deaminase deficiency, which causes accumulation of the preceding prophyrin, porphobilinogen, as well as delta-aminolevulinic acid.

References: Butterworth JF IV, Mackey DC, Wasnick JD, eds. *Morgan & Mikhail's Clinical Anesthesiology*. 7th ed. New York, NY: McGraw Hill; 2022: Chapter 9.

Hines RL, Marschall KE. *Stoelting's Anesthesia and Co-existing Disease*. 7th ed. Philadelphia, PA: Elsevier Saunders; 2018: Chapter 15.

356. Which are secreted by tumors in carcinoid syndrome?

    (A) Ocotreotide
    (B) Serotonin, kallikrein, histamine
    (C) Interferon alpha
    (D) Capecitabine

    Rationale: Octreotide, capecitabine, and interferon alpha represent treatment options.
    References: Butterworth JF IV, Mackey DC, Wasnick JD, eds. *Morgan & Mikhail's Clinical Anesthesiology*. 7th ed. New York, NY: McGraw Hill; 2022: Chapter 34.

    Elisha S, Heiner JS, Nagelhout JJ. *Nurse Anesthesia*. 7th ed. St. Louis, MO: Elsevier Saunders; 2023: Chapter 33.

357. What is the most likely location of a carcinoid tumor?

    (A) Kidney
    (B) Lung
    (C) Ovary
    (D) Appendix

    Rationale: More than half of carcinoid tumors occur in the gastrointestinal tract with the appendix being the most common location.
    References: Butterworth JF IV, Mackey DC, Wasnick JD, eds. *Morgan & Mikhail's Clinical Anesthesiology*. 7th ed. New York, NY: McGraw Hill; 2022: Chapter 34.

    Elisha S, Heiner JS, Nagelhout JJ. *Nurse Anesthesia*. 7th ed. St. Louis, MO: Elsevier Saunders; 2023: Chapter 33.

358. What is the typical progression of Guillain-Barré syndrome?

    (A) Descending paralysis
    (B) Unilateral hemiparesis
    (C) Ascending paralysis
    (D) Concurrent upper and lower extremity weakness

    Rationale: Guillain-Barré syndrome progresses from the feet up.
    References: Butterworth JF IV, Mackey DC, Wasnick JD, eds. *Morgan & Mikhail's Clinical Anesthesiology*. 7th ed. New York, NY: McGraw Hill; 2022: Chapter 28.

    Hines RL, Marschall KE. *Stoelting's Anesthesia and Co-existing Disease*. 7th ed. Philadelphia, PA: Elsevier Saunders; 2018: Chapter 12.

359. Which neuromuscular blocking agent is most appropriate for use in severe cirrhosis?

    (A) Cisatracurium
    (B) Rocuronium
    (C) Vecuronium
    (D) Pancuronium

    Rationale: Cisatracurium metabolism is not dependent upon normal liver function.
    References: Butterworth JF IV, Mackey DC, Wasnick JD, eds. *Morgan & Mikhail's Clinical Anesthesiology*. 7th ed. New York, NY: McGraw Hill; 2022: Chapter 33.

    Hemmings HC Jr, Egan TD, eds. *Pharmacology and Physiology for Anesthesia: Foundations and Clinical Application*. 2nd ed. Philadelphia, PA: Elsevier Saunders; 2019: Chapter 19.

360. Which drugs will be prolonged in the glaucoma patient treated with echothiophate?

    (A) Cocaine and succinylcholine
    (B) Succinylcholine and chloroprocaine
    (C) Glycopyrrolate and succinylcholine
    (D) Chloroprocaine and glycopyrrolate

    Rationale: Echothiophate is a cholinesterase inhibitor. Drugs dependent upon this enzyme, like succinylcholine and ester local anesthetics, will be prolonged. Cocaine is an ester but is dependent upon the liver for metabolism.
    References: Butterworth JF IV, Mackey DC, Wasnick JD, eds. *Morgan & Mikhail's Clinical Anesthesiology*. 7th ed. New York, NY: McGraw Hill; 2022: Chapter 36.

    Hemmings HC Jr, Egan TD, eds. *Pharmacology and Physiology for Anesthesia: Foundations and Clinical Application*. 2nd ed. Philadelphia, PA: Elsevier Saunders; 2019: Chapter 17.

361. What causes Eaton-Lambert syndrome?

    (A) Autoimmune destruction of calcium channels
    (B) Atypical pseudocholinesterase
    (C) Autoimmune destruction of cholinergic receptors
    (D) Autoimmune destruction of thyroid tissue

    Rationale: Eaton-Lambert, or Lambert-Eaton Myasthenic Syndrome, is caused by destruction of calcium channels.
    References: Butterworth JF IV, Mackey DC, Wasnick JD, eds. *Morgan & Mikhail's Clinical Anesthesiology*. 7th ed. New York, NY: McGraw Hill; 2022: Chapter 11.

Hemmings HC Jr, Egan TD, eds. *Pharmacology and Physiology for Anesthesia: Foundations and Clinical Application.* 2nd ed. Philadelphia, PA: Elsevier Saunders; 2019: Chapter 18.

362. Which abnormality is associated with syringomyelia?

   (A) Craniosynostosis

   (B) Crouzon's syndrome

   (C) Arnold-Chiari malformation

   (D) Apert syndrome

Rationale: There is increased incidence of Arnold-Chiari malformation in patients with cysts within the spinal cord.

References: Butterworth JF IV, Mackey DC, Wasnick JD, eds. *Morgan & Mikhail's Clinical Anesthesiology.* 7th ed. New York, NY: McGraw Hill; 2022: Chapter 28.

Hines RL, Marschall KE. *Stoelting's Anesthesia and Co-existing Disease.* 7th ed. Philadelphia, PA: Elsevier Saunders; 2018: Chapter 11.

363. Which causes Zollinger-Ellison syndrome?

   (A) Gastrinoma

   (B) Pheochromocytoma

   (C) Pituitary adenoma

   (D) Osteosarcoma

Rationale: Hypersecretion of gastrin due to a gastrinoma causes increased stomach acid secretion.

References: Butterworth JF IV, Mackey DC, Wasnick JD, eds. *Morgan & Mikhail's Clinical Anesthesiology.* 7th ed. New York, NY: McGraw Hill; 2022: Chapter 17.

Hines RL, Marschall KE. *Stoelting's Anesthesia and Co-existing Disease.* 7th ed. Philadelphia, PA: Elsevier Saunders; 2018: Chapter 14.

364. A patient's cardiac assessment reveals a functional capacity of four metabolic equivalents. What activity can she most likely perform?

   (A) Walk one to two blocks on level ground

   (B) Singles tennis

   (C) Cross-country skiing

   (D) Swimming

Rationale: A patient with four metabolic equivalents has the capacity to walk on level ground for a short at 4 mph or run a short distance. (B), (C), and (D) are associated with a functional capacity of 10 or more.

References: Butterworth JF IV, Mackey DC, Wasnick JD, eds. *Morgan & Mikhail's Clinical Anesthesiology.* 7th ed. New York, NY: McGraw Hill; 2022: Chapter 21.

Elisha S, Heiner JS, Nagelhout JJ. *Nurse Anesthesia.* 7th ed. St. Louis, MO: Elsevier Saunders; 2023: Chapter 20.

365. What factors may cause a flow volume loop to change?

   (A) Pulmonary and airway compliance

   (B) Airway compliance and increased fluid volume

   (C) Increased fluid volume and pulmonary compliance

   (D) Patent airways

Rationale: Pulmonary or airway compliance or a combination will change the configuration of the flow volume loop. Airway obstruction or a circuit disconnect may be causative factors.

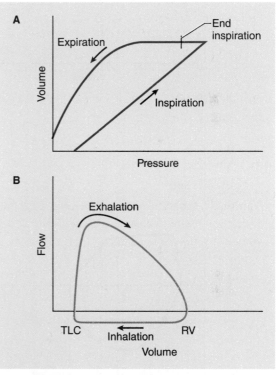

FIG. 1-9. A: Normal volume–pressure loop. **B:** Normal flow–volume loop. (Reproduced with permission from Butterworth JF IV, Mackey DC, Wasnick JD, eds. *Morgan & Mikhail's Clinical Anesthesiology.* 7th ed. New York, NY: McGraw Hill; 2022.)

References: Butterworth JF IV, Mackey DC, Wasnick JD, eds. *Morgan & Mikhail's Clinical Anesthesiology.* 7th ed. New York, NY: McGraw Hill; 2022: Chapter 6.

Butterworth JF IV, Mackey DC, Wasnick JD, eds. *Morgan & Mikhail's Clinical Anesthesiology.* 7th ed. New York, NY: McGraw Hill; 2022: Chapter 25.

Longnecker DE, Mackey SC, Newman MF, Sandberg WS, Zapol WM, eds. *Anesthesiology.* 3rd ed. McGraw Hill; 2018: Chapter 49.

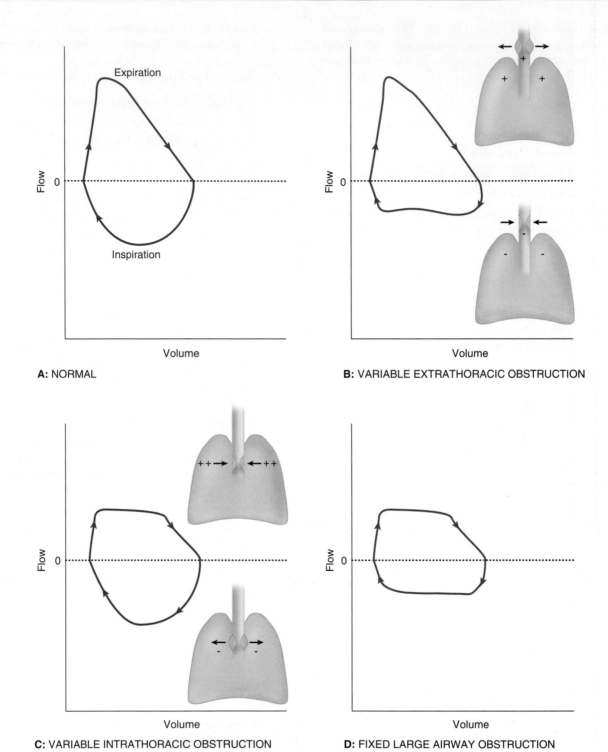

FIG. 1-10. A–D: Flow–volume loops. (Reproduced with permission from Butterworth JF IV, Mackey DC, Wasnick JD, eds. *Morgan & Mikhail's Clinical Anesthesiology*. 7th ed. New York, NY: McGraw Hill; 2022.)

366. Meperidine's effectiveness in reducing postoperative shivering is due to its action on _____ receptors in the hypothalamus.

(A) Kappa

(B) Delta

(C) GABA

(D) Mu$_1$

Rationale: Meperidine is effective in reducing shivering from diverse causes, including general and epidural anesthesia. The action is due to Kappa receptor stimulation.

Reference: Elisha S, Heiner JS, Nagelhout JJ. *Nurse Anesthesia.* 7th ed. St. Louis, MO: Elsevier Saunders; 2023: Chapter 11.

367. Which opioid may cause delayed respiratory depression 8 to 12 hours following subarachnoid administration?

(A) Fentanyl

(B) Morphine

(C) Sufentanil

(D) Alfentanil

Rationale: A later phase of respiratory depression occurs with subarachnoid administration of morphine. This later phase can occur 8 to 12 hours following injection.

Reference: Elisha S, Heiner JS, Nagelhout JJ. *Nurse Anesthesia.* 7th ed. St. Louis, MO: Elsevier Saunders; 2023: Chapter 11.

368. Which drug provides analgesia at the level of the spinal cord by binding to pre- and postsynaptic alpha-2 receptors?

(A) Nortriptyl

(B) Clonidine

(C) Venlafaxine

(D) Duloxetine

Rationale: Alpha-2 agonists exhibit their effect by interacting with the G-coupled alpha-2 receptors in the dorsal horn of the spinal cord. Presynaptically, this inhibits the release of neurotransmitters. Postsynaptically, this activates K+ channels hyperpolarizing the secondary afferent neuron.

Reference: Elisha S, Heiner JS, Nagelhout JJ. *Nurse Anesthesia.* 7th ed. St. Louis, MO: Elsevier Saunders; 2023: Chapter 56.

369. Substance P primarily works on which receptor?

(A) Neurokinin-1

(B) 5 HT

(C) Interleukin-1

(D) NMDA

Rationale: The primary afferent neuron releases Substance P in response to an action potential reaching its terminal. Substance P binds to NK-1 type receptors on the dendrite of the secondary afferent neuron within the dorsal horn of the spinal cord.

Reference: Elisha S, Heiner JS, Nagelhout JJ. *Nurse Anesthesia.* 7th ed. St. Louis, MO: Elsevier Saunders; 2023: Chapter 56.

370. What type of pain is well localized, sharp in nature, and generally hurts at the point or area of the stimulus?

(A) Visceral

(B) Musculoskeletal

(C) Neuropathic

(D) Somatic

Rationale: Somatic pain is well localized, sharp in nature, and generally hurts at the point or area of the stimulus.

Reference: Elisha S, Heiner JS, Nagelhout JJ. *Nurse Anesthesia.* 7th ed. St. Louis, MO: Elsevier Saunders; 2023: Chapter 56.

371. Within the pain pathway, what region of the brain does secondary afferent neurons synapse with third-order neurons?

(A) Thalamus

(B) Periaqueductal gray area

(C) Cerebral cortex

(D) Amygdala

Rationale: In the lateral thalamus and the intralaminar nuclei, second-order neurons synapse with third-order neurons, which then send projections to the cerebral cortex.

Reference: Elisha S, Heiner JS, Nagelhout JJ. *Nurse Anesthesia.* 7th ed. St. Louis, MO: Elsevier Saunders; 2023: Chapter 56.

372. Which fibers are primarily responsible for nociception?

    (A) A-alpha fibers

    (B) Beta fibers

    (C) A-delta and C fibers

    (D) C-delta fibers

Rationale: The primary afferent nociceptive neurons (A-delta and C fibers) have cell bodies located in the dorsal root ganglia of the spinal cord.

Reference: Elisha S, Heiner JS, Nagelhout JJ. *Nurse Anesthesia.* 7th ed. St. Louis, MO: Elsevier Saunders; 2023: Chapter 56.

373. What is physiologic process where a noxious mechanical, chemical, or thermal stimulus is converted into an electrical impulse called an action potential?

    (A) Transmission

    (B) Transduction

    (C) Perception

    (D) Modulation

Rationale: Transduction is the transformation of a noxious stimulus (chemical, mechanical, or thermal) into an action potential.

Reference: Elisha S, Heiner JS, Nagelhout JJ. *Nurse Anesthesia.* 7th ed. St. Louis, MO: Elsevier Saunders; 2023: Chapter 56.

CHAPTER 2

Equipment, Instrumentation, and Technology
Questions

1. What is the maximum allowable current leakage in the operating room?

   (A) 10 μA
   (B) 20 μA
   (C) <1 μA
   (D) 100 mA

2. What monitor alarms when a high current flow to the ground exists?

   (A) Isolation transformer monitor
   (B) Line isolation monitor
   (C) Leak current monitor
   (D) Electrical overload monitor

3. What humidity levels are appropriate for the operating room?

   (A) <20%
   (B) Between 20 and 60%
   (C) >60%
   (D) No specific humidity level required

4. Which of the following is true about heat and moisture exchangers?

   (A) Dead space increases in the breathing circuit.
   (B) Heat and moisture exchangers increase heat loss.
   (C) Dead space decreases in the breathing circuit.
   (D) Heat and moisture exchangers increase water loss.

5. What is the most effective method to minimize the initial phase (phase I) of perioperative unintentional hypothermia?

   (A) Heat and moisture exchangers
   (B) Head wrapping
   (C) Forced air warming beginning in the preoperative area
   (D) Heated intraoperative warming blankets

6. During infusion of multiple units of packed red blood cells, what infusion temperature is needed to avoid hypothermia?

   (A) 37°C
   (B) 36°C
   (C) 35°C
   (D) 34°C

7. What is the capacity of nitrous oxide in a full E-cylinder?

   (A) 1,590 L
   (B) 700 L
   (C) 625 L
   (D) 950 L

8. What is the cylinder color designation for air in the United States?

   (A) Blue
   (B) Black
   (C) Green
   (D) Yellow

9. What is the only reliable way to determine residual volume of nitrous oxide in an E-cylinder?

   (A) Calculate the pressure constant.
   (B) Measure the amount of liquid.
   (C) Calculate the gas flow.
   (D) Weigh the cylinder.

10. Which statement is true regarding the pin index safety system (PISS)?

    (A) Avoid incorrect attachment of H-cylinders to the yoke.
    (B) Pin configuration consists of three pins.
    (C) Pin configurations may be converted to accommodate cylinder gas.
    (D) The use of multiple washers may defeat the purpose of the system.

11. Which statement is true regarding the fail-safe valve?

    (A) Part of the low-pressure system
    (B) Prevents delivery of a hypoxic gas mixture
    (C) Shuts off when pressure in oxygen supply circuit exceeds 35 psi
    (D) Prevents flowmeter tube leaks

12. Which principle is not included in radiation safety?

    (A) Time
    (B) Distance
    (C) Shielding
    (D) Temperature

13. What component is not included in a Mapleson circuit?

    (A) Fresh gas inlet
    (B) Adjustable pressure-limiting valve
    (C) Reservoir bag
    (D) Inspiratory unidirectional valve

14. What component of the circle system is not present in a Mapleson circuit?

    (A) CO_2 absorber
    (B) Reservoir bag
    (C) Fresh gas inlet
    (D) APL valve

15. Which breathing circuit affords rebreathing?

    (A) Mapleson A
    (B) Mapleson D
    (C) Circle system
    (D) Bain circuit

16. Which statement is true regarding soda lime as a carbon dioxide (CO_2) absorbent?

    (A) CO_2 absorption capability can be regenerated during periods of unuse.
    (B) Optimal granule size ranges 10 to 14 mesh.
    (C) The activators (NaOH or KOH) are regenerated with the component calcium hydroxide ($Ca(OH)_2$).
    (D) If the absorbent is not colored at the beginning of the day, it has full CO_2 absorbing capacity.

17. The operating room lost electrical supply. Which device does not require wall-outlet electrical power?

    (A) Scavenging system
    (B) Digital flow meter displays
    (C) Mechanical ventilators
    (D) Gas/vapor blenders

18. Which safety device on the anesthesia workstation does not sense oxygen supply pressure (psi)?

    (A) Fail-safe
    (B) Balance regulator
    (C) Oxygen failure protection device
    (D) Oxygen analyzer

19. Which step indicates the difference in the pre-procedural vaporizer check of the TEC 6 compared to a variable-bypass vaporizer?

    (A) Confirmation that the vaporizer is in the OFF position
    (B) Checking the level of fullness
    (C) Checking the alarm battery low indicator
    (D) Verification of a functioning interlock system

20. What type of vaporizer is used with desflurane?

    (A) Vernitrol
    (B) Measured-flow
    (C) Electronic
    (D) Copper kettle

21. What adverse or unexpected effect may result from compressing the oxygen flush valve while the circuit is connected to a patient?

    (A) Barotrauma
    (B) Ventricular fibrillation
    (C) Concentrated inhaled agent
    (D) Increased anesthetic depth

22. Which oxygen analyzer is self-calibrating?

    (A) Galvanic
    (B) Polarographic
    (C) Clark
    (D) Paramagnetic

23. Following intubation, you connect the endotracheal tube to the breathing circuit. The machine is in manual ventilation mode and the APL valve is nearly closed. What patient condition is most likely to result if no adjustment is made to the APL valve?

    (A) Tachycardia
    (B) Hypertension
    (C) Hypotension
    (D) Increased cardiac output

24. What agency(s) recommends safe levels of waste gas exposure?

    (A) U.S. Food and Drug Administration (USDA)
    (B) National Institute for Occupational Safety and Health (NIOSH) and Occupational Safety and Health Administration (OSHA)
    (C) U.S. Food and Drug Administration (USDA) and Occupational Safety and Health Administration (OSHA)
    (D) U.S. Food and Drug Administration (USDA) and National Institute for Occupational Safety and Health (NIOSH)

25. Which anesthesia check procedure is repeated before each case?

    (A) Scavenger system check
    (B) Flow control valve check
    (C) Pipeline gas pressure check
    (D) Breathing circuit leak check

26. After inducing a patient, you are unable to ventilate with a mask. What should you do first?

    (A) Proceed with two-hand mask ventilation
    (B) Awaken the patient
    (C) Consider using a strap
    (D) Reposition the patient's head

27. What nerve injury may result from prolonged pressure involving bag mask ventilation?

    (A) Trigeminal and facial nerves
    (B) Greater auricular
    (C) Anterior cutaneous nerve of the neck
    (D) Lesser Occipital

28. Following induction of general anesthesia, you are unable to intubate the patient. Facemask ventilation is inadequate. What should you do next?

    (A) Consider placing an LMA
    (B) Cricothyrotomy
    (C) Wake the patient up
    (D) Reintubate

29. Where is the distal end of the combitube positioned?

    (A) Trachea
    (B) Esophagus
    (C) Hyperpharynx
    (D) Supraglottic

30. How do you determine the proper position of the fiberoptic bronchoscope when performing a fiberoptic intubation?

    (A) Visualization of the esophagus
    (B) Visualization of the arytenoid cartilages
    (C) Visualization of the tracheal rings and carina
    (D) Visualization of the epiglottis

31. You plan to intubate a patient with an unstable cervical spine injury. What is the best airway management approach?

    (A) One attempt at gentle laryngoscopy
    (B) Placement of an LMA
    (C) Lighted stylet
    (D) Flexible fiberoptic bronchoscope

32. You have trouble visualizing the glottic opening but can see the posterior arytenoid cartilages during laryngoscopy. What airway device combined with direct laryngoscopy may be useful for intubation in this situation?

    (A) LMA
    (B) Eschmann Stylet
    (C) Fastrach LMA
    (D) Proseal LMA

33. When using the MacIntosh laryngoscope, where is the tip of the blade placed?

    (A) Vallecula
    (B) Hyoepiglottic ligament
    (C) Posterior to the epiglottis
    (D) Posterior pharynx

34. What statement is true about jet ventilation?

    (A) Considered in "Cannot intubate, mask ventilation adequate" scenarios
    (B) Inspiratory pressures should be <50 psi
    (C) Use with low-pressure oxygen source
    (D) Inspiratory pressure should be >50 psi

35. In which patient condition is a nasal airway used with caution?

    (A) Obesity
    (B) Basilar skull fracture
    (C) Hemodynamic instability
    (D) Coronary artery disease

36. When comparing sites for placement of a central venous catheter, which site carries the greatest risk for pneumothorax?

    (A) Right internal jugular vein
    (B) Subclavian vein
    (C) Left internal jugular vein
    (D) Right external jugular vein

37. What does the "a" wave represent in a CVP tracing?

    (A) Atrial contraction
    (B) Tricuspid valve elevation
    (C) Venous return
    (D) Tricuspid valve opening

38. What type of ventilator bellow rises during expiration?

    (A) Ascending
    (B) Descending
    (C) Hanging
    (D) Pneumatic

39. In which patient would you avoid using an esophageal stethoscope?

    (A) 50-year-old with gastroesophageal reflux disease
    (B) 70-year-old with congestive heart failure
    (C) 70-year-old with advanced alcoholic liver disease
    (D) 50-year-old with gastrointestinal polyps

40. Which statement is true regarding pulse oximetry?

    (A) Pulse oximetry artifact is due to excessive ambient light, motion, and methylene blue dye.
    (B) Pulse oximetry requires calibration.
    (C) Pulse oximetry artifact is due to hyperthermia and increased cardiac output.
    (D) Oxyhemoglobin and deoxyhemoglobin absorb red and infrared light equally.

41. During the course of a general anesthesia there is a sudden cessation of the end-tidal CO_2 waveform. What is the most likely cause?

    (A) Esophageal intubation
    (B) Circuit disconnects
    (C) Bronchial intubation
    (D) Malignant hyperthermia

42. The patient is surgically anesthetized. What is the corresponding Bispectral Index (BIS) value?

    (A) 96
    (B) 90
    (C) 78
    (D) 56

43. When using evoked potentials which of the following agents would you avoid?

    (A) Zemuron
    (B) Nitrous oxide
    (C) Sufenta
    (D) Isoflurane

44. What monitoring modality does not reflect core body temperature?

    (A) Tympanic membrane
    (B) Esophageal
    (C) Liquid crystal skin adhesives
    (D) Pulmonary artery

45. What is the motor response when stimulating the ulnar nerve?

    (A) Contraction of the abductor pollicis
    (B) Contraction of the orbicularis oculi
    (C) Contraction of the adductor pollicis
    (D) Contraction of the facial nerve

46. Which concept is accurate regarding neuromuscular blockade (NMB) and monitoring using a peripheral nerve stimulation?

    (A) Peripheral nerve stimulators are only effective when administering nondepolarizing muscle relaxants.
    (B) Atrophied muscles may appear refractory to NMB and may lead to potential overdosing.
    (C) Muscle relaxants only affect post-synaptic acetylcholine receptors.
    (D) The concept of fade represents complete reversal of neuromuscular blockade.

47. What statement is true about the accuracy of blood pressure measurement?

    (A) The cuff's bladder should extend at least 40% around the extremity.
    (B) The width of the cuff should be 20 to 25% greater than the diameter of the extremity.
    (C) Blood pressure is a measure of perfusion.
    (D) The Doppler probe is the preferred noninvasive blood pressure measuring technique.

48. What is the normal range in the left ventricular end diastolic pressure?

    (A) 1 to 10
    (B) 10 to 20
    (C) 5 to 15
    (D) 4 to 12

49. When monitoring central venous pressure (CVP), what causes the loss of a-waves?

    (A) Atrial fibrillation
    (B) Tricuspid regurgitation
    (C) PVCs
    (D) Myocardial ischemia

50. In the normal capnograph, what does phase III indicate?

    (A) Decreased CO_2
    (B) Dead space
    (C) Dead space and alveolar gas
    (D) Alveolar gas plateau

51. Which condition may cause an increased end-tidal carbon dioxide?

    (A) CNS depression
    (B) Decreased cardiac output
    (C) Hypotension
    (D) VQ mismatching

52. What factor results in a shift to the right in an oxyhemoglobin dissociation curve?

    (A) Decreased CO_2
    (B) Elevated temperature
    (C) Alkalosis
    (D) Decreased temperature

53. What statement about pressure-controlled ventilation is false?

    (A) Limited peak inspiratory pressure exists.
    (B) Inspiratory pressure is controlled.
    (C) Tidal volume is uncontrolled.
    (D) Tidal volume is controlled.

54. Which Mapleson circuit is the most efficient for controlled ventilation?

    (A) Mapleson D
    (B) Mapleson A
    (C) Mapleson B
    (D) Mapleson C

55. What mechanism facilitates heat loss through air currents?

    (A) Radiation
    (B) Convection
    (C) Conduction
    (D) Evaporation

56. When is cell salvage contraindicated?

    (A) Sepsis
    (B) Benign tumors
    (C) Connective tissue disorders
    (D) Orthopedic procedures

57. How much blood loss is recommended for the use of cell salvage?

    (A) <250 mL
    (B) 250 to 500 mL
    (C) 500 to 750 mL
    (D) >1,000 mL

58. Where is the best location to monitor blood pressure for patients undergoing right shoulder arthroscopy in the beach chair position?

    (A) Right lower extremity
    (B) Left lower extremity
    (C) Left upper extremity
    (D) Right upper extremity

59. What is the first step in the management of a suspected oxygen pipeline cross-connection of another gas after opening the backup oxygen cylinder?

    (A) Recalibrate the oxygen analyzer
    (B) Institute high flows of oxygen
    (C) Use controlled ventilation with the ventilator
    (D) Disconnect pipeline supply

60. Which is not a task of oxygen in the anesthesia workstation?

    (A) Pressurizing the closed waste gas scavenger system
    (B) Powering the oxygen flush
    (C) Activating fail-safe mechanisms
    (D) Compressing the bellows of mechanical ventilator

61. What is a disadvantage of the Bain circuit?

    (A) Increases circuit bulk
    (B) Partial warming of inspiratory gas
    (C) Kinking or disconnection of the fresh gas inlet tube
    (D) Requires low fresh gas flow

62. What are the pin positions for oxygen, nitrous oxide, and air in the pin index safety system?

    (A) Oxygen 1 and 5, nitrous oxide 2 and 5, air 3 and 5
    (B) Oxygen 3 and 5, nitrous oxide 1 and 5, air 2 and 5
    (C) Oxygen 2 and 5, nitrous oxide 3 and 5, air 1 and 5
    (D) Oxygen 2 and 5, nitrous oxide 1 and 5, air 3 and 5

63. The E-cylinder oxygen gauge pressure reads 850 psi: How many liters are remaining presuming that the E-cylinder was full at 2,000 psi?

    (A) 300 L
    (B) 660 L
    (C) 240 L
    (D) 280 L

64. How many liters of CO_2 per 100 g of absorbent can soda lime absorb?

    (A) 23 L
    (B) 32 L
    (C) 44 L
    (D) 18 L

65. What does the National Institute for Occupational Safety and Health (NIOSH) recommend limiting the room concentration of a halogenated agent when nitrous oxide is used?

    (A) 25 ppm
    (B) 2 ppm
    (C) 0.5 ppm
    (D) 2.5 ppm

66. Which selection most accurately describes the components of a closed waste gas scavenging system with an active disposal/suctioning system?

    (A) Must have a negative pressure relief valve
    (B) Must have both a negative and positive pressure relief valve
    (C) Must have a positive pressure relief valve
    (D) Requires no pressure relief valves

67. What is the approximate pipeline pressure delivered to the anesthesia machine?

    (A) 35 psi
    (B) 50 psi
    (C) 1,900 psi
    (D) 745 psi

68. How many liters per minute will the oxygen flush valve provide to the common gas outlet?

    (A) 10 L/min
    (B) 80 to 100 L/min
    (C) 20 to 30 L/min
    (D) 35 to 75 L/min

69. What is the outer diameter of the scavenger transfer tubing?

    (A) 22 mm
    (B) 15 mm
    (C) 19 mm
    (D) 32 mm

70. Which Mapleson circuit is most efficient for spontaneous ventilation?

    (A) Mapleson D
    (B) Mapleson A
    (C) Mapleson B
    (D) Mapleson C

71. What is a benefit of the Bain circuit?

    (A) Decreases the circuit bulk and retains heat and humidity
    (B) Decreases resistance
    (C) Decrease in fresh gas flow
    (D) Able to scavenge waste gas

72. What is the granule size commonly used in CO_2 absorbent?

    (A) 2 to 4 mesh
    (B) 6 to 8 mesh
    (C) 4 to 8 mesh
    (D) 1 to 2 mesh

73. What does the AANA Foundation Closed Claims Research Team (CCRT) identify as the sentinel, contributory practice pattern in every hypoventilation claim?

    (A) Failure of the anesthesia delivery equipment
    (B) Faulty ventilator
    (C) Inaccurate calibration of the oxygen analyzer
    (D) Failure to optimally monitor ventilation

74. What are three functions of the hanger yoke?

    (A) Shuts off nitrous oxide when oxygen pressure falls below 20 psi, provides a gas tight seal, and ensures unidirectional flow
    (B) Monitors inspired oxygen level, reduces pressure to around 45 to 47 psi, and ensures unidirectional flow
    (C) Orients cylinders, provides a tight gas seal, and ensures unidirectional flow
    (D) Ensures at least 25% oxygen is given when using nitrous oxide, provides a gas tight seal, and ensures unidirectional flow

75. Which oxygen analyzer works by using the oxygen molecules' unique attraction into magnetic fields?

    (A) Electrogalvanic cell
    (B) Polarographic electrode
    (C) Paramagnetic oxygen sensor
    (D) Fluorescence quenching

76. Which classification of breathing circuits has complete rebreathing?

    (A) Open
    (B) Semi-open
    (C) Semi-closed
    (D) Closed

77. How many liters does a full oxygen E-cylinder tank hold?

    (A) 660 L
    (B) 1,590 L
    (C) 625 L
    (D) 750 L

78. What are appropriate measures to reduce the amount of oxygen consumed and prolong the duration of your backup oxygen supply when the pipeline oxygen supply fails?

    (A) Turn off the ventilator and ventilate manually through the circle system.
    (B) Set oxygen flows to 5 L/min.
    (C) Place the patient on pressure control ventilation.
    (D) Reduce tidal volume and increase respiratory rate on the ventilator.

79. What is the function of the fail-safe device on the anesthesia machine?

    (A) Prevents a hypoxic mixture of gas
    (B) Reduces cylinder pressure to around 45 to 47 psi
    (C) Ensures unidirectional flow from the gas supply into the anesthesia workstation
    (D) Closes the supply of nitrous oxide when the oxygen pipeline pressure falls below 25 psi

80. When the pressure gauge initially drops below 745 psig on a nitrous oxide E-cylinder at room temperature, how much nitrous oxide is approximately remaining in the tank?

    (A) 1,590 L
    (B) 660 L
    (C) 400 L
    (D) 625 L

81. What is the only device that will ensure that oxygen is present in the pipelines or cylinder?

    (A) Oxygen analyzer
    (B) Hypoxic guard
    (C) Oxygen failsafe device
    (D) Cylinder gauge

82. In a closed scavenging system, what component protects the patient from barotrauma if the scavenging suction fails or the hose distal to the system becomes kinked?

    (A) No component is available for protection and is the reason these systems are used anymore.
    (B) The design allows for waste gases to exit into the OR environment.
    (C) The negative pressure relief valve becomes kinked.
    (D) The positive pressure relief valve becomes kinked.

83. Which type of waste-gas scavenger interface requires negative and positive pressure relief valves?

    (A) Passive open interface
    (B) Passive closed interface
    (C) Active closed interface
    (D) Active open interface

84. Which organization published a generic checkout procedure for anesthesia gas machines and breathing circuits?

    (A) American Association of Nurse Anesthetist (AANA)
    (B) Department of Transportation (DOT)
    (C) Food and Drug Administration (FDA)
    (D) American Society for Testing and Materials (ASTM)

85. What component of the high-pressure system provides unidirectional flow to prevent transfilling or leakage of gases into the OR environment?

    (A) Pressure relief valve
    (B) Pressure regulator valve
    (C) Hypoxic guard
    (D) Check/unidirectional valve

86. After opening your oxygen E-cylinder on the back of the anesthesia workstation to determine the pressure, what is the next step?

    (A) Leave open in case of pipeline failure
    (B) The oxygen E-cylinder is only for an emergency
    (C) Leave partly open
    (D) Close the cylinder

87. Which circuit design incorporates a fresh gas inlet tube (inspiratory limb) inside the breathing circuit?

    (A) Mapelson D
    (B) Bain circuit
    (C) Mapelson A
    (D) Mapelson B

88. During which phase of an anesthetic is the most precipitous heat loss in the patient?

    (A) During the first perioperative hour
    (B) Maintenance (second to fourth hours)
    (C) Emergence
    (D) Postoperative

89. The formation of carbon monoxide by the degradation of volatile anesthetics due to dry soda lime is greatest with which agent?

    (A) Desflurane
    (B) Isoflurane
    (C) Sevoflurane
    (D) Nitrous oxide

90. Compound A is one of the by-products of degradation of which volatile anesthetic?

    (A) Desflurane
    (B) Isoflurane
    (C) Sevoflurane
    (D) Nitrous oxide

91. What is the end product of the soda lime reaction?

    (A) CO_2
    (B) Carbonic acid
    (C) Calcium carbonate
    (D) Ethyl violet

92. When should the LMA be removed?

    (A) When the patient moves
    (B) When the patient regains airway reflexes
    (C) When the surgery is completed
    (D) In the postanesthesia care unit

93. Which Mapleson circuit is a modification of the Mapleson D?

    (A) Jackson-Reese
    (B) Mapleson A
    (C) Bain
    (D) Mapleson C

94. Which statement is the most accurate description of the Diameter-Index Safety System (DISS)?

    (A) Allows for orientation of gas cylinders to the yoke
    (B) Prevents attaching wrong gas cylinders to anesthesia machine
    (C) Avoids attaching a nongrounded electrical supply to anesthesia machine
    (D) Prevents connection of the wrong pipeline gas supply hose to the anesthesia machine

95. What is your greatest concern when inflating the pulmonary artery balloon?

    (A) Conduction abnormalities
    (B) Pulmonary artery rupture
    (C) Catheter knotting
    (D) Bacteremia

96. Following intubation you are unable to palpate the tracheal tube cuff in the sternal notch. The breathing bag compliance is decreased. Breath sounds are unilateral. Where is the endotracheal tube most likely positioned?

    (A) Hypopharynx
    (B) Esophageal
    (C) Supraglottic
    (D) Right mainstem bronchus

97. What ultrasound (US) principle describes the manually adjusted amplification of US echoes returning from different depths of the tissue being scanned?

    (A) Depth
    (B) Focus
    (C) Acoustic enhancement
    (D) Time-gain compensation

98. What type of artifact refers to the loss of ultrasound echoes returning from tissue deep to a strong reflector such as a metal implant or bone?

    (A) Acoustic enhancement
    (B) Shadowing
    (C) Mirror
    (D) Reverberation

99. Which ultrasound mode will produce the best depiction of ventricular wall motion over time for the purpose of quantitative measurement?

    (A) A mode
    (B) B mode
    (C) M mode
    (D) Color Doppler

100. What ultrasound principle describes the change in frequency of the echoes reflecting from fluid either moving away or toward the transducer?

    (A) Doppler shift
    (B) Spectral analysis
    (C) Acoustic impedance
    (D) Refraction

101. At what angle of incidence/insonation produces the greatest reflection of ultrasound waves from a tissue target?

    (A) 0 degrees
    (B) 45 degrees
    (C) 60 degrees
    (D) 90 degrees

Answers and Explanations: Equipment, Instrumentation, and Technology

1. What is the maximum allowable current leakage in the operating room?

   (A) 10 μA
   (B) 20 μA
   (C) <1 μA
   (D) 50 mA

   Rationale: The maximum allowable current leakage in the operating room is 10 μA. Less than 1 μA is typically not felt whereas 50 mA is the fibrillation threshold and may be fatal.
   Reference: Butterworth JF IV, Mackey DC, Wasnick JD, eds. *Morgan & Mikhail's Clinical Anesthesiology*. 7th ed. New York, NY: McGraw Hill; 2022: Chapter 2.

2. What monitor alarms when a potential for a high electrical current flow to the ground exists?

   (A) Isolation transformer
   (B) Line isolation monitor
   (C) Leak current
   (D) High-efficiency particulate filter

   Rationale: The line isolation monitor affords protection from electrical shocks in the operating room. The isolation transformer affords isolation between the power supply in the operating room and the ground. High efficiency particulate filter (HEPA) is used to maintain air quality in the operating room.

   Line-isolated power systems commonly contain a line isolation monitor, or LIM, which monitors the current that *could* flow if one of the two isolated lines became electrically connected to ground. This potential leakage current is displayed prominently on the front of the line isolation panel within the isolated room. Each piece of equipment attached to the isolated system, including the built-in LIM, contributes to the cumulative potential leakage current. If the predicted leakage current rises to a set level (commonly 5 mA), the LIM sounds an audible alarm to indicate that a potentially unsafe state has been detected. It is important to note that an LIM alarm does not indicate that leakage current is flowing, but rather the potential exists for unsafe current to flow if an occupant was contacted with either line 1 or line 2. LIMs also have no automated mechanism for disconnecting power, which is convenient when critical monitoring or life support equipment is plugged into the distribution system. OR and ICU personnel should be familiar with the location of LIMs in their ORs and bed spaces and basic LIM troubleshooting procedures.
   References: Butterworth JF IV, Mackey DC, Wasnick JD, eds. *Morgan & Mikhail's Clinical Anesthesiology*. 7th ed. New York, NY: McGraw Hill; 2022: Chapter 2.
   Longnecker DE, Mackey SC, Newman MF, Sandberg WS, Zapol WM, eds. *Anesthesiology*. 3rd ed. McGraw Hill; 2018: Chapter 24.

3. What humidity levels are appropriate for the operating room?

   (A) <20%
   (B) Between 20 and 60%
   (C) >60%
   (D) No specific humidity level required

   Rationale: Humidity levels between 20 and 60% foster infection control in the operating room. Sterile drapes may be affected by high humidity causing dampness whereas low humidity may accelerate movement of particulate matter. Below this range the dry air facilitates airborne mobility of particulate matter, which can be a vector for infection. At high humidity, dampness can affect the integrity of barrier devices such as sterile cloth drapes and pan liners.
   Reference: Butterworth JF IV, Mackey DC, Wasnick JD, eds. *Morgan & Mikhail's Clinical Anesthesiology*. 7th ed. New York, NY: McGraw Hill; 2022: Chapter 2.

4. Which of the following is true about heat and moisture exchangers?

    (A) Dead space increases in the breathing circuit.

    (B) Heat and moisture exchangers increase heat loss.

    (C) Dead space decreases in the breathing circuit.

    (D) Heat and moisture exchanges increase water loss.

    Rationale: When using a heat and moisture exchanges, dead space increases. These passive devices do not add heat or vapor but rather contain a hygroscopic material that traps exhaled humidification and heat, which is released upon subsequent inhalation. Depending on the design, they may substantially increase apparatus dead space (more than 60 mL^3), which can cause significant rebreathing in pediatric patients. They can also increase breathing-circuit resistance and the work of breathing during spontaneous respirations. Excessive saturation of an HME with water or secretions can obstruct the breathing circuit.

    References: Butterworth JF IV, Mackey DC, Wasnick JD, eds. *Morgan & Mikhail's Clinical Anesthesiology.* 7th ed. New York, NY: McGraw Hill; 2022: Chapter 4.

    Pardo MC Jr, ed. *Basics of Anesthesia.* 8th ed. Philadelphia, PA: Elsevier Saunders; 2023: Chapter 15.

5. What is the most effective method to minimize the initial phase (phase I) of perioperative unintentional hypothermia?

    (A) Heat and moisture exchangers

    (B) Head wrapping

    (C) Preoperative forced-air warming

    (D) Heated intraoperative warming blankets

    Rationale: All methods in combination help conserve body heat during the perioperative period. Active warming fosters greater heat conservation than passive methods. "Prewarming the patient for half an hour with convective, forced-air warming blankets reduces the phase one decline in core temperature by reducing the central–peripheral temperature gradient."

    Reference: Butterworth JF IV, Mackey DC, Wasnick JD, eds. *Morgan & Mikhail's Clinical Anesthesiology.* 7th ed. New York, NY: McGraw Hill; 2022: Chapters 4 and 52.

6. During infusion of multiple units of packed red blood cells, what temperature is needed to avoid hypothermia?

    (A) 37°C

    (B) 36°C

    (C) 35°C

    (D) 34°C

    Rationale: Hypothermia results with multiple transfusions when the infused products are not warmed. Warming fluids (37°C) assists in minimizing body temperature loss. Massive blood transfusion is an absolute indication for warming all blood products and intravenous fluids to normal body temperature. Ventricular arrhythmias progressing to fibrillation often occur at temperatures close to 30°C, and hypothermia will hamper cardiac resuscitation. The customary use of rapid infusion devices with efficient heat transfer capability has decreased the incidence of transfusion-related hypothermia.

    Reference: Butterworth JF IV, Mackey DC, Wasnick JD, eds. *Morgan & Mikhail's Clinical Anesthesiology.* 7th ed. New York, NY: McGraw Hill; 2022: Chapter 52.

7. What is the capacity of nitrous oxide in an E-cylinder?

    (A) 1,590 L

    (B) 700 L

    (C) 625 L

    (D) 950 L

    Rationale: The capacity of nitrous oxide in an E-cylinder is 1,590 L as compared to an H-cylinder (15,900 L). The capacity of oxygen, air and nitrogen in an E-cylinder is 625 to 700 L at 1,800 to 2,200 psi.

    References: Butterworth JF IV, Mackey DC, Wasnick JD, eds. *Morgan & Mikhail's Clinical Anesthesiology.* 7th ed. New York, NY: McGraw Hill; 2022: Chapter 2.

TABLE 2-1. Characteristics of medical gas cylinders.

Gas	E-Cylinder Capacity[1] (L)	H-Cylinder Capacity[1] (L)	Pressure[1] (psig at 20°C)	Color (USA)	Color (International)	Form
O_2	625-700	6,000-8,000	1,800-2,200	Green	White	Gas
Air	625-700	6,000-8,000	1,800-2,200	Yellow	White and black	Gas
N_2O	1,590	15,900	745	Blue	Blue	Liquid
N_2	625-700	6,000-8,000	1,800-2,200	Black	Black	Gas

[1]Depending on the manufacturer.

N_2O, nitrous oxide; O_2, oxygen.

(Reproduced with permission from Butterworth JF IV, Mackey DC, Wasnick JD, eds. *Morgan & Mikhail's Clinical Anesthesiology.* 7th ed. New York, NY: McGraw Hill; 2022.)

Elisha S, Heiner JS, Nagelhout JJ. *Nurse Anesthesia.* 7th ed. St. Louis, MO: Elsevier Saunders; 2023: Chapter 16.

8. What is the cylinder color designation for air in the United States?

(A) Blue
(B) Black
(C) Green
(D) Yellow

Rationale: Air cylinders are yellow; oxygen is green; nitrous oxide, blue and nitrogen is black.

References: Butterworth JF IV, Mackey DC, Wasnick JD, eds. *Morgan & Mikhail's Clinical Anesthesiology.* 7th ed. New York, NY: McGraw Hill; 2022: Chapter 2.

Elisha S, Heiner JS, Nagelhout JJ. *Nurse Anesthesia.* 7th ed. St. Louis, MO: Elsevier Saunders; 2023: Chapter 16.

9. What is the only reliable way to determine the residual volume of nitrous oxide in a tank?

(A) Calculate the pressure constant.
(B) Measure the amount of liquid.
(C) Calculate the gas flow over time.
(D) Weigh the cylinder.

Rationale: Weighing the cylinder is the most reliable method to determine the residual volume of nitrous oxide. The liquid volume of nitrous oxide is not proportional to the pressure in the cylinder. Nitrous oxide is stored as a liquid. As the liquid vaporizes within the tank, the gaseous form creates a pressure (745 psi). This pressure remains constant if there is nitrous oxide in the liquid form. Only when the liquid form is used up (approximately 25% of the original contents—400 L), will the pressure in the tank decrease as the gaseous form is used.

References: Butterworth JF IV, Mackey DC, Wasnick JD, eds. *Morgan & Mikhail's Clinical Anesthesiology.* 7th ed. New York, NY: McGraw Hill; 2022: Chapter 4.

Longnecker DE, Mackey SC, Newman MF, Sandberg WS, Zapol WM, eds. *Anesthesiology.* 3rd ed. McGraw Hill; 2018: Chapter 35.

10. Which statement is true regarding the pin index safety system (PISS)?

(A) Avoids incorrect attachment of H-cylinders to the yoke.
(B) Pin configuration consists of three pins.
(C) Pin configurations may be converted to accommodate multiple gases.

(D) Use of multiple washers may defeat purpose of the system.

Rationale: The PISS is designed to ensure the correct attachment of E-cylinders to the yoke. A two-pin system connects the correct E-cylinder to the correct holes on the yoke. E-cylinders are never attached or forced into reconfigured holes on the yoke. The use of multiple washers may prevent proper engagement of pins into cylinder holes, mitigating the safety system.

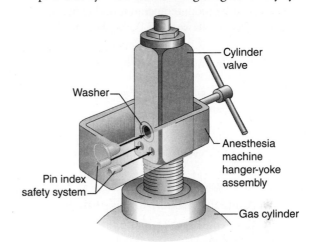

FIG. 2-1. Pin index safety system interlink between the anesthesia machine and gas cylinder. (Reproduced with permission from Butterworth JF IV, Mackey DC, Wasnick JD, eds. *Morgan & Mikhail's Clinical Anesthesiology.* 7th ed. New York, NY: McGraw Hill; 2022.)

References: Butterworth JF IV, Mackey DC, Wasnick JD, eds. *Morgan & Mikhail's Clinical Anesthesiology.* 7th ed. New York, NY: McGraw Hill; 2022: Chapter 4.

Elisha S, Heiner JS, Nagelhout JJ. *Nurse Anesthesia.* 7th ed. St. Louis, MO: Elsevier Saunders; 2023: Chapter 16.

11. Which statement is true regarding the fail-safe valve?

(A) Component of the low-pressure system
(B) Prevents delivery of a hypoxic gas mixture
(C) Shuts off when pressure in oxygen supply circuit is >30 psi
(D) Prevents flow meter tube leaks

Rationale: The fail-safe valve, part of the high-pressure system, prevents delivery of a hypoxic gas mixture. The valve shuts off or decreases gas flow when oxygen pressure decreases to less than 30 psi. Flow meters are part of the low-pressure system.

References: Butterworth JF IV, Mackey DC, Wasnick JD, eds. *Morgan & Mikhail's Clinical Anesthesiology.* 7th ed. New York, NY: McGraw Hill; 2022: Chapter 4.

Longnecker DE, Mackey SC, Newman MF, Sandberg WS, Zapol WM, eds. *Anesthesiology.* 3rd ed. McGraw Hill; 2018: Chapter 35.

12. Which principle is not included in radiation safety?

(A) Time

(B) Distance

(C) Shielding

(D) Temperature

Rationale: Time, distance, and shielding guide the need for anesthesia providers to avoid the hazards of radiation in the operating room. No relationship exists between the operating room temperature and radiation safety.

References: Butterworth JF IV, Mackey DC, Wasnick JD, eds. *Morgan & Mikhail's Clinical Anesthesiology.* 7th ed. New York, NY: McGraw Hill; 2022: Chapter 2.

Longnecker DE, Mackey SC, Newman MF, Sandberg WS, Zapol WM, eds. *Anesthesiology.* 3rd ed. McGraw Hill; 2018: Chapter 24.

13. What component is not included in a Mapleson circuit?

(A) Fresh gas inlet

(B) Adjustable pressure-limiting valve

(C) Reservoir bag

(D) Inspiratory unidirectional valve

Rationale: Inspiratory and expiratory unidirectional valves are included in the circle systems but are not a part of the Mapleson circuits.

References: Butterworth JF IV, Mackey DC, Wasnick JD, eds. *Morgan & Mikhail's Clinical Anesthesiology.* 7th ed. New York, NY: McGraw Hill; 2022: Chapter 3.

Longnecker DE, Mackey SC, Newman MF, Sandberg WS, Zapol WM, eds. *Anesthesiology.* 3rd ed. McGraw Hill; 2018: Chapter 35.

14. What component of the circle system is not present in a Mapleson circuit?

(A) CO_2 absorber

(B) Reservoir

(C) Fresh gas inlet

(D) APL valve

Rationale: CO_2 absorbers are present in the circle system but not the Mapleson circuit. Also included in circle system, but not the Mapleson system are an inspiratory unidirectional valve and breathing tube, Y-connector and an expiratory unidirectional valve, and breath tube.

References: Butterworth JF IV, Mackey DC, Wasnick JD, eds. *Morgan & Mikhail's Clinical Anesthesiology.* 7th ed. New York, NY: McGraw Hill; 2022: Chapter 3.

Longnecker DE, Mackey SC, Newman MF, Sandberg WS, Zapol WM, eds. *Anesthesiology.* 3rd ed. McGraw Hill; 2018: Chapter 35.

15. What breathing circuit affords rebreathing?

(A) Mapleson A

(B) Mapleson D

(C) Circle System

(D) Bain circuit

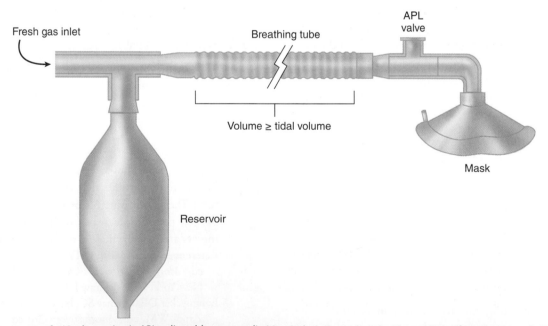

FIG. 2-2. Components of a Mapleson circuit. APL, adjustable pressure-limiting (valve). (Reproduced with permission from Butterworth JF IV, Mackey DC, Wasnick JD, eds. *Morgan & Mikhail's Clinical Anesthesiology.* 7th ed. New York, NY: McGraw Hill; 2022.)

Rationale: There is no rebreathing with the Mapleson or Bain circuits. Rebreathing occurs with circle systems specifically with low fresh gas flows.
References: Butterworth JF IV, Mackey DC, Wasnick JD, eds. *Morgan & Mikhail's Clinical Anesthesiology.* 7th ed. New York, NY: McGraw Hill; 2022: Chapter 3.
Longnecker DE, Mackey SC, Newman MF, Sandberg WS, Zapol WM, eds. *Anesthesiology.* 3rd ed. McGraw Hill; 2018: Chapter 35.

16. Which statement is true regarding soda lime as a carbon dioxide (CO_2) absorbent?

   (A) CO_2 absorption capability can be regenerated during periods of unuse.

   (B) Optimal granule size ranges 10 to 14 mesh.

   (C) The activators (NaOH or KOH) are regenerated with calcium hydroxide ($Ca(OH)_2$).

   (D) If the absorbent is not colored at the beginning of the day, it has full CO_2 absorbing capacity and does not need to be changed out.

   Rationale: Calcium hydroxide ($Ca(OH)_2$) combines with Na_2CO_3 or K_2CO_3 to regenerate NaOH or KOH. The indicator will exhibit some color reversion (back to white) during rest periods. The color of the absorbent at the beginning of the day may not reflect its remaining CO_2 absorbent capacity. Optimal mesh size is 4 to 8. The absorbent does not regain its ability to absorb CO_2 to any extent after periods when it is not in use.
   References: Longnecker DE, Mackey SC, Newman MF, Sandberg WS, Zapol WM, eds. *Anesthesiology.* 3rd ed. McGraw Hill; 2018: Chapters 34-35.
   Elisha S, Heiner JS, Nagelhout JJ. *Nurse Anesthesia.* 7th ed. St. Louis, MO: Elsevier Saunders; 2023: Chapter 16.

17. The operating room lost electrical supply. Which device does not require wall-outlet or battery electrical power?

   (A) Scavenging system

   (B) Digital flow meter displays

   (C) Mechanical ventilators

   (D) Gas/vapor blenders

   Rationale: Electrical wall outlet power is required for most physiologic monitors, mechanical ventilators, gas/vapor blenders in the operating room. Digital flow meter displays require electric power for electronic flow meters. Anesthesia machines do have battery backup systems which can be exhausted during periods of prolonged power outages. Items not requiring electric power include the scavenging system, variable bypass vaporizers, and mechanical flow meters.

Reference: Elisha S, Heiner JS, Nagelhout JJ. *Nurse Anesthesia.* 7th ed. St. Louis, MO: Elsevier Saunders; 2023: Chapter 16.

18. Which safety device on the anesthesia workstation does not sense oxygen supply pressure (psi)?

   (A) Fail-safe

   (B) Balance regulator

   (C) Oxygen failure protection device

   (D) Oxygen analyzer

   Rationale: To prevent delivery of a hypoxic mixture, safety devices sense the oxygen pressure. When the oxygen pressure falls below 20 to 30 psi, the oxygen safety devices shut off or proportionally decrease all gas flow. Traditional terms including fail-safe and nitrous cut-off have been replaced by proportioning devices called oxygen failure protection device or balance regulator. The oxygen analyzer detects the oxygen partial pressure in the sample gas.
   Reference: Butterworth JF IV, Mackey DC, Wasnick JD, eds. *Morgan & Mikhail's Clinical Anesthesiology.* 7th ed. New York, NY: McGraw Hill; 2022: Chapter 4.

19. Which step indicates the difference in the pre-procedural vaporizer check of the Tec 6 compared to a variable-bypass vaporizers?

   (A) Confirmation the vaporizer is in the off position

   (B) Checking the level of fullness

   (C) Checking the alarm battery low indicator

   (D) Verification of a functioning interlock

   Rationale: As compared to other variable-bypass type vaporizers, the Tec 6 vaporizer contains an alarm battery low indicator light. Confirmation that the vaporizer is turned off, checking the level of fullness, and verification of a functioning interlock are steps that should be completed for all vaporizers during the pre-procedural check.
   Reference: Elisha S, Heiner JS, Nagelhout JJ. *Nurse Anesthesia.* 7th ed. St. Louis, MO: Elsevier Saunders; 2023: Chapter 16.

20. What type of vaporizer is used with desflurane?

   (A) Vernitrol

   (B) Measured flow

   (C) Electronic

   (D) Copper kettle

Rationale: Unlike the vapor pressures of the other inhalational agents, desflurane's high vapor pressure requires a special electronically controlled vaporizer. Measured-flow vaporizers include the copper kettle and vernitrol.

References: Butterworth JF IV, Mackey DC, Wasnick JD, eds. *Morgan & Mikhail's Clinical Anesthesiology.* 7th ed. New York, NY: McGraw Hill; 2022: Chapter 4.

Pardo MC Jr, ed. *Basics of Anesthesia.* 8th ed. Philadelphia, PA: Elsevier Saunders; 2023: Chapter 15.

Elisha S, Heiner JS, Nagelhout JJ. *Nurse Anesthesia.* 7th ed. St. Louis, MO: Elsevier Saunders; 2023: Chapter 16.

21. What adverse or unexpected effect may result from compressing the oxygen flush valve while the circuit is connected to a patient?

    (A) Barotrauma
    (B) Ventricular fibrillation
    (C) Concentrated inhaled agent
    (D) Increased anesthetic depth

    Rationale: Compressing the oxygen flush valve (35-75 L/min) results in filling the breathing circuit. If the circuit is connected to the endotracheal tube during general anesthesia, barotrauma may result. The oxygen flush dilutes the inhaled agent and promotes the likelihood of decreased anesthetic depth.

    References: Butterworth JF IV, Mackey DC, Wasnick JD, eds. *Morgan & Mikhail's Clinical Anesthesiology.* 7th ed. New York, NY: McGraw Hill; 2022: Chapter 4.

    Elisha S, Heiner JS, Nagelhout JJ. *Nurse Anesthesia.* 7th ed. St. Louis, MO: Elsevier Saunders; 2023: Chapter 16.

22. Which oxygen analyzer is self-calibrating?

    (A) Galvanic
    (B) Polarographic
    (C) Clark
    (D) Paramagnetic

    Rationale: Galvanic and polarographic (Clark) oxygen analyzers are electrochemical sensors requiring calibration. Components of the electrochemical sensors include anode and cathode electrodes, electrolyte gel, and an oxygen-permeable membrane. Quick oxygen analysis, no additional components, and self-calibration serve as advantages of paramagnetic oxygen analyzers.

    Reference: Butterworth JF IV, Mackey DC, Wasnick JD, eds. *Morgan & Mikhail's Clinical Anesthesiology.* 7th ed. New York, NY: McGraw Hill; 2022: Chapter 4.

23. Following intubation, you connect the endotracheal tube to the breathing circuit. The machine is in manual mode and the APL valve is nearly closed. What patient condition is most likely to result if no adjustment is made to the APL valve?

    (A) Tachycardia
    (B) Hypertension
    (C) Hypotension
    (D) Increased cardiac output

    Rationale: Hypotension and pneumothorax (late) may result from increased pressure when the APL valve is nearly closed or closed completely.

    References: Butterworth JF IV, Mackey DC, Wasnick JD, eds. *Morgan & Mikhail's Clinical Anesthesiology.* 7th ed. New York, NY: McGraw Hill; 2022: Chapter 4.

    Pardo MC Jr, ed. *Basics of Anesthesia.* 8th ed. Philadelphia, PA: Elsevier Saunders; 2023: Chapter 15.

24. What agency(s) recommends safe levels of waste gas exposure?

    (A) U.S. Food and Drug Administration (USDA)
    (B) National Institute for Occupational Safety and Health (NIOSH) and Occupational Safety and Health Administration (OSHA)
    (C) U.S. Food and Drug Administration (USDA) and Occupational Safety and Health Administration (OSHA)
    (D) U.S. Food and Drug Administration and National Institute for Occupational Safety and Health Administration (OSHA)

    Rationale: NIOSH and OSHA recommend that the concentration of nitrous oxide in the operating room is less than 25 ppm and 2 ppm for halogenated agents (0.5 ppm if nitrous oxide is also being used).

    References: Butterworth JF IV, Mackey DC, Wasnick JD, eds. *Morgan & Mikhail's Clinical Anesthesiology.* 7th ed. New York, NY: McGraw Hill; 2022: Chapters 2 and 4.

    Elisha S, Heiner JS, Nagelhout JJ. *Nurse Anesthesia.* 7th ed. St. Louis, MO: Elsevier Saunders; 2023: Chapter 16.

25. Which anesthesia check procedure is repeated before each case?

    (A) Scavenger system check
    (B) Flow control valve check
    (C) Pipeline gas pressure check
    (D) Breathing circuit leak check

TABLE 2-2. Anesthesia apparatus checkout recommendations.[1]

This checkout, or a reasonable equivalent, should be conducted before the administration of anesthesia. These recommendations are valid only for an anesthesia system that conforms to current and relevant standards and includes an ascending bellows ventilator and at least the following monitors: capnograph, pulse oximeter, oxygen analyzer, respiratory volume monitor (spirometer), and breathing-system pressure monitor with high- and low-pressure alarms. Users are encouraged to modify this guideline to accommodate differences in equipment design and variations in local clinical practice. Such local modifications should have appropriate peer review. Users should refer to the appropriate operator manuals for specific procedures and precautions.

Emergency Ventilation Equipment

*1. Verify that backup ventilation equipment is available and functioning.

High-Pressure System

*2. Check the O_2 cylinder supply.
 a. Open the O_2 cylinder, and verify it is at least half full (about 1,000 psig).
 b. Close the cylinder.

*3. Check central pipeline supplies; check that hoses are connected and pipeline gauges read about 50 psig.

Low-Pressure System

*4. Check the initial status of the low-pressure system.
 a. Close flow control valves and turn vaporizers off.
 b. Check the fill level and tighten vaporizers' filler caps.

*5. Perform a leak check of the machine's low-pressure system.
 a. Verify that the machine master switch and flow control valves are off.
 b. Attach the suction bulb to the common (fresh) gas outlet.
 c. Squeeze the bulb repeatedly until fully collapsed.
 d. Verify the bulb stays *fully* collapsed for at least 10 seconds.
 e. Open one vaporizer at a time, and repeat steps c and d.
 f. Remove the suction bulb, and reconnect the fresh gas hose.

*6. Turn on the machine master switch and all other necessary electrical equipment.

*7. Test flowmeters.
 a. Adjust the flow of all gases through their full range, checking for smooth operation of floats and undamaged flow tubes.
 b. Attempt to create a hypoxic O_2/N_2O mixture, and verify the correct changes in the flow or alarm.

Scavenging System

*8. Adjust and check the scavenging system.
 a. Ensure proper connections between the scavenging system and both the APL (pop-off) valve and the ventilator relief valve.
 b. Adjust the waste-gas vacuum (if possible).
 c. Fully open the APL valve and occlude the Y-piece.
 d. With minimum O_2 flow, allow the scavenger reservoir bag to collapse completely, and verify that the absorber pressure gauge reads about zero.
 e. With the O_2 flush activated, allow the scavenger reservoir bag to distend fully, and then verify that the absorber pressure gauge reads <10 cm H_2O.

Breathing System

*9. Calibrate the O_2 monitor.
 a. Ensure the monitor reads 21% in room air.
 b. Verify that the low-O_2 alarm is enabled and functioning.
 c. Reinstall the sensor in the circuit and flush the breathing system with O_2.
 d. Verify that the monitor now reads greater than 90%.

10. Check the initial status breathing system.
 a. Set the selector switch to Bag mode.
 b. Check that the breathing circuit is complete, undamaged, and unobstructed.
 c. Verify that CO_2 absorbent is adequate.
 d. Install the breathing-circuit accessory equipment (e.g., humidifier, PEEP valve) to be used during the case.

11. Perform a leak check of the breathing system.
 a. Set all gas flows to zero (or minimum).
 b. Close the APL (pop-off) valve, and occlude the Y-piece.
 c. Pressurize the breathing system to about 30 cm H_2O with O_2 flush.
 d. Ensure that the pressure remains fixed for at least 10 seconds.
 e. Open the APL (pop-off) valve and ensure that pressure decreases.

Manual and Automatic Ventilation Systems

12. Test ventilation systems and unidirectional valves.
 a. Place a second breathing bag on the Y-piece.
 b. Set appropriate ventilator parameters for the next patient.
 c. Switch to automatic-ventilation (ventilator) mode.
 d. Turn the ventilator on, and fill the bellows and breathing bag with O_2 flush.
 e. Set O_2 flow to minimum and other gas flows to zero.
 f. Verify that during inspiration the bellows delivers the appropriate tidal volume and that during expiration the bellows fills completely.
 g. Set the fresh gas flow to about 5 L min^{-1}.
 h. Verify that the ventilator bellows and simulated lungs fill and empty appropriately without sustained pressure at end expiration.
 i. Check for proper action of unidirectional valves.
 j. Exercise breathing circuit accessories to ensure proper function.
 k. Turn the ventilator off, and switch to manual ventilation (Bag/APL) mode.
 l. Ventilate manually, and ensure inflation and deflation of artificial lungs and appropriate feel of system resistance and compliance.
 m. Remove the second breathing bag from the Y-piece.

Monitors

13. Check, calibrate, or set alarm limits of all monitors: capnograph, pulse oximeter, O_2 analyzer, respiratory-volume monitor (spirometer), and pressure monitor with high and low airway-pressure alarms.

Final Position

14. Check the final status of the machine.
 a. Vaporizers off.
 b. APL valve open.
 c. Selector switch to Bag mode.
 d. All flowmeters to zero (or minimum).
 e. Patient suction level adequate.
 f. Breathing system ready to use.

[1]Data from the U.S. Food and Drug Administration and the U.S. Department of Health and Human Services.
*If an anesthesia provider uses the same machine in successive cases, these steps need not be repeated, or they can be abbreviated after the initial checkout.
APL, adjustable pressure-limiting; CO_2, carbon dioxide; H_2O, water; O_2, oxygen; PEEP, positive end-expiratory pressure.
(Reproduced with permission from Butterworth JF IV, Mackey DC, Wasnick JD, eds. *Morgan & Mikhail's Clinical Anesthesiology*. 7th ed. New York, NY: McGraw Hill; 2022.)

Rationale: While the scavenger, flow control valve, and pipeline gas pressure are checked daily prior to conducting any anesthetic case, the breathing system leak check is conducted prior to each anesthetic.

References: Butterworth JF IV, Mackey DC, Wasnick JD, eds. *Morgan & Mikhail's Clinical Anesthesiology.* 7th ed. New York, NY: McGraw Hill; 2022: Chapter 4.

Elisha S, Heiner JS, Nagelhout JJ. *Nurse Anesthesia.* 7th ed. St. Louis, MO: Elsevier Saunders; 2023: Chapter 16.

26. After inducing a patient you are unable to ventilate with a mask. What should you do first?

    (A) Proceed with two-hand mask ventilation
    (B) Awaken the patient
    (C) Consider using a strap
    (D) Reposition the patient's head

    Rationale: Each of the options will assist with proper bag mask ventilation. Repositioning the patient's head will optimize the ability to ventilate. If after repositioning it remains difficult to ventilate using a head strap, placing an oropharyngeal airway, use two-hand mask ventilation or using an alternative airway may be considered.

    References: Butterworth JF IV, Mackey DC, Wasnick JD, eds. *Morgan & Mikhail's Clinical Anesthesiology.* 7th ed. New York, NY: McGraw Hill; 2022: Chapter 19.

    Elisha S, Heiner JS, Nagelhout JJ. *Nurse Anesthesia.* 7th ed. St. Louis, MO: Elsevier Saunders; 2023: Chapter 24.

27. What nerve injury may result from prolonged pressure involving bag mask ventilation?

    (A) Trigeminal and facial nerves
    (B) Greater auricular
    (C) Anterior cutaneous nerve of the neck
    (D) Lesser Occipital

    Rationale: Nerve injuries result from improper positioning. In addition, pressure may result in nerve injury from devices including the facemask.

    References: Butterworth JF IV, Mackey DC, Wasnick JD, eds. *Morgan & Mikhail's Clinical Anesthesiology.* 7th ed. New York, NY: McGraw Hill; 2022: Chapter 19.

    Elisha S, Heiner JS, Nagelhout JJ. *Nurse Anesthesia.* 7th ed. St. Louis, MO: Elsevier Saunders; 2023: Chapter 24.

28. Following induction of general anesthesia, you are unable to intubate the patient. Facemask ventilation is inadequate. What should you do next?

    (A) Consider placing an LMA
    (B) Cricothyrotomy

    (C) Wake the patient up
    (D) Reintubate

    Rationale: The American Association of Anesthesiologists Difficult Airway Algorithm informs how to manage difficult airway scenarios. For this case, calling for help, returning the patient to spontaneous ventilation or awakening the patient is considered. If inadequate mask ventilation persists, consider, or attempt LMA placement. If an LMA attempt fails, proceed to the emergency airway pathway.

    References: Butterworth JF IV, Mackey DC, Wasnick JD, eds. *Morgan & Mikhail's Clinical Anesthesiology.* 7th ed. New York, NY: McGraw Hill; 2022: Chapter 19.

    Elisha S, Heiner JS, Nagelhout JJ. *Nurse Anesthesia.* 7th ed. St. Louis, MO: Elsevier Saunders; 2023: Chapter 24.

29. Where is the distal end of the combitube positioned?

    (A) Trachea
    (B) Esophagus
    (C) Hyperpharynx
    (D) Supraglottic

    Rationale: The double lumen combitube is a supraglottic alternative airway device that is blindly placed in the hypopharynx. The tip is placed in the esophagus.

    References: Butterworth JF IV, Mackey DC, Wasnick JD, eds. *Morgan & Mikhail's Clinical Anesthesiology.* 7th ed. New York, NY: McGraw Hill; 2022: Chapter 19.

    Elisha S, Heiner JS, Nagelhout JJ. *Nurse Anesthesia.* 7th ed. St. Louis, MO: Elsevier Saunders; 2023: Chapter 24.

30. How do you determine the proper position of the fiberoptic bronchoscope when performing a fiberoptic intubation?

    (A) Visualization of the esophagus
    (B) Visualization of the arytenoid cartilages
    (C) Visualization of the tracheal rings and carina
    (D) Visualization of the epiglottis

    Rationale: Successful fiberoptic intubation is dependent on identification of airway structures. Once the glottis opening is identified, the fiberoptic bronchoscope is advanced. Visualization of the tracheal rings and carina inform proper placement.

    References: Butterworth JF IV, Mackey DC, Wasnick JD, eds. *Morgan & Mikhail's Clinical Anesthesiology.* 7th ed. New York, NY: McGraw Hill; 2022: Chapter 19.

    Elisha S, Heiner JS, Nagelhout JJ. *Nurse Anesthesia.* 7th ed. St. Louis, MO: Elsevier Saunders; 2023: Chapter 24.

31. You plan to intubate a patient with an unstable cervical spine injury. What is the best airway management approach?

    (A) One attempt at gentle laryngoscopy
    (B) Placement of an LMA
    (C) Lighted stylet
    (D) Flexible fiberoptic bronchoscope

    Rationale: For patients where an awake intubation is indicated, a flexible fiberoptic bronchoscope facilitates intubation. Patients with conditions including cervical spine injuries, congenital abnormalities or certain temporomandibular joint conditions benefit from this approach.
    References: Butterworth JF IV, Mackey DC, Wasnick JD, eds. *Morgan & Mikhail's Clinical Anesthesiology.* 7th ed. New York, NY: McGraw Hill; 2022: Chapter 19.
    Elisha S, Heiner JS, Nagelhout JJ. *Nurse Anesthesia.* 7th ed. St. Louis, MO: Elsevier Saunders; 2023: Chapter 24.

32. You have trouble visualizing the glottic opening but can see the posterior arytenoid cartilages during laryngoscopy. What airway device combined with direct laryngoscopy may be useful for intubation?

    (A) LMA
    (B) Eschmann Stylet
    (C) Fastrach LMA
    (D) Proseal LMA

    Rationale: Alternative airway devices include each of the options. As compared to the variety of LMAs, the Eschmann stylet uses direct laryngoscopy to facilitate intubation.
    References: Butterworth JF IV, Mackey DC, Wasnick JD, eds. *Morgan & Mikhail's Clinical Anesthesiology.* 7th ed. New York, NY: McGraw Hill; 2022: Chapter 19.
    Elisha S, Heiner JS, Nagelhout JJ. *Nurse Anesthesia.* 7th ed. St. Louis, MO: Elsevier Saunders; 2023: Chapter 24.

33. When using the MacIntosh laryngoscope, where is the tip of the blade placed?

    (A) Vallecula
    (B) Hyoepiglottic ligament
    (C) Posterior to the epiglottis
    (D) Posterior pharynx

    Rationale: The tip of the curved MacIntosh laryngoscope is place in the vallecula. The straight Miller blade is positioned posterior to the epiglottis.

References: Butterworth JF IV, Mackey DC, Wasnick JD, eds. *Morgan & Mikhail's Clinical Anesthesiology.* 7th ed. New York, NY: McGraw Hill; 2022: Chapter 19.
Elisha S, Heiner JS, Nagelhout JJ. *Nurse Anesthesia.* 7th ed. St. Louis, MO: Elsevier Saunders; 2023: Chapter 24.

34. What statement is true about jet ventilation?

    (A) Considered in "Cannot intubate, mask ventilation adequate" scenarios
    (B) Inspiratory pressures should be <50 psi
    (C) Use with low-pressure oxygen source
    (D) Inspiratory pressure should be >50 psi

    Rationale: Transtracheal jet ventilation is accomplished through a high-pressure oxygen source. High pressure oxygen source is needed. The inspiratory pressure should not exceed 25 to 50 psi. Higher inspiratory pressures may result in barotrauma.
    References: Butterworth JF IV, Mackey DC, Wasnick JD, eds. *Morgan & Mikhail's Clinical Anesthesiology.* 7th ed. New York, NY: McGraw Hill; 2022: Chapter 19.
    Elisha S, Heiner JS, Nagelhout JJ. *Nurse Anesthesia.* 7th ed. St. Louis, MO: Elsevier Saunders; 2023: Chapter 24.

35. In which patient condition is a nasal airway used with caution?

    (A) Obesity
    (B) Basilar skull fracture
    (C) Hemodynamic instability
    (D) Coronary artery disease

    Rationale: Nasal airways are used with caution for patients receiving anticoagulation therapy, thrombocytopenia, and basilar skull fracture.
    Reference: Butterworth JF IV, Mackey DC, Wasnick JD, eds. *Morgan & Mikhail's Clinical Anesthesiology.* 7th ed. New York, NY: McGraw Hill; 2022: Chapter 19.

36. When comparing sites for placement of a central venous catheter, which site carries the greatest risk for pneumothorax?

    (A) Right internal jugular vein
    (B) Subclavian vein
    (C) Left internal jugular vein
    (D) Right external jugular vein

    Rationale: Each of the sites may be used for central venous catheter placement. The right internal jugular vein provides easy access and safety. Increased risk of pleural effusion and chylothorax is linked to the

left internal jugular vein. Due to the anatomy of the external jugular veins, placement may be challenging.
Reference: Butterworth JF IV, Mackey DC, Wasnick JD, eds. *Morgan & Mikhail's Clinical Anesthesiology.* 7th ed. New York, NY: McGraw Hill; 2022: Chapter 5.

37.   What does the "a" wave represent in a CVP tracing?

(A)   Atrial contraction

(B)   Tricuspid valve elevation

(C)   Venous return

(D)   Tricuspid valve opening

Rationale: C waves represent tricuspid valve elevation; v waves represent venous return; x and y waves represent downward tricuspid valve replacement and valve opening during diastole.

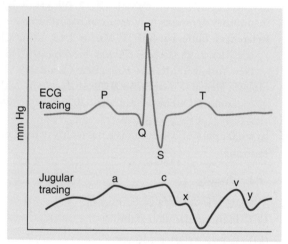

FIG. 2-3. The upward waves (*a, c, v*) and the downward descents (*x, y*) of a central venous tracing in relation to the electrocardiogram (ECG). (Reproduced with permission from Butterworth JF IV, Mackey DC, Wasnick JD, eds. *Morgan & Mikhail's Clinical Anesthesiology.* 7th ed. New York, NY: McGraw Hill; 2022.)

References: Butterworth JF IV, Mackey DC, Wasnick JD, eds. *Morgan & Mikhail's Clinical Anesthesiology.* 7th ed. New York, NY: McGraw Hill; 2022: Chapter 5.
Elisha S, Heiner JS, Nagelhout JJ. *Nurse Anesthesia.* 7th ed. St. Louis, MO: Elsevier Saunders; 2023: Chapter 17.

38.   What type of ventilator bellow that rises during expiration?

(A)   Ascending

(B)   Descending

(C)   Hanging

(D)   Pneumatic

Rationale: A standing (ascending) bellow rises during expiration and collapse during inspiration. A standing

(ascending) bellow is preferred as it readily draws attention to a circuit disconnection by collapsing.
References: Butterworth JF IV, Mackey DC, Wasnick JD, eds. *Morgan & Mikhail's Clinical Anesthesiology.* 7th ed. New York, NY: McGraw Hill; 2022: Chapter 4.
Elisha S, Heiner JS, Nagelhout JJ. *Nurse Anesthesia.* 7th ed. St. Louis, MO: Elsevier Saunders; 2023: Chapter 18.

39.   In which patient would you avoid using an esophageal stethoscope?

(A)   50-year-old with gastroesophageal reflux disease

(B)   70-year-old with congestive heart failure

(C)   70-year-old with advanced alcoholic liver disease

(D)   50-year-old with gastrointestinal polyps

Rationale: Contraindications for using an esophageal stethoscope include patients with esophageal conditions including strictures or varices. The pathophysiology of advanced liver disease includes the presence of varices.
Reference: Butterworth JF IV, Mackey DC, Wasnick JD, eds. *Morgan & Mikhail's Clinical Anesthesiology.* 7th ed. New York, NY: McGraw Hill; 2022: Chapter 6.

40.   Which statement is true regarding pulse oximetry?

(A)   Pulse oximetry artifact is due to excessive ambient light, motion, and methylene blue dye.

(B)   Pulse oximetry requires calibration.

(C)   Pulse oximetry artifact is due to hyperthermia and increased cardiac output.

(D)   Oxyhemoglobin and deoxyhemoglobin absorb red and infrared light equally.

Rationale: No calibration is required for pulse oximetry. Low output states including any condition decreasing cardiac output will affect pulse oximetry. Oxyhemoglobin absorbs a greater amount of infrared light as compared to deoxyhemoglobin which absorbs a greater amount of red light.
References: Butterworth JF IV, Mackey DC, Wasnick JD, eds. *Morgan & Mikhail's Clinical Anesthesiology.* 7th ed. New York, NY: McGraw Hill; 2022: Chapter 6.
Elisha S, Heiner JS, Nagelhout JJ. *Nurse Anesthesia.* 7th ed. St. Louis, MO: Elsevier Saunders; 2023: Chapter 18.

41.   During the course of a general anesthetic there is a sudden cessation of the end-tidal CO_2 waveform. What is the most likely cause?

(A)   Esophageal intubation

(B)   Circuit disconnects

(C) Bronchial intubation

(D) Malignant hyperthermia

Rationale: When the CO_2 wave form stops, a circuit disconnect is the most likely cause. During induction of anesthesia, incorrect placement of the endotracheal tube results in little to no end-tidal CO_2. An increased $ETCO_2$ is a heralding sign of malignant hyperthermia.

Reference: Butterworth JF IV, Mackey DC, Wasnick JD, eds. *Morgan & Mikhail's Clinical Anesthesiology.* 7th ed. New York, NY: McGraw Hill; 2022: Chapter 6.

42. The patient is surgically anesthetized. What is the corresponding Bispectral Index (BIS) value?

(A) 96

(B) 90

(C) 78

(D) 56

Rationale: The BIS values for patients undergoing sedation are 65-85. BIS values for general anesthesia are 40-65. A BIS of 90 and 96 represents an awake or near awake patient.

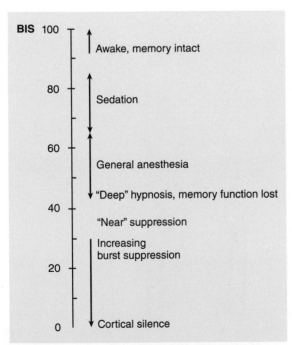

FIG. 2-4. The bispectral index (BIS versions 3.0 and higher) is a dimensionless scale from 0 (complete cortical electroencephalographic suppression) to 100 (awake). BIS values of 65 to 85 have been recommended for sedation, whereas values of 40 to 65 have been recommended for general anesthesia. At BIS values lower than 40, cortical suppression becomes discernible in a raw electroencephalogram as a burst suppression pattern. (Reproduced with permission from Johansen JW et al: Development and clinical application of electroencephalographic bispectrum monitoring. *Anesthesiology.* 2000;93(5):1337-1344.)

References: Butterworth JF IV, Mackey DC, Wasnick JD, eds. *Morgan & Mikhail's Clinical Anesthesiology.* 7th ed. New York, NY: McGraw Hill; 2022: Chapter 6.

Elisha S, Heiner JS, Nagelhout JJ. *Nurse Anesthesia.* 7th ed. St. Louis, MO: Elsevier Saunders; 2023: Chapter 19.

43. When using evoked potentials, which of the following agents would you avoid?

(A) Zemuron

(B) Nitrous oxide

(C) Sufenta

(D) Isoflurane

Rationale: Neuromuscular blockers, narcotics, and nitrous oxide result in small changes for evoked potentials. While low dose volatile anesthetic agents are permissible, avoiding inhalational agents is best.

References: Butterworth JF IV, Mackey DC, Wasnick JD, eds. *Morgan & Mikhail's Clinical Anesthesiology.* 7th ed. New York, NY: McGraw Hill; 2022: Chapter 6.

Elisha S, Heiner JS, Nagelhout JJ. *Nurse Anesthesia.* 7th ed. St. Louis, MO: Elsevier Saunders; 2023: Chapter 19.

44. What monitoring modality does not reflect core body temperature?

(A) Tympanic membrane

(B) Esophageal

(C) Liquid crystal skin adhesives

(D) Pulmonary artery

Rationale: Each of the modalities except skin temperature measurements reflect the core body temperature.

References: Butterworth JF IV, Mackey DC, Wasnick JD, eds. *Morgan & Mikhail's Clinical Anesthesiology.* 7th ed. New York, NY: McGraw Hill; 2022: Chapter 6.

Elisha S, Heiner JS, Nagelhout JJ. *Nurse Anesthesia.* 7th ed. St. Louis, MO: Elsevier Saunders; 2023: Chapter 17.

45. What is the motor response when stimulating the ulnar nerve?

(A) Contraction of the abductor pollicis

(B) Contraction of the orbicularis oculi

(C) Contraction of the adductor pollicis

(D) Contraction of the facial nerve

Rationale: When using a nerve stimulator, stimulation of the facial nerve results in contraction of the orbicularis oculi. Stimulation of the ulnar nerve results in adductor pollicis muscle contraction.

References: Butterworth JF IV, Mackey DC, Wasnick JD, eds. *Morgan & Mikhail's Clinical Anesthesiology*. 7th ed. New York, NY: McGraw Hill; 2022: Chapter 6.
Elisha S, Heiner JS, Nagelhout JJ. *Nurse Anesthesia*. 7th ed. St. Louis, MO: Elsevier Saunders; 2023: Chapter 19.

46. Which concept is accurate regarding neuromuscular blockade (NMB) and monitoring using a peripheral nerve stimulator?

    (A) Peripheral nerve stimulators are only effective when administering nondepolarizing relaxants.

    (B) Atrophied muscles may appear refractory to NMB and may lead to potential overdosing.

    (C) Muscle relaxants affect only post-synaptic acetylcholine receptors.

    (D) The concept of fade represents complete reversal of neuromuscular blockade.

Rationale: Atrophied muscles due to nerve damage experience a proliferation of receptors which many lead to an appearance of being refractory to NMB. NMB monitoring is effective for both depolarizing and nondepolarizing relaxants. NMB agents work on both pre-synaptic and post-synaptic Ach receptors. Fade represents incomplete NMB reversal.

References: Butterworth JF IV, Mackey DC, Wasnick JD, eds. *Morgan & Mikhail's Clinical Anesthesiology*. 7th ed. New York, NY: McGraw Hill; 2022: Chapter 6.
Elisha S, Heiner JS, Nagelhout JJ. *Nurse Anesthesia*. 7th ed. St. Louis, MO: Elsevier Saunders; 2023: Chapter 19.

47. What statement is true about the accuracy of blood pressure measurement?

    (A) The cuff's bladder should extend at least 40% around the extremity.

    (B) The width of the cuff should be 20 to 25% greater than the diameter of the extremity.

    (C) Blood pressure is a measure of perfusion.

    (D) The Doppler probe is the preferred noninvasive blood pressure measuring technique.

Rationale: The bladder of the blood pressure cuff should extend at least half-way around the extremity. The width should be 20 to 50% greater than the diameter of the extremity. The blood pressure is an indicator of perfusion rather than a measure of perfusion. Oscillometric devices are the preferred noninvasive blood pressure measuring technique.

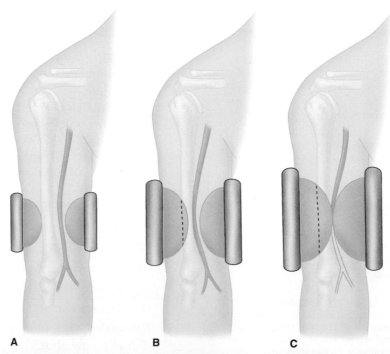

A   **B**   **C**

FIG. 2-5. Blood pressure cuff width influences the pressure readings. The narrowest cuff **(A)** will require more pressure and the widest cuff **(B)** normal cuff size **(C)** will require less pressure to occlude the brachial artery for the determination of systolic pressure. Too narrow a cuff may produce a large overestimation of systolic pressure. Whereas the wider cuff may underestimate the systolic pressure, the error with a cuff 20% too wide is not as significant as the error with a cuff 20% too narrow. (Reproduced with permission from Gravenstein JS, Paulus DA. *Clinical Monitoring Practice*. 2nd ed. Philadelphia, PA: Lippincott Williams & Wilkins; 1987.)

References: Butterworth JF IV, Mackey DC, Wasnick JD, eds. *Morgan & Mikhail's Clinical Anesthesiology.* 7th ed. New York, NY: McGraw Hill; 2022: Chapter 5.

Elisha S, Heiner JS, Nagelhout JJ. *Nurse Anesthesia.* 7th ed. St. Louis, MO: Elsevier Saunders; 2023: Chapter 17.

48. What is the normal range of the left ventricular end diastolic pressure?

(A) 1 to 10

(B) 10 to 20

(C) 5 to 15

(D) 4 to 12

Rationale: Ranges are as follows: Mean right atrial pressure (1-10); Mean pulmonary artery pressure (10-20); Pulmonary artery occlusive pressure (5-15).

References: Butterworth JF IV, Mackey DC, Wasnick JD, eds. *Morgan & Mikhail's Clinical Anesthesiology.* 7th ed. New York, NY: McGraw Hill; 2022: Chapter 5.

Elisha S, Heiner JS, Nagelhout JJ. *Nurse Anesthesia.* 7th ed. St. Louis, MO: Elsevier Saunders; 2023: Chapter 17.

49. When monitoring central venous pressure (CVP), what causes the loss of "*a*" waves?

(A) Atrial fibrillation

(B) Tricuspid regurgitation

(C) PVCs

(D) Myocardial ischemia

Rationale: The loss of *a* waves is due to atrial fibrillation or ventricular pacing during asystole. Large *v* waves may be caused by tricuspid or mitral regurgitation as well as increased intravascular volume. Cannon *a*-waves result from myocardial ischemia and numerous arrhythmias.

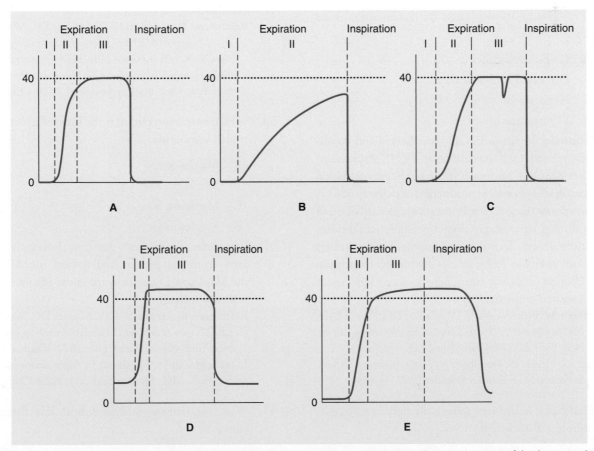

FIG. 2-6. A: A normal capnograph demonstrating the three phases of expiration: phase I—dead space; phase II—a mixture of dead space and alveolar gas; phase III—alveolar gas plateau. **B**: Capnograph of a patient with severe chronic obstructive pulmonary disease. No plateau is reached before the next inspiration. The gradient between end-tidal carbon dioxide (CO_2) and arterial CO_2 is increased. **C**: Depression during phase III indicates spontaneous respiratory effort. **D**: Failure of the inspired CO_2 to return to zero may represent an incompetent expiratory valve or exhausted CO_2 absorbent. **E**: The persistence of exhaled gas during part of the inspiratory cycle signals the presence of an incompetent inspiratory valve. (Reproduced with permission from Butterworth JF IV, *Mackey DC, Wasnick JD, eds. Morgan & Mikhail's Clinical Anesthesiology.* 7th ed. New York, NY: McGraw Hill; 2022.)

References: Butterworth JF IV, Mackey DC, Wasnick JD, eds. *Morgan & Mikhail's Clinical Anesthesiology.* 7th ed. New York, NY: McGraw Hill; 2022: Chapter 5.

Elisha S, Heiner JS, Nagelhout JJ. *Nurse Anesthesia.* 7th ed. St. Louis, MO: Elsevier Saunders; 2023: Chapter 17.

50. In the normal capnograph, what does phase III indicate?

    (A) Decreased CO_2

    (B) Dead space

    (C) Dead space and alveolar gas

    (D) Alveolar gas plateau

    Rationale: Phases of capnography include Phase I—dead space; Phase II—dead space and alveolar gas; Phase III—alveolar gas plateau; Final phase—rapid decrease in CO_2

    References: Butterworth JF IV, Mackey DC, Wasnick JD, eds. *Morgan & Mikhail's Clinical Anesthesiology.* 7th ed. New York, NY: McGraw Hill; 2022: Chapter 6.

    Elisha S, Heiner JS, Nagelhout JJ. *Nurse Anesthesia.* 7th ed. St. Louis, MO: Elsevier Saunders; 2023: Chapter 18.

51. Which condition may cause an increased end-tidal carbon dioxide?

    (A) CNS depression

    (B) Decreased cardiac output

    (C) Hypotension

    (D) VQ mismatching

    Rationale: Increases in CO_2 production and conditions related to hypoventilation (CNS depression) increase CO_2. Conditions related to hyperventilation decrease CO_2 as well as production or delivery of CO_2 (tourniquet release; bicarbonate; sepsis; instillation of gas during laparoscopy; hypermetabolic conditions; seizures; fever). Technical or equipment malfunctions including airway leaks, circuit disconnect esophageal intubation or airway equipment kinks or leaks result in deceased end-tidal CO_2.

    References: Butterworth JF IV, Mackey DC, Wasnick JD, eds. *Morgan & Mikhail's Clinical Anesthesiology.* 7th ed. New York, NY: McGraw Hill; 2022: Chapter 6.

    Elisha S, Heiner JS, Nagelhout JJ. *Nurse Anesthesia.* 7th ed. St. Louis, MO: Elsevier Saunders; 2023: Chapter 18.

52. What factor results in a shift to the right in an oxyhemoglobin dissociation curve?

    (A) Decreased CO_2

    (B) Elevated temperature

    (C) Alkalosis

    (D) Decreased temperature

    Rationale: Elevated temperature; 2,3-DPG; increased CO_2 and acidosis (decreased pH) shift the oxyhemoglobin dissociation curve to the right. Alkalosis (increased pH), decreased 2,3-DPG, decreased CO_2 and decreased temperature shift the oxyhemoglobin dissociation curve to the left.

    References: Butterworth JF IV, Mackey DC, Wasnick JD, eds. *Morgan & Mikhail's Clinical Anesthesiology.* 7th ed. New York, NY: McGraw Hill; 2022: Chapter 23.

    Elisha S, Heiner JS, Nagelhout JJ. *Nurse Anesthesia.* 7th ed. St. Louis, MO: Elsevier Saunders; 2023: Chapter 17.

53. What statement about pressure-controlled ventilation is false?

    (A) Limited peak inspiratory pressure exists.

    (B) Inspiratory pressure is controlled.

    (C) Tidal volume is uncontrolled.

    (D) Tidal volume is controlled.

    Rationale: Tidal volume is controlled with volume-controlled ventilation rather than pressure-controlled ventilation.

    References: Butterworth JF IV, Mackey DC, Wasnick JD, eds. *Morgan & Mikhail's Clinical Anesthesiology.* 7th ed. New York, NY: McGraw Hill; 2022: Chapters 3 and 58.

    Elisha S, Heiner JS, Nagelhout JJ. *Nurse Anesthesia.* 7th ed. St. Louis, MO: Elsevier Saunders; 2023: Chapter 16.

54. Which Mapleson circuit is the most efficient for controlled ventilation?

    (A) Mapleson D

    (B) Mapleson A

    (C) Mapleson B

    (D) Mapleson C

    Rationale: Since fresh gas flow forces alveolar air away from the patient and toward the APL valve, the Mapleson D circuit is the most efficient for controlled ventilation.

    References: Butterworth JF IV, Mackey DC, Wasnick JD, eds. *Morgan & Mikhail's Clinical Anesthesiology.* 7th ed. New York, NY: McGraw Hill; 2022: Chapter 3.

    Elisha S, Heiner JS, Nagelhout JJ. *Nurse Anesthesia.* 7th ed. St. Louis, MO: Elsevier Saunders; 2023: Chapter 16.

55. What mechanism facilitates heat loss through air currents?

    (A) Radiation

    (B) Convection

    (C) Conduction

    (D) Evaporation

Rationale: Evaporative heat loss results fluid loss through the skin and respiratory system. Conductive heat loss occurs when direct contact between cold and warm objects. Radiation involves the transfer of heat from infrared rays. Convective heat loss requires currents and is dependent on thermal gradients.

References: Butterworth JF IV, Mackey DC, Wasnick JD, eds. *Morgan & Mikhail's Clinical Anesthesiology.* 7th ed. New York, NY: McGraw Hill; 2022: Chapter 52.

Elisha S, Heiner JS, Nagelhout JJ. *Nurse Anesthesia.* 7th ed. St. Louis, MO: Elsevier Saunders; 2023: Chapter 15.

56. When is cell salvage contraindicated?

    (A) Sepsis
    (B) Benign tumors
    (C) Connective tissue disorders
    (D) Orthopedic procedures

    Rationale: Relative contraindications for the use of cell saver include sepsis, malignancies, pharmacologic agents, and hematologic conditions. Cell salvage is used in orthopedic and cardiac procedures.

    References: Butterworth JF IV, Mackey DC, Wasnick JD, eds. *Morgan & Mikhail's Clinical Anesthesiology.* 7th ed. New York, NY: McGraw Hill; 2022: Chapter 51.

    Elisha S, Heiner JS, Nagelhout JJ. *Nurse Anesthesia.* 7th ed. St. Louis, MO: Elsevier Saunders; 2023: Chapter 21.

57. How much blood loss is recommended for the use of cell salvage?

    (A) <250 mL
    (B) 250 to 500 mL
    (C) 500 to 750 mL
    (D) >1,000 mL

    Rationale: Cell salvage is used in large blood loss surgeries (1,000 mL or greater).

    References: Butterworth JF IV, Mackey DC, Wasnick JD, eds. *Morgan & Mikhail's Clinical Anesthesiology.* 7th ed. New York, NY: McGraw Hill; 2022: Chapter 51.

    Elisha S, Heiner JS, Nagelhout JJ. *Nurse Anesthesia.* 7th ed. St. Louis, MO: Elsevier Saunders; 2023: Chapter 21.

58. Where is the best location to monitor blood pressure for patients undergoing right shoulder arthroscopy in the beach chair position?

    (A) Right lower extremity
    (B) Left lower extremity
    (C) Left upper extremity
    (D) Right upper extremity

Rationale: The upper extremity is used to monitor noninvasive blood pressure for this case. There is a significant difference (40 mmHg) when using the lower extremity. Hypotension, although common for this procedure and position, needs to be minimized to avoid low cerebral perfusion.

References: Butterworth JF IV, Mackey DC, Wasnick JD, eds. *Morgan & Mikhail's Clinical Anesthesiology.* 7th ed. New York, NY: McGraw Hill; 2022: Chapter 38.

Elisha S, Heiner JS, Nagelhout JJ. *Nurse Anesthesia.* 7th ed. St. Louis, MO: Elsevier Saunders; 2023: Chapter 23.

59. What is the first step in the management of a suspected oxygen pipeline cross-connection of another gas after opening the backup oxygen cylinder?

    (A) Recalibrate the oxygen analyzer
    (B) Institute high flows of oxygen
    (C) Use controlled ventilation with the ventilator
    (D) Disconnect pipeline supply

    Rationale: After opening the backup oxygen cylinder, disconnecting the pipeline will prevent gas from the pipeline from continuing to be delivered. If the pipeline supply is still connected, gas will be preferentially drawn from that supply before the cylinder.

    References: Butterworth JF IV, Mackey DC, Wasnick JD, eds. *Morgan & Mikhail's Clinical Anesthesiology.* 7th ed. New York, NY: McGraw Hill; 2022: Chapter 4.

    Longnecker DE, Mackey SC, Newman MF, Sandberg WS, Zapol WM, eds. *Anesthesiology.* 3rd ed. McGraw Hill; 2018: Chapter 35.

60. Which is not a task of oxygen in the anesthesia workstation?

    (A) Pressurizing the closed waste gas scavenger system
    (B) Powering the oxygen flush
    (C) Activating fail-safe mechanisms
    (D) Compressing the bellows of mechanical ventilators

    Rationale: Oxygen has five tasks in the anesthesia workstation: (1) proceeds to the fresh gas flowmeter, (2) powers the oxygen flush, (3) activates the fail-safe mechanism, (4) activates oxygen low-pressure alarms, and (5) compresses the bellows of mechanical ventilators. The waste-gas scavenger systems are not pressurized.

    References: Butterworth JF IV, Mackey DC, Wasnick JD, eds. *Morgan & Mikhail's Clinical Anesthesiology.* 7th ed. New York, NY: McGraw Hill; 2022: Chapter 4.

Elisha S, Heiner JS, Nagelhout JJ. *Nurse Anesthesia.* 7th ed. St. Louis, MO: Elsevier Saunders; 2023: Chapter 16.

61. What is a disadvantage of the Bain circuit?

(A) Increases circuit bulk

(B) Partial warming of inspiratory gas

(C) Kinking or disconnection of the fresh gas inlet tube

(D) Requires low fresh gas flow

Rationale: A disadvantage of this circuit is the chance of kinking or disconnection of the fresh gas inlet. Periodic check of the inner tubing is set to prevent this complication.

References: Butterworth JF IV, Mackey DC, Wasnick JD, eds. *Morgan & Mikhail's Clinical Anesthesiology.* 7th ed. New York, NY: McGraw Hill; 2022: Chapter 3.

Elisha S, Heiner JS, Nagelhout JJ. *Nurse Anesthesia.* 7th ed. St. Louis, MO: Elsevier Saunders; 2023: Chapter 16.

62. What are the pin positions for oxygen, nitrous oxide, and air in the pin index safety system?

(A) Oxygen 1 and 5, nitrous oxide 2 and 5, air 3 and 5

(B) Oxygen 3 and 5, nitrous oxide 1 and 5, air 2 and 5

(C) Oxygen 2 and 5, nitrous oxide 3 and 5, air 1 and 5

(D) Oxygen 2 and 5, nitrous oxide 1 and 5, air 3 and 5

Rationale: Pin position placement for each E-cylinder the pin index safety system prevents accidental connection of a wrong gas cylinder.

References: Butterworth JF IV, Mackey DC, Wasnick JD, eds. *Morgan & Mikhail's Clinical Anesthesiology.* 7th ed. New York, NY: McGraw Hill; 2022: Chapter 2.

Elisha S, Heiner JS, Nagelhout JJ. *Nurse Anesthesia.* 7th ed. St. Louis, MO: Elsevier Saunders; 2023: Chapter 16.

63. The E-cylinder oxygen gauge pressure reads 850 psi: How many liters are remaining presuming that the E-cylinder was full at 2,000 psi?

(A) 300 L

(B) 660 L

(C) 240 L

(D) 280 L

Rationale: $\dfrac{Capacity\ L}{Service\ Pressure\ psi} = \dfrac{Contents\ Remaining\ L}{Gauge\ Pressure\ psi}$

References: Butterworth JF IV, Mackey DC, Wasnick JD, eds. *Morgan & Mikhail's Clinical Anesthesiology.* 7th ed. New York, NY: McGraw Hill; 2022: Chapter 4.

Elisha S, Heiner JS, Nagelhout JJ. *Nurse Anesthesia.* 7th ed. St. Louis, MO: Elsevier Saunders; 2023: Chapter 16.

64. How many liters of CO_2 per 100g of absorbent can soda lime absorb?

(A) 23 L

(B) 32 L

(C) 44 L

(D) 18 L

Rationale: Soda lime is the more common absorbent and can absorb up to 23 L of CO_2 per 100 g of absorbent.

References: Butterworth JF IV, Mackey DC, Wasnick JD, eds. *Morgan & Mikhail's Clinical Anesthesiology.* 7th ed. New York, NY: McGraw Hill; 2022: Chapter 4.

Pardo MC Jr, ed. *Basics of Anesthesia.* 8th ed. Philadelphia, PA: Elsevier Saunders; 2023: Chapter 15.

65. What does the National Institute for Occupational Safety and Health (NIOSH) recommend limiting the room concentration of a halogenated agent when nitrous oxide is used?

(A) 25 ppm

(B) 2 ppm

(C) 0.5 ppm

(D) 2.5 ppm

Rationale: The National institute for Occupational Safety and Health (NIOSH) recommend limiting the room concentration of nitrous oxide to 25 ppm and halogenated agent to 2 ppm and 0.5 ppm when nitrous oxide is also used.

References: Butterworth JF IV, Mackey DC, Wasnick JD, eds. *Morgan & Mikhail's Clinical Anesthesiology.* 7th ed. New York, NY: McGraw Hill; 2022: Chapter 4.

Elisha S, Heiner JS, Nagelhout JJ. *Nurse Anesthesia.* 7th ed. St. Louis, MO: Elsevier Saunders; 2023: Chapter 47.

66. Which selection most accurately describes the components of a closed waste gas scavenging system with an active disposal (suctioning) system?

(A) Must have a negative-pressure relief valve

(B) Must have both a negative and positive pressure relief valve

(C) Must have a positive-pressure relief valve

(D) Requires no pressure relief valves

Rationale: A closed waste gas scavenging system is closed to the outside atmosphere and requires negative and positive pressure relief valves that shield the patient from the negative pressure of the vacuum system and positive pressure from an impediment in the scavenging tubing.

References: Butterworth JF IV, Mackey DC, Wasnick JD, eds. *Morgan & Mikhail's Clinical Anesthesiology.* 7th ed. New York, NY: McGraw Hill; 2022: Chapter 4.

Elisha S, Heiner JS, Nagelhout JJ. *Nurse Anesthesia.* 7th ed. St. Louis, MO: Elsevier Saunders; 2023: Chapter 16.

67. What is the approximate pipeline pressure delivered to the anesthesia machine?

(A) 35 psi

(B) 50 psi

(C) 1,900 psi

(D) 745 psi

Rationale: The approximate pipeline pressure delivered to the anesthesia machine is 50 psi; 35 psi is too low. 1,900 psi is the approximate psi for a full O_2 E-cylinder, and 745 is the psi for N_2O E-cylinder.

References: Butterworth JF IV, Mackey DC, Wasnick JD, eds. *Morgan & Mikhail's Clinical Anesthesiology.* 7th ed. New York, NY: McGraw Hill; 2022: Chapter 4.

Elisha S, Heiner JS, Nagelhout JJ. *Nurse Anesthesia.* 7th ed. St. Louis, MO: Elsevier Saunders; 2023: Chapter 16.

68. How many liters per minute will the oxygen flush valve provide to the common gas outlet?

(A) 10 L/min

(B) 80 to 100 L/min

(C) 20 to 30 L/min

(D) 35 to 75 L/min

Rationale: The oxygen flush valve provides a high flow of oxygen directly to the common gas outlet at 35 to 75 L/minute.

References: Butterworth JF IV, Mackey DC, Wasnick JD, eds. *Morgan & Mikhail's Clinical Anesthesiology.* 7th ed. New York, NY: McGraw Hill; 2022: Chapter 4.

Elisha S, Heiner JS, Nagelhout JJ. *Nurse Anesthesia.* 7th ed. St. Louis, MO: Elsevier Saunders; 2023: Chapter 16.

69. What is the outer diameter of the scavenger transfer tubing?

(A) 22 mm

(B) 15 mm

(C) 19 mm

(D) 32 mm

Rationale: The outer diameter of the scavenger transfer tubing is 19 mm; the outer diameter for the common gas outlet is 22 mm.

References: Butterworth JF IV, Mackey DC, Wasnick JD, eds. *Morgan & Mikhail's Clinical Anesthesiology.* 7th ed. New York, NY: McGraw Hill; 2022: Chapter 4.

Pardo MC Jr, ed. *Basics of Anesthesia.* 8th ed. Philadelphia, PA: Elsevier Saunders; 2023: Chapter 15.

70. Which Mapleson circuit is most efficient for spontaneous ventilation?

(A) Mapleson D

(B) Mapleson A

(C) Mapleson B

(D) Mapleson C

Rationale: Because the fresh gas flow is equal to minute ventilation, the Mapleson A circuit is the most efficient for spontaneous ventilation.

Reference: Butterworth JF IV, Mackey DC, Wasnick JD, eds. *Morgan & Mikhail's Clinical Anesthesiology.* 7th ed. New York, NY: McGraw Hill; 2022: Chapter 3.

71. What is a benefit of the Bain circuit?

(A) Decreases the circuit bulk and retains heat and humidity

(B) Decreases resistance

(C) Decrease in fresh gas flow

(D) Able to scavenge waste gas

Rationale: The Bain circuit incorporates the fresh gas inlet tubing inside the breathing tube which decreases the circuit bulk and retains heat and humidity.

References: Butterworth JF IV, Mackey DC, Wasnick JD, eds. *Morgan & Mikhail's Clinical Anesthesiology.* 7th ed. New York, NY: McGraw Hill; 2022: Chapter 3.

Elisha S, Heiner JS, Nagelhout JJ. *Nurse Anesthesia.* 7th ed. St. Louis, MO: Elsevier Saunders; 2023: Chapter 16.

72. What is the granule size commonly used in CO_2 absorbent?

(A) 2 to 4 mesh

(B) 6 to 8 mesh

(C) 4 to 8 mesh

(D) 1 to 2 mesh

Rationale: Granule size is a compromise between the higher absorptive surface area of small granules and the lower resistance to gas flow of larger granules. The granule size commonly used in CO_2 absorbent is between 4 and 8 mesh.

References: Butterworth JF IV, Mackey DC, Wasnick JD, eds. *Morgan & Mikhail's Clinical Anesthesiology.* 7th ed. New York, NY: McGraw Hill; 2022: Chapter 3.

Elisha S, Heiner JS, Nagelhout JJ. *Nurse Anesthesia.* 7th ed. St. Louis, MO: Elsevier Saunders; 2023: Chapter 16.

73. What does the AANA Foundation Closed-Claims research team (CCRT) identify as a sentinel, contributory practice pattern in every hypoventilation claim?

    (A) Failure of the anesthesia delivery equipment

    (B) Faulty ventilator

    (C) Inaccurate calibration of the oxygen analyzer

    (D) Failure to optimally monitor ventilation

    Rationale: The AANA Foundation CCRT found: In every hypoventilation claim, a failure to optimally monitor the patient's ventilation was identified as a sentinel, contributory practice pattern.

    Reference: Elisha S, Heiner JS, Nagelhout JJ. *Nurse Anesthesia.* 7th ed. St. Louis, MO: Elsevier Saunders; 2023: Chapter 18.

74. What are three functions of the hanger yoke?

    (A) Shuts off nitrous oxide when oxygen pressure falls below 20 psi, provides a gas tight seal, and ensures unidirectional flow.

    (B) Monitors inspired oxygen level, reduces pressure to around 45 to 47 psi, and ensures unidirectional flow.

    (C) Orients cylinders, provides a tight gas seal, and ensures unidirectional flow.

    (D) Ensures at least 25% oxygen is given when using nitrous oxide, provides a gas tight seal, and ensures unidirectional flow.

    Rationale: Part one of A refers to the oxygen shut off valve, part one and two of B refer to the oxygen analyzer and the pressure regulator, part one of D refers to the hypoxic guard.

    References: Butterworth JF IV, Mackey DC, Wasnick JD, eds. *Morgan & Mikhail's Clinical Anesthesiology.* 7th ed. New York, NY: McGraw Hill; 2022: Chapter 4.

    Elisha S, Heiner JS, Nagelhout JJ. *Nurse Anesthesia.* 7th ed. St. Louis, MO: Elsevier Saunders; 2023: Chapter 16.

75. Which oxygen analyzer works by using the oxygen molecules' unique attraction into magnetic fields?

    (A) Electrogalvanic cell

    (B) Polarographic electrode

    (C) Paramagnetic oxygen sensor

    (D) Fluorescence quenching

    Rationale: (A)—Creates its own electric current by using a lead anode and either a gold or silver anode. (B)—Creates its own electric current by using a silver anode and platinum cathode. (D)—Uses the fluorescence caused by a molecule emitting light in response to being energized.

    References: Butterworth JF IV, Mackey DC, Wasnick JD, eds. *Morgan & Mikhail's Clinical Anesthesiology.* 7th ed. New York, NY: McGraw Hill; 2022: Chapter 4.

    Elisha S, Heiner JS, Nagelhout JJ. *Nurse Anesthesia.* 7th ed. St. Louis, MO: Elsevier Saunders; 2023: Chapter 16.

76. Which classification of breathing circuits has complete rebreathing?

    (A) Open

    (B) Semi-open

    (C) Semi-closed

    (D) Closed

    Rationale: Open and semi-open have no rebreathing; semi-closed has partial rebreathing.

    References: Butterworth JF IV, Mackey DC, Wasnick JD, eds. *Morgan & Mikhail's Clinical Anesthesiology.* 7th ed. New York, NY: McGraw Hill; 2022: Chapter 4.

    Elisha S, Heiner JS, Nagelhout JJ. *Nurse Anesthesia.* 7th ed. St. Louis, MO: Elsevier Saunders; 2023: Chapter 16.

77. How many liters does a full oxygen E-cylinder tank hold?

    (A) 660 L

    (B) 1,590 L

    (C) 625 L

    (D) 750 L

    Rationale: B is nitrous oxide; C is air.

    References: Butterworth JF IV, Mackey DC, Wasnick JD, eds. *Morgan & Mikhail's Clinical Anesthesiology.* 7th ed. New York, NY: McGraw Hill; 2022: Chapter 2.

    Elisha S, Heiner JS, Nagelhout JJ. *Nurse Anesthesia.* 7th ed. St. Louis, MO: Elsevier Saunders; 2023: Chapter 16.

TABLE 2-3. Characteristics of medical gas cylinders.

Gas	E-Cylinder Capacity[1] (L)	H-Cylinder Capacity[1] (L)	Pressure[1] (psig at 20°C)	Color (USA)	Color (International)	Form
O_2	625-700	6,000-8,000	1,800-2,200	Green	White	Gas
Air	625-700	6,000-8,000	1,800-2,200	Yellow	White and black	Gas
N_2O	1,590	15,900	745	Blue	Blue	Liquid
N_2	625-700	6,000-8,000	1,800-2,200	Black	Black	Gas

[1]Depending on the manufacturer.
N_2O, nitrous oxide; O_2, oxygen.
(Reproduced with permission from Butterworth JF IV, Mackey DC, Wasnick JD, eds. *Morgan & Mikhail's Clinical Anesthesiology*. 7th ed. New York, NY: McGraw Hill; 2022.)

78. What are appropriate measures to reduce the amount of oxygen used and prolong the duration of your backup oxygen supply when the pipeline oxygen supply fails?

    (A) Turn off the ventilator and ventilate manually through the circle system.
    (B) Set oxygen flows to 5 L/min.
    (C) Place the patient on pressure control ventilation.
    (D) Reduce tidal volume and increase respiratory rate on the ventilator.

    Rationale: Most anesthesia machines utilize oxygen as the driving gas to power the ventilator. By reducing fresh oxygen flow rates and eliminating the use of the ventilator by allowing the patient to breathe spontaneously or ventilating via the reservoir bag, you will prolong the backup oxygen supply.
    References: Butterworth JF IV, Mackey DC, Wasnick JD, eds. *Morgan & Mikhail's Clinical Anesthesiology*. 7th ed. New York, NY: McGraw Hill; 2022: Chapter 4.
    Elisha S, Heiner JS, Nagelhout JJ. *Nurse Anesthesia*. 7th ed. St. Louis, MO: Elsevier Saunders; 2023: Chapter 16.

79. What is the function of the fail-safe device on the anesthesia machine?

    (A) Prevents a hypoxic mixture of gas
    (B) Reduces cylinder pressure to around 45 to 47 psi
    (C) Ensures unidirectional flow
    (D) Closes the supply of nitrous oxide and other gases when the oxygen pressure falls below 25 psi

    Rationale: The fail-safe device triggers an alarm and closes the supply of nitrous oxide and other gases when the oxygen pressure falls below 25 psi. Even though the other gases are shut off, the supply of oxygen could still be hypoxic in nature due to a cross-connection scenario in which a gas other than oxygen was connected to the oxygen pipeline system.
    References: Butterworth JF IV, Mackey DC, Wasnick JD, eds. *Morgan & Mikhail's Clinical Anesthesiology*. 7th ed. New York, NY: McGraw Hill; 2022: Chapter 4.
    Elisha S, Heiner JS, Nagelhout JJ. *Nurse Anesthesia*. 7th ed. St. Louis, MO: Elsevier Saunders; 2023: Chapter 16.

80. When the pressure gauge initially drops below 745 psig on a nitrous oxide E-cylinder at room temperature, approximately how many liters of nitrous oxide are approximately remaining in the tank?

    (A) 1,590 L
    (B) 660 L
    (C) 400 L
    (D) 625 L

    Rationale: E-cylinder nitrous oxide tanks contain nitrous oxide in the liquid and gas state. The only accurate way to determine the amount of gas left in the tank is by weighing it. A full E-cylinder tank will hold 1,590 liters of nitrous oxide. When the liquid form is consumed and the tank pressure begins to drop below 745 psig, the amount of nitrous oxide in the gas phase is about 400 liters.
    References: Butterworth JF IV, Mackey DC, Wasnick JD, eds. *Morgan & Mikhail's Clinical Anesthesiology*. 7th ed. New York, NY: McGraw Hill; 2022: Chapter 4.
    Elisha S, Heiner JS, Nagelhout JJ. *Nurse Anesthesia*. 7th ed. St. Louis, MO: Elsevier Saunders; 2023: Chapter 16.

81. What is the only device that will ensure that oxygen is present in the pipelines or cylinder?

    (A) Oxygen analyzer
    (B) Hypoxic guard
    (C) Oxygen failsafe device
    (D) Cylinder gauge

    Rationale: The oxygen analyzer is the only device of the anesthesia workstation that will detect that oxygen is present in the machine. B, C, and D only detect pressure which does not necessarily denote which gas is present.

References: Butterworth JF IV, Mackey DC, Wasnick JD, eds. *Morgan & Mikhail's Clinical Anesthesiology*. 7th ed. New York, NY: McGraw Hill; 2022: Chapter 4.

Elisha S, Heiner JS, Nagelhout JJ. *Nurse Anesthesia*. 7th ed. St. Louis, MO: Elsevier Saunders; 2023: Chapter 16.

82. In a closed scavenging system, what component protects the patient from barotrauma if the scavenging suction fails or the hose distal to the system becomes kinked?

    (A) No component is available for protection and is the reason these systems are used anymore.

    (B) The design allows for waste gases to exit into the OR environment.

    (C) The negative pressure relief valve becomes kinked.

    (D) The positive pressure relief valve becomes kinked.

    Rationale: The positive pressure relief valve will open and allow waste gases to enter the OR environment if the suction is disrupted. The negative pressure relief valve opens if too much suction is applied. B refers to the open system.

    References: Butterworth JF IV, Mackey DC, Wasnick JD, eds. *Morgan & Mikhail's Clinical Anesthesiology*. 7th ed. New York, NY: McGraw Hill; 2022: Chapter 4.

    Elisha S, Heiner JS, Nagelhout JJ. *Nurse Anesthesia*. 7th ed. St. Louis, MO: Elsevier Saunders; 2023: Chapter 16.

83. Which type of waste-gas scavenger interface requires negative and positive pressure relief valves?

    (A) Passive open interface

    (B) Passive closed interface

    (C) Active closed interface

    (D) Active open interface

    Rationale: An active closed interface is closed to the outside atmosphere and requires negative and positive pressure relief valves that protect the patient from the negative pressure of the vacuum system and positive pressure from an obstruction in the disposal tubing.

    References: Butterworth JF IV, Mackey DC, Wasnick JD, eds. *Morgan & Mikhail's Clinical Anesthesiology*. 7th ed. New York, NY: McGraw Hill; 2022: Chapter 4.

    Elisha S, Heiner JS, Nagelhout JJ. *Nurse Anesthesia*. 7th ed. St. Louis, MO: Elsevier Saunders; 2023: Chapter 16.

84. Which organization published a generic checkout procedure for anesthesia gas machines and breathing circuits?

    (A) American Association of Nurse Anesthetist (AANA)

    (B) Department of Transportation (DOT)

    (C) Food and Drug Administration (FDA)

    (D) American Society for Testing and Materials (ASTM)

    Rationale: The Food and Drug Administration (FDA) published a generic checkout procedure for anesthesia gas machines and breathing circuits.

    References: Butterworth JF IV, Mackey DC, Wasnick JD, eds. *Morgan & Mikhail's Clinical Anesthesiology*. 7th ed. New York, NY: McGraw Hill; 2022: Chapter 4.

    Elisha S, Heiner JS, Nagelhout JJ. *Nurse Anesthesia*. 7th ed. St. Louis, MO: Elsevier Saunders; 2023: Chapter 16.

85. What component of the high-pressure system provides unidirectional flow to prevent transfilling or leakage of gases into the OR environment?

    (A) Pressure relief valve

    (B) Pressure regulator valve

    (C) Hypoxic guard

    (D) Check/unidirectional valve

    Rationale: The check valve of the cylinder hanger yoke (high pressure system) provides unidirectional flow to prevent transfilling or leakage of gases from the anesthesia machine to the atmosphere.

    References: Butterworth JF IV, Mackey DC, Wasnick JD, eds. *Morgan & Mikhail's Clinical Anesthesiology*. 7th ed. New York, NY: McGraw Hill; 2022: Chapter 4.

    Elisha S, Heiner JS, Nagelhout JJ. *Nurse Anesthesia*. 7th ed. St. Louis, MO: Elsevier Saunders; 2023: Chapter 16.

86. After opening the oxygen E-cylinder on the back of the anesthesia workstation to determine the pressure, what is the next step?

    (A) Leave open in case of pipeline failure

    (B) The oxygen E-cylinder is only for an emergency

    (C) Leave partly open

    (D) Close the cylinder

    Rationale: The oxygen E-cylinder should be closed because in the event pipeline pressure fails the anesthetist may not become aware until the emergency E oxygen cylinders are empty.

References: Butterworth JF IV, Mackey DC, Wasnick JD, eds. *Morgan & Mikhail's Clinical Anesthesiology.* 7th ed. New York, NY: McGraw Hill; 2022: Chapter 4.

Elisha S, Heiner JS, Nagelhout JJ. *Nurse Anesthesia.* 7th ed. St. Louis, MO: Elsevier Saunders; 2023: Chapter 16.

87. Which circuit design incorporates a fresh gas inlet tube (inspiratory limb) inside the breathing circuit?

(A) Mapleson D

(B) Bain circuit

(C) Mapleson A

(D) Mapleson B

Rationale: The Bain circuit is a modification of the Mapleson D breathing system. The circuit contains a fresh gas inlet tube inside the breathing tube (coaxial). Because of the modification, heat conservation and humidity exist. The circuit is less bulky. The lack modification of the Mapleson A is a coaxial system although the inner tube is the expiratory limb.

References: Butterworth JF IV, Mackey DC, Wasnick JD, eds. *Morgan & Mikhail's Clinical Anesthesiology.* 7th ed. New York, NY: McGraw Hill; 2022: Chapter 3.

Pardo MC Jr, ed. *Basics of Anesthesia.* 8th ed. Philadelphia, PA: Elsevier Saunders; 2023: Chapter 15.

88. During which phase of an anesthetic is the most precipitous heat loss in the patient?

(A) During the first perioperative hour

(B) Maintenance (second to fourth hours)

(C) Emergence

(D) Postoperative

Rationale: The greatest amount of heat loss occurs during the first hour in the perioperative setting. It begins in the preoperative setting and extends into the initial phase of the anesthetic. Afterward, hear loss continues unless effective warming measures are applied but at a reduced rate.

References: Butterworth JF IV, Mackey DC, Wasnick JD, eds. *Morgan & Mikhail's Clinical Anesthesiology.* 7th ed. New York, NY: McGraw Hill; 2022: Chapter 52.

Elisha S, Heiner JS, Nagelhout JJ. *Nurse Anesthesia.* 7th ed. St. Louis, MO: Elsevier Saunders; 2023: Chapter 18.

89. The formation of carbon monoxide by the degradation of volatile anesthetic due to dry soda lime is greatest with which agent?

(A) Desflurane

(B) Isoflurane

(C) Sevoflurane

(D) Nitrous oxide

Rationale: The drier the soda lime, the more likely that it absorbs and degrades volatile anesthetics. Volatile anesthetics can be broken down to carbon monoxide by dry absorbent to the extent that it can cause clinically significant carbon monoxide poisoning. The formation of carbon monoxide is highest with Desflurane.

References: Butterworth JF IV, Mackey DC, Wasnick JD, eds. *Morgan & Mikhail's Clinical Anesthesiology.* 7th ed. New York, NY: McGraw Hill; 2022: Chapter 3.

Elisha S, Heiner JS, Nagelhout JJ. *Nurse Anesthesia.* 7th ed. St. Louis, MO: Elsevier Saunders; 2023: Chapter 8.

90. Compound A is one of the by-products of degradation of which volatile anesthetic?

(A) Desflurane

(B) Isoflurane

(C) Sevoflurane

(D) Nitrous oxide

Rationale: Compound A is one of the by-products of degradation of sevoflurane by absorbent. Higher concentrations of sevoflurane, prolonged exposure, and low-flow anesthetic technique seem to increase the formation of Compound A. Compound A has been shown to produce nephrotoxicity in animals.

References: Butterworth JF IV, Mackey DC, Wasnick JD, eds. *Morgan & Mikhail's Clinical Anesthesiology.* 7th ed. New York, NY: McGraw Hill; 2022: Chapter 8.

Elisha S, Heiner JS, Nagelhout JJ. *Nurse Anesthesia.* 7th ed. St. Louis, MO: Elsevier Saunders; 2023: Chapter 8.

91. What is the end product of the soda lime reaction?

(A) CO_2

(B) Carbonic acid

(C) Calcium carbonate

(D) Ethyl violet

Rationale: Soda lime contains hydroxide salts that are capable of neutralizing carbonic acid. Reaction end products include heat, water, and calcium carbonate.

References: Butterworth JF IV, Mackey DC, Wasnick JD, eds. *Morgan & Mikhail's Clinical Anesthesiology.* 7th ed. New York, NY: McGraw Hill; 2022: Chapter 3.

Elisha S, Heiner JS, Nagelhout JJ. *Nurse Anesthesia.* 7th ed. St. Louis, MO: Elsevier Saunders; 2023: Chapter 16.

92. When should the LMA be removed?

(A) When the patient moves

(B) When the patient regains airway reflexes

(C) When the surgery is completed

(D) In the postanesthesia care unit

Rationale: Because the LMA is not fully protective of pharyngeal secretions, risk of aspiration remains. For this reason, ensure that the patient's airway reflexes have returned prior to removal.

Reference: Butterworth JF IV, Mackey DC, Wasnick JD, eds. *Morgan & Mikhail's Clinical Anesthesiology*. 7th ed. New York, NY: McGraw Hill; 2022: Chapter 56.

93. Which Mapleson circuit is a modification of the Mapleson D?

(A) Jackson-Reese

(B) Mapleson A

(C) Bain

(D) Mapleson C

Rationale: The Bain circuit is a coaxial adaptation of the Mapleson D system that incorporates the fresh gas inlet tubing inside the breathing tube. This modification decreases the circuit's bulkiness and preserves heat and humidity more effectively. A disadvantage of this circuit is the chance of kinking or detachment of the fresh gas inlet tubing.

References: Butterworth JF IV, Mackey DC, Wasnick JD, eds. *Morgan & Mikhail's Clinical Anesthesiology*. 7th ed. New York, NY: McGraw Hill; 2022: Chapter 3.
Elisha S, Heiner JS, Nagelhout JJ. *Nurse Anesthesia*. 7th ed. St. Louis, MO: Elsevier Saunders; 2023: Chapter 16.

94. Which statement is the most accurate description of the Diameter-Index Safety System (DISS)?

(A) Allows for orientation of gas cylinder to the yoke

(B) Prevents attaching wrong gas cylinders to anesthesia machine

(C) Avoids attaching a nongrounded electrical supply to anesthesia machine

(D) Prevents connection of the wrong pipeline gas supply hose to the anesthesia machine

Rationale: The DISS describes different size diameter fittings for each pipeline gas supply hose to the back of the anesthesia machine. A and B refer to the PISS.

References: Butterworth JF IV, Mackey DC, Wasnick JD, eds. *Morgan & Mikhail's Clinical Anesthesiology*. 7th ed. New York, NY: McGraw Hill; 2022: Chapter 4.
Elisha S, Heiner JS, Nagelhout JJ. *Nurse Anesthesia*. 7th ed. St. Louis, MO: Elsevier Saunders; 2023: Chapter 16.

95. What is your greatest concern when inflating the pulmonary artery balloon?

(A) Conduction abnormalities

(B) Pulmonary artery rupture

(C) Catheter knotting

(D) Bacteremia

Rationale: Each of the concerns is linked to complications associated with pulmonary artery catheters. Balloon over inflation and frequent wedge readings may be result in pulmonary artery rupture leading to death.

Reference: Butterworth JF IV, Mackey DC, Wasnick JD, eds. *Morgan & Mikhail's Clinical Anesthesiology*. 7th ed. New York, NY: McGraw Hill; 2022: Chapter 22.

96. Following intubation you are unable to palpate the tracheal tube cuff in the sternal notch. The breathing bag compliance is decreased. Breath sounds are unilateral. Where is the endotracheal tube most likely positioned?

(A) Hypopharynx

(B) Esophageal

(C) Supraglottic

(D) Right mainstem bronchus

Rationale: Bronchial intubation results in unilateral breath sounds, falling pulse oximetry values, inability to feel the tracheal tube, and high peak inspiratory pressures.

Reference: Butterworth JF IV, Mackey DC, Wasnick JD, eds. *Morgan & Mikhail's Clinical Anesthesiology*. 7th ed. New York, NY: McGraw Hill; 2022: Chapter 19.

97. What ultrasound (US) principle describes the manually adjusted amplification of US echoes returning from different depths of the tissue being scanned?

(A) Depth

(B) Focus

(C) Acoustic enhancement

(D) Time-gain compensation

Rationale: Time-gain compensation refers to the manual amplification of US echoes returning from tissues at different depths. This is achieved by the computer determining the time it takes for the echoes to return depending on the depth of the tissues.

Reference: Farag E, Mounir-Soliman L, Brown DL. *Brown's Atlas of Regional Anesthesia.* 6th ed. Philadelphia, PA: Elsevier; 2021: Chapter 3.

98. What type of artifact refers to the loss of ultrasound echoes returning from tissue deep to a strong reflector such as a metal implant or bone?

   (A) Acoustic enhancement

   (B) Shadowing

   (C) Mirror

   (D) Reverberation

   Rationale: US waves do not penetrate well through strong reflectors (dense tissues such as bone or metal implants). As a result, there will be little to none reflected echoes deep to the strong reflector. Acoustic enhancement is the enhancement of returning echoes of tissue deep to a fluid-filled structure like the bladder or a blood vessel.

   References: Farag E, Mounir-Soliman L, Brown DL. *Brown's Atlas of Regional Anesthesia.* 6th ed. Philadelphia, PA: Elsevier; 2021: Chapter 3.

   Gropper MA, Cohen NH, Eriksson LI, et al, eds. *Miller's Anesthesia.* 9th ed. Philadelphia, PA: Churchill Livingstone Elsevier; 2020; Chapter 37.

99. Which ultrasound mode will produce the best depiction of ventricular wall motion over time for the purpose of quantitative measurement?

   (A) A mode

   (B) B mode

   (C) M mode

   (D) Color Doppler

   Rationale: M mode refers to the display of the motion of tissues (cardiac wall motion) relative to time. A mode is not used. B mode is the two-dimensional imaging of tissues real time. Color Doppler assigns a color to the movement of blood through vessels.

   Reference: Gropper MA, Cohen NH, Eriksson LI, et al, eds. *Miller's Anesthesia.* 9th ed. Philadelphia, PA: Churchill Livingstone Elsevier; 2020; Chapter 37.

100. What ultrasound principle describes the change in frequency of the echoes reflecting from fluid either moving away or toward the transducer?

   (A) Doppler shift

   (B) Spectral analysis

   (C) Acoustic impedance

   (D) Refraction

   Rationale: If an ultrasound pulse is sent out and strikes moving red blood cells, the ultrasound that is reflected to the transducer will have a frequency that is different from the original emitted frequency. This change in frequency is known as the *Doppler shift.*

   References: Gropper MA, Cohen NH, Eriksson LI, et al, eds. *Miller's Anesthesia.* 9th ed. Philadelphia, PA: Churchill Livingstone Elsevier; 2020: Chapter 37.

   Farag E, Mounir-Soliman L, Brown DL. *Brown's Atlas of Regional Anesthesia.* 6th ed. Philadelphia, PA: Elsevier; 2021: Chapter 3.

101. At what angle of incidence/insonation produces the greatest reflection of ultrasound waves from a tissue target?

   (A) 0 degrees

   (B) 45 degrees

   (C) 60 degrees

   (D) 90 degrees

   Rationale: The angle of incidence/insonation refers to the angle (in degrees) of the transmitted ultrasound beam as it contacts the target. The angle producing the greatest number of reflected US waves is perpendicular to the target (90 degrees). At angles greater or less than 90 degrees, more US waves will be refracted.

   References: Gropper MA, Cohen NH, Eriksson LI, et al, eds. *Miller's Anesthesia.* 9th ed. Philadelphia, PA: Churchill Livingstone Elsevier; 2020; Chapter 37.

   Farag E, Mounir-Soliman L, Brown DL. *Brown's Atlas of Regional Anesthesia.* 6th ed. Philadelphia, PA: Elsevier; 2021: Chapter 3.

CHAPTER 3

Basic Principles
Questions

1. When do symptoms of ischemic optic neuropathy that result in postoperative vision loss typically first occur?

   (A) Immediately postoperatively
   (B) 2 hours postoperatively
   (C) 2 days postoperatively
   (D) 2 weeks postoperatively

2. During a general anesthetic you suspect an episode of MH. What will you do first?

   (A) Call the MHAUS hotline.
   (B) Administer dantrolene.
   (C) Inform the surgeon.
   (D) Turn off inhalational agents.

3. When is body temperature loss the greatest?

   (A) During the preoperative preparation
   (B) During the first hour in the operating room
   (C) During the second and third hour in the operating room
   (D) During the fourth hour in the operating room

4. For an awake fiberoptic intubation, anesthesia for the posterior 1/3 of the tongue, vallecula, anterior epiglottis, walls of the pharynx, and tonsils can be performed by injecting local anesthetic into which of the following structures?

   (A) Base of the frenulum
   (B) Palatoglossal arch
   (C) Thyroid membrane
   (D) Cricothyroid membrane

5. Which is an example of sensation without stimulus?

   (A) Temporal summation
   (B) Dynamic allodynia

   (C) Paresthesia
   (D) Analgesia

6. Which statement about stored blood is correct?

   (A) The amount of extracellular potassium transfused per unit is 10 mEq per unit.
   (B) Stored blood typically has a pH less than 7.45.
   (C) Stored blood contains factors V and VIII.
   (D) Stored blood can contain as much as 150 mEq/L of potassium.

7. Which patient is least likely to aspirate?

   (A) Second trimester parturient
   (B) Gastroesophageal reflux
   (C) First trimester parturient
   (D) NPO < 6 hours

8. What percent of the total body water is extracellular?

   (A) 67%
   (B) 33%
   (C) 25%
   (D) 100%

9. Which drug is not a trigger for malignant hyperthermia?

   (A) Halothane
   (B) Sevoflurane
   (C) Brevital
   (D) Succinylcholine

10. How is the brachial plexus formed?

    (A) Roots, divisions, trunks, cords, branches
    (B) Divisions, trunks, cords, branches
    (C) Cords, divisions, roots, branches
    (D) Trunks, divisions, cords, branches

11. Which laboratory test provides the most comprehensive assessment of coagulation in a patient with severe cirrhosis?

(A) International normalized ratio
(B) Prothrombin time
(C) Partial thromboplastin time
(D) Thromboelastography

12. Where does the spinal cord end in adults?

(A) L_1
(B) L_2
(C) L_3
(D) L_4

13. A 25-kg infant has a preoperative hematocrit of 40%. What volume of blood loss will decrease the hematocrit from 36% to 30%?

(A) 250 mL
(B) 360 mL
(C) 400 mL
(D) 450 mL

14. Which cranial nerve (CN) provides sensation to the posterior one-third of the tongue?

(A) CN I
(B) CN V
(C) CN IX
(D) CN X

15. Which patient is more likely to experience complications when using a hypotensive technique?

(A) Uncontrolled glaucoma
(B) Myesthenia gravis
(C) Multiple sclerosis
(D) Osteoarthritis

16. What is the smallest volume of infused ABO-incompatible donor blood that will cause an acute hemolytic reaction?

(A) 40 to 60 mL
(B) 25 to 30 mL
(C) 10 to 15 mL
(D) 1 to 3 mL

17. Which risk factor does not predispose patients to lower extremity neuropathy?

(A) Hypertension
(B) Surgery <2 hours
(C) Thin body habitus
(D) Cigarette smoking

18. What is the mechanism of action of a transcutaneous electrical nerve stimulation (TENS) unit?

(A) TENS stimulation of large diameter afferent nerve fibers competitively blocks pain signals from smaller fibers.
(B) TENS stimulation of small diameter afferent nerve fibers competitively blocks pain signals from larger fibers.
(C) TENS stimulation damages the small afferent fibers conducting the pain signals.
(D) TENS stimulation induces a signal conduction interruption in large diameter fibers.

19. What are the primary adductors of the vocal cords?

(A) Lateral cricoarytenoid muscles
(B) Recurrent laryngeal nerve
(C) Posterior cricoarytenoid muscles
(D) External laryngeal nerve

20. Which group lists the vitamin K–dependent clotting factors?

(A) II, VII, IX, X
(B) II, IV, IX, XII
(C) III, VII, X, XI
(D) I, VII, IX, XI

21. Which of the following chemical mediators is released from peripheral afferent C fibers resulting in dull pain?

(A) Substance P
(B) Glutamate
(C) Histamine
(D) Serotonin

22. To supplement a brachial plexus block to cover the anterior shoulder, the cervical plexus can be blocked at which of the following locations?

(A) Anterior to the mastoid process
(B) The posterior border of the sternocleidomastoid

(C) At the interscalene groove

(D) Posterior to the angle of the mandible

23. Following general endotracheal anesthesia the patient is in respiratory distress and is unable to speak. What nerve(s) may be injured?

(A) Unilateral recurrent laryngeal nerve

(B) Bilateral superior laryngeal nerve

(C) Unilateral superior laryngeal nerve

(D) Bilateral vagus nerves

24. A patient's serum potassium level is 7.2 mEq/L. In which sequential order will cardiac manifestations of hyperkalemia progress?

(A) Peaked T waves, loss of P wave, widened QRS complex, sine wave

(B) Peaked T waves, widened QRS complex, loss of P wave, sine wave

(C) Loss of R-wave amplitude, peaked T waves, widened QRS complex, sine wave

(D) Prolonged P-R interval, peaked T waves, widened QRS complex, asystole

25. Which of the following is not a physiologic response to pain?

(A) Increased peripheral vascular resistance

(B) Decreased tidal volume

(C) Increased platelet aggregation

(D) Decreased urinary sphincter tone

26. What is the treatment of choice for hyponatremic patients with decreased total body sodium content?

(A) 0.9% NS

(B) D5. ½NS

(C) 0.5 NS

(D) 3% NS

27. What statement is false regarding nasal airways?

(A) Nasal airways are 2 to 4 cm shorter than oral airways.

(B) Thrombocytopenia is a contraindication.

(C) Nasal airways are 2 to 4 cm longer than oral airways.

(D) Basilar skull fracture is a contraindication.

28. A patient-controlled analgesia order is written. What is the lockout interval for morphine?

(A) 8 to 20 minutes

(B) 5 to 10 minutes

(C) 10 to 15 minutes

(D) 15 to 18 minutes

29. A patient taking duloxetine for chronic neuropathic pain is scheduled for a cholecystectomy. How is duloxetine classified?

(A) Tricyclic antidepressant

(B) Selective serotonin reuptake inhibitor

(C) Serotonin-norepinephrine reuptake inhibitor

(D) Non-selective serotonin reuptake inhibitor

30. What is the rationale for rapidly freezing plasma for the purpose of making fresh frozen plasma?

(A) Rapid freezing prevents the inactivation of factors VIII and I.

(B) Rapid freezing prevents the inactivation of factors V and VIII.

(C) Rapid freezing prevents the inactivation of all the factors.

(D) Rapid freezing prevents the inactivation of antithrombin III.

31. Which of the following is not a risk factor for developing cauda equine syndrome?

(A) 5% lidocaine spinal anesthesia

(B) Use of glucose to increase baricity of neuraxial anesthetics

(C) Epidural anesthesia

(D) Continuous spinal anesthesia (CSA)

32. How soon must fresh frozen plasma be transfused once thawed?

(A) Within 4 hours

(B) Within 8 hours

(C) Within 12 hours

(D) Within 24 hours

33. Preoxygenation/denitrogenation results in how many minutes of oxygen reserve?

    (A) 1 to 3 minutes
    (B) 3 to 6 minutes
    (C) 5 to 8 minutes
    (D) >8 minutes

34. Which patient should receive a type and crossmatch instead of a type and screen prior to surgery?

    (A) A 48-year-old female scheduled for an endovascular stent of an aortic aneurysm
    (B) An obese 12-year male undergoing an emergency tonsillectomy
    (C) A 22-year-old male with no history of multiple blood transfusions
    (D) A pregnant Rh-positive patient with Rh-negative baby undergoing emergency surgery

35. A 150-kg male patient has a serum sodium concentration of 110 mEq/L. How much sodium would be needed to bring the serum sodium to 125 mEq/L?

    (A) 750 mEq
    (B) 1,350 mEq
    (C) 2,400 mEq
    (D) 3,200 mEq

36. How much blood does a fully soaked laparotomy "lap" pad contain?

    (A) 10 to 20 mL
    (B) 25 to 50 mL
    (C) 50 to 100 mL
    (D) 100 to 150 mL

37. Six hours after a patient received transfusion with 2 units of fresh frozen plasma and 1 unit of platelets, she presents with hypoxia, fever, and noncardiogenic pulmonary edema. What complication do you suspect?

    (A) Post-transfusion purpura
    (B) Transfusion-related acute lung injury
    (C) Delayed hemolytic reaction
    (D) Transfusion-related immunomodulation

38. A 44-year-old 50-kg male received 750 mL of fresh frozen plasma. What percent of normal would you expect his clotting factor concentration to achieve post-transfusion?

    (A) 100%
    (B) 75%
    (C) 60%
    (D) 30%

39. For which infectious diseases is donor blood tested after it is collected, typed, and screened?

    (A) Hepatitis A, hepatitis B, and hepatitis C
    (B) Hepatitis B, hepatitis C, and hepatitis D
    (C) Hepatitis C, syphilis, and human immunodeficiency virus
    (D) Hepatitis C, cytomegalovirus (CMV), and syphilis

40. Which is not an indication for cryoprecipitate administration?

    (A) Fibrinogen levels <80 to 100 mg/dL
    (B) Factor XIII deficiency
    (C) Antithrombin deficiency
    (D) Pre-op prophylaxis for patient with von Willebrand disease

41. Which factor is not a complication associated with massive blood transfusion?

    (A) Serum K^+ 5.5
    (B) Core temperature 35.5°C
    (C) Increased 2,3-DPG
    (D) Decreased 2,3-DPG

42. What is the approximate half-life of serum albumin?

    (A) 12 hours
    (B) 6 days
    (C) 10 days
    (D) 21 days

43. Which of the following nerves must be separately blocked during an axillary approach to the brachial plexus?

    (A) Musculocutaneous
    (B) Ulnar
    (C) Medial Brachial Cutaneous
    (D) Median

44. What is the most effective initial treatment of symptomatic hypercalcemia?

    (A) Hydration with IV normal saline followed by furosemide

    (B) Thiazide followed by IV normal saline hydration

    (C) Hydration with IV normal saline followed by bisphosphonates

    (D) Glucocorticoids followed by IV normal saline hydration

45. Caudal anesthesia involves needle penetration of the sacrococcygeal ligament covering the sacral hiatus created by which unfused laminae?

    (A) S_1 and S_2

    (B) S_2 and S_3

    (C) S_3 and S_4

    (D) S_4 and S_5

46. A 154 lb female has a serum sodium level 120 mEq/L. To correct the sodium level to 128 mEq, how many milliequivalents of sodium are required?

    (A) 280 mEq

    (B) 336 mEq

    (C) 616 mEq

    (D) 739 mEq

47. C fibers transmit what type of sensation?

    (A) Proprioception

    (B) Touch-pressure

    (C) Somatic pain

    (D) Visceral pain

48. Which nerve provides sensory innervation to the lateral thigh?

    (A) Lateral femoral cutaneous

    (B) Saphenous

    (C) Femoral

    (D) Posterior femoral cutaneous

49. An axillary block is performed for a surgical procedure on the right forearm and hand. The patient begins to experience pain at the tip of the index finger during the procedure. An effective rescue block would involve injecting local into which of the following sites?

    (A) Antecubital space at the lateral aspect of the biceps tendon

    (B) Antecubital crease medial to the biceps insertion

    (C) One finger breadth proximal to the arcuate ligament

    (D) Immediately lateral to the flexor carpi ulnaris

50. Which of the following is associated with slow pain?

    (A) Myelinated A-delta primary efferents

    (B) Action potential 0.5 to 2 m/s

    (C) Myelinated A-delta primary afferents

    (D) Action potential 6 to 30 m/s

51. A patient is having pain on the dorsum of the foot and the lateral aspect of the knee. What nerve root is involved?

    (A) L_3

    (B) L_5

    (C) L_4

    (D) S_1

52. Which of the following patients are at greatest risk for postdural puncture headaches?

    (A) Obese

    (B) Elderly

    (C) Pregnant

    (D) Pediatric

53. While performing an axillary block utilizing the transarterial approach, a paresthesia is elicited after passing through the artery. Which nerve is posterior to the artery?

    (A) Ulnar

    (B) Radial

    (C) Median

    (D) Intercostobrachial

54. A patient receives large volumes of 0.9% normal saline during a case. What is the risk associated with this?

    (A) Hypochloremic alkalosis

    (B) Hyperchloremic alkalosis

    (C) Hypochloremic acidosis

    (D) Hyperchloremic acidosis

55. What causes hypocalcemia?

(A) Hypoparathyroidism
(B) Paget's disease (hypercalcemia)
(C) Fat embolism
(D) Rapid infusion of 1,000 mL normal saline

56. Which of the following local anesthetics should be avoided in a glucose-6-phosphate dehydrogenase (G₆PD) deficiency?

(A) Ropivacaine
(B) Etidocaine
(C) Prilocaine
(D) Tetracaine

57. You plan to use an intravenous regional technique for hand surgery. What is your greatest concern?

(A) Duration of the case
(B) Using the dual tourniquet system
(C) Tourniquet discomfort
(D) Tourniquet failure

58. Removal of epidural catheters should be delayed for a minimum of how many hours following the administration of prophylactic low molecular weight heparin (LMWH)?

(A) 1
(B) 12
(C) 3
(D) 6

59. When performing an ankle block, which of the following nerves is located by identifying the groove formed proximally by the extensor hallucis longus tendon and the extensor digitorum longus tendon?

(A) Saphenous
(B) Deep peroneal
(C) Posterior tibial
(D) Sural

60. Which of the following terms is defined as perception of an ordinary non-noxious stimulus as pain?

(A) Hyperalgesia
(B) Allodynia
(C) Hyperesthesia
(D) Dysesthesia

61. What is your main anesthetic concern when caring for a patient taking anabolic steroids?

(A) Myocardial infarction
(B) Hepatotoxicity
(C) Hypercoagulopathy
(D) Stroke

62. Injecting local anesthetic at which site is associated with the greatest risk of systemic absorption?

(A) Brachial plexus
(B) Paracervical
(C) Intercostal
(D) Caudal

63. Which topical local anesthetic may cause methemoglobinemia?

(A) Bupivacaine
(B) Procaine
(C) Mepivacaine
(D) Benzocaine

64. Which of the following factors has the greatest effect on the level of spinal anesthesia?

(A) Age
(B) Patient height
(C) Position of patient during injection
(D) Drug volume

65. A female patient's preoperative hematocrit is 42%. How much blood could a 90-kg patient lose and still maintain a hematocrit of 30%?

(A) 702 mL
(B) 2,106 mL
(C) 2,457 mL
(D) 5,850 mL

66. Interruption of pain impulses can be accomplished through the administration of intrathecal opioids. These opioids act by binding to which of the following sites?

(A) Periaqueductal gray
(B) Dorsal root ganglia
(C) Anterior horn
(D) Dorsal horn

67. Epidural morphine was administered for postoperative pain control. What is the duration of action?

    (A) 12 to 24 hours
    (B) 4 to 6 hours
    (C) 24 to 48 hours
    (D) 2 to 6 hours

68. A 20-kg child is scheduled for a urology procedure. What is the appropriate dose for a caudal anesthetic?

    (A) 10 mL
    (B) 5 mL
    (C) 3 mL
    (D) 25 mL

69. Which of the following peripheral nerve blocks would provide the most effective analgesia for a total knee arthroplasty?

    (A) Femoral nerve block
    (B) Femoral nerve block and obturator nerve block
    (C) Sciatic nerve block and psoas block
    (D) Sciatic and popliteal block

70. Which mechanisms of action are common among nonsteroidal anti-inflammatory drugs?

    (A) Inhibition of cyclooxygenase and prostaglandin synthesis
    (B) Promotes release of serotonin
    (C) Inhibition of lipoxygenase
    (D) Inhibition of leukotriene synthesis

71. What factor is not associated with postoperative pulmonary complications?

    (A) ASA III
    (B) Cigarette smoking
    (C) Aortic aneurysm repair
    (D) Surgery lasting 2 hours

72. Which muscle is likely to be unaffected by an axillary brachial plexus block?

    (A) Abductor pollicis brevis
    (B) Interosseous
    (C) Brachialis
    (D) Pronator teres

73. Which of the following does not define somatic nociceptive pain?

    (A) Transduction
    (B) Transmission
    (C) Thermal
    (D) Modulation

74. During an unremarkable spinal anesthetic a bilateral T_2 level in a healthy parturient results in cardiac arrest. Which of the following is most likely responsible?

    (A) Decreased preload
    (B) Effect of local anesthetic on the medulla
    (C) Blockade of the carotid sinus
    (D) Cardiogenic hypertensive chemoreflex

75. Which medication should be held on the day of surgery?

    (A) Beta-adrenergic blockers
    (B) Tricyclic antidepressants
    (C) Selective serotonin reuptake inhibitors
    (D) Beta-adrenergic blocker combinations

76. What nerve injury results most often with the lithotomy position?

    (A) Common peroneal
    (B) Sciatic
    (C) Obturator
    (D) Saphenous

77. Which of the following explains the rapid onset of 2-chloroprocaine when used for epidural anesthesia?

    (A) It is activated by ester hydrolysis.
    (B) It is administered in high concentrations.
    (C) It has high potency and lipid solubility.
    (D) It has relatively low pKa.

78. A patient taking furosemide is scheduled for a total knee arthroscopy. What statement is true?

    (A) Continue in patients with chronic renal failure
    (B) Discontinue
    (C) Continue in patients with diabetes
    (D) Discontinue in the elderly

79. What discontinuation issues may result for patients who take angiotensin converting enzyme (ACE) inhibitors?

    (A) Potential clotting abnormalities
    (B) Cholinergic symptoms and psychosis
    (C) Rebound hypertension
    (D) Reduced atrial compliance

80. What is the preexisting fluid deficit for a 13-kg patient fasting for 6 hours?

    (A) 46 mL/h
    (B) 53 mL/h
    (C) 138 mL/h
    (D) 276 mL/h

81. Which of the following elements in the postoperative note is not required by the Center for Medicare and Medicaid Services (CMS)?

    (A) Mental status
    (B) Temperature
    (C) Pain
    (D) Urine output

82. Which nerve is blocked by injection through the thyrohyoid membrane to anesthetize the area between the vocal cords and the epiglottis?

    (A) Hypoglossal
    (B) Recurrent laryngeal
    (C) Superior laryngeal
    (D) Glossopharyngeal

83. Tachycardia, euphoria, delirium, and excitement are noted when conducting the preoperative evaluation in the emergency department. Which of the following is probably not related to the symptoms?

    (A) Narcotics
    (B) Cocaine
    (C) Hallucinogens
    (D) Marijuana

84. Which of the following may cause prolonged sedation?

    (A) Echinacea and garlic
    (B) Ephedra and garlic
    (C) Garlic and kava kava
    (D) Kava kava and valerian

85. Calculate the ideal body weight (BW) for a 6', 90-kg male.

    (A) 80 kg
    (B) 177 kg
    (C) 72 kg
    (D) 145 kg

86. A morbidly obese male patient is scheduled for a bariatric surgery. Which of the following diagnostic tests should be ordered?

    (A) Chest x-ray and coagulation studies
    (B) 12 lead EKG and hCG
    (C) Coagulation studies and glucose tolerance test
    (D) hCG

87. A patient with two peripheral intravenous (PIV) lines is undergoing GETA for an orthopedic procedure. A recent lab value reveals a serum potassium level of 2.9 mEq/L. Which intervention is appropriate for this patient?

    (A) Administer IV replacement K^+ in dextrose solutions
    (B) Maintain $ETCO_2$ levels between 25 and 30 mmHg
    (C) Reduce the rocuronium redose by 25 to 50%
    (D) Administer IV replacement K^+ 20 mEq IV in 0.9% NS over 1 hour

88. What is the primary innervation of the lumbar facet joint?

    (A) The spinal nerve at the level of the joint
    (B) The spinal nerve superior to the joint
    (C) Both the nerve at the joint level and the nerve immediately superior
    (D) Neither the superior nor the inferior spinal nerve

89. What is the gold standard diagnostic test for obstructive sleep apnea?

    (A) Polysomnography
    (B) STOP-bang questionnaire
    (C) STOP questionnaire
    (D) Bang questionnaire

90. A patient with rheumatoid arthritis is undergoing a total knee replacement. What is the recommended glucocorticoid dosing regimen?

    (A) Usual corticosteroid dose + hydrocortisone 25 mg

    (B) Usual corticosteroid dose + hydrocortisone 100 mg

    (C) Usual corticosteroid dose + 150 mg

    (D) Usual corticosteroid dose + 50 mg

91. Which diagnostic finding is consistent with intracranial hypertension?

    (A) MRI with a 0.5-mm midline brain shift

    (B) CT with a 0.5-cm midline brain shift

    (C) CT with contrast with a 0.4-cm midline brain shift

    (D) MRI with a 0.4-cm midline brain shift

92. Which surgical procedure poses the lowest risk for myocardial infarction within 30 days of surgery?

    (A) Liver transplant

    (B) Prostatectomy

    (C) Liver resection

    (D) Cataract

93. What is the most common cause of nonsurgical bleeding following massive blood transfusion?

    (A) Dilutional thrombocytopenia

    (B) Citrate toxicity

    (C) Dilution of factors V and X

    (D) Dilution of factors II and VIII

94. The patient weighs 120 kg. The ideal body weight is 60 kg. What is the patient's classification?

    (A) Obese

    (B) Morbidly obese

    (C) Overweight

    (D) Moderate obesity

95. An adult patient's platelet count is 25,000/μL. After transfusing the patient with 2 units of apheresis platelets, what would you expect the platelet count to be?

    (A) 30,000 to 35,000/μL

    (B) 55,000 to 85,000/μL

    (C) 85,000 to 145,000/μL

    (D) 145,000 to 165,000/μL

96. During the preoperative interview the patient shares that they perform light housework, play golf once a week and walk to the grocery store to get the newspaper. What is their metabolic equivalent (METs)?

    (A) 1 MET

    (B) 2 METs

    (C) 3 METs

    (D) 4 METs

97. What AANA Standard guides the practice of providing postanesthesia report?

    (A) Standard I

    (B) Standard III

    (C) Standard V

    (D) Standard XI

98. Which statement about fresh frozen plasma (FFP) administration is correct?

    (A) Each unit of FFP will increase the level of each clotting factor by 2 to 3% in adults.

    (B) The initial therapeutic dose is 1 to 5 mL/kg.

    (C) It should be ABO-compatible.

    (D) It must be Rh-compatible.

99. Which of the following are risk factors for postoperative nausea and vomiting?

    (A) Male gender

    (B) History of motion sickness and opioids

    (C) Opioids and laser retinal surgery

    (D) Cataract surgery

100. Which of the following statements is true regarding airway blocks?

    (A) Topical lidocaine may produce methemoglobinemia.

    (B) 4% lidocaine is injected into the trachea upon inspiration.

    (C) Nerve blocks of the airway pose risk for aspiration.

    (D) Local anesthesia to the mouth and pharynx blocks nerve transmission from the superior laryngeal nerve.

101. A patient is admitted to the postanesthesia care unit with shallow, rapid respirations, diaphoresis, and tachycardia. What is the most likely cause?

(A) Delayed awakening

(B) Hypothermia

(C) Emergence delirium

(D) Inadequate oxygenation

102. The anesthesia plan includes using topical cocaine for nasal surgery. What is the maximum dose?

(A) 50 mg

(B) 200 mg

(C) 400 mg

(D) 40 mg

103. What factors are associated with hypotension in the postanesthesia care unit?

(A) Hypervolemia

(B) Nausea

(C) Shivering

(D) Pain

104. What constitutes the eutectic mixture of local anesthetic?

(A) Benzocaine and prilocaine

(B) Prilocaine and tetracaine

(C) Lidocaine and prilocaine

(D) Prilocaine and lidocaine

105. During postanesthesia recovery the patient is snoring and use of the accessory muscle for ventilation are noted. What is the most likely cause?

(A) Airway obstruction

(B) Hypoventilation

(C) Hypoxemia

(D) Bronchospasm

106. Gabapentin is most helpful in treating which type of pain?

(A) Acute somatic pain

(B) Deep visceral pain

(C) Neuropathic pain

(D) Chronic arthritic joint pain

107. When using EMLA cream, what is the maximum total dose for children >20 kg?

(A) 20 g

(B) 10 g

(C) 2 g

(D) 1 g

108. Which peripheral nerve block provides complete anesthesia for ankle surgery?

(A) Femoral

(B) Sciatic

(C) Obturator

(D) Popliteal

109. Which nerve block results in the highest blood level of local anesthetic?

(A) Sciatic

(B) Intercostal

(C) Paravertebral

(D) Cervical plexus

110. What are the fluid requirements for redistribution and evaporative surgical fluid losses during a bowl resection?

(A) 0 to 2 mL/kg

(B) 2 to 4 mL/kg

(C) 4 to 8 mL/kg

(D) 10 to 14 mL/kg

111. Which airway block provides anesthesia below the vocal cords?

(A) Superior laryngeal nerve block and transtracheal block

(B) Tonsillar block

(C) Glossopharyngeal block

(D) Instilling local anesthetic onto the vocal cords

112. Which of the following landmarks form the lumbar plexus?

(A) L1–3 and T-10

(B) L1–4 and T-10

(C) L1–4 and T-12

(D) L1–3 and T-12

113. What results when placing a femoral block with nerve stimulation?

    (A) Thigh adduction
    (B) Quadriceps twitch
    (C) Sciatic nerve block posterior approach
    (D) Sciatic nerve block anterior approach

114. Which phrase describes radiculopathy?

    (A) Abnormal sensation with or without a stimulus
    (B) Pain linked to noxious stimulation
    (C) Nerve distribution pain
    (D) Abnormal function of nerve roots

115. Which of the following is not a pain modulating excitatory neurotransmitters?

    (A) Glycine
    (B) Calcitonin
    (C) Adenosine
    (D) Asparate

116. Which of the following physiological effects results from acute pain stimulation?

    (A) Increased myocardial workload
    (B) Increased vital capacity
    (C) Increased gastric emptying
    (D) Decreased platelet aggregation

117. Vocal cord paralysis occurred following intubation. What is the most likely cause?

    (A) Recurrent laryngeal nerve damage
    (B) Epiglottic damage
    (C) Esophageal damage
    (D) Superior laryngeal nerve

118. A patient with a history of hiatal hernia, diabetes mellitus, and peripheral neuropathy is scheduled for a bowel resection. Which fasting guideline applies?

    (A) NPO for 8 hours
    (B) Clear fluids up to 2 hours
    (C) Light meal up to 6 hours
    (D) NPO for 4 hours

119. A 40-year-old male with a history of well-controlled hypertension is scheduled for a carpal tunnel release. How will you classify the patient?

    (A) ASA-PS IV
    (B) ASA-PS III
    (C) ASA-PS II
    (D) ASA-PS I

120. During the preoperative airway exam, you visualize the soft palate, faces, and uvula. How would you classify the patient's airway?

    (A) Mallampati I
    (B) Mallampati III
    (C) Mallampati II
    (D) Mallampati IV

121. A patient's lab values reveal digoxin toxicity and hyperkalemia. Which option for treating hyperkalemia will you need to avoid in this patient?

    (A) 10 units regular insulin with 30 to 50 g dextrose 50% IV
    (B) 3 to 5 mL of 10% calcium chloride IV
    (C) 45 mEq sodium bicarbonate IV
    (D) 30 g kayexalate PR

122. A patient is scheduled for knee arthroscopy. The blood glucose is markedly elevated along with the A_{1c}. What will you do first?

    (A) Notify the surgeon that the surgery will be delayed.
    (B) Proceed with the surgery.
    (C) Cancel the surgery.
    (D) Call the endocrinologist.

123. What is the primary intracellular cation?

    (A) Potassium
    (B) Sodium
    (C) Calcium
    (D) Chloride

124. What mechanism results in the greatest amount of heat loss in the operating room?

    (A) Convection
    (B) Evaporation
    (C) Radiation
    (D) Conduction

125. What is the average blood volume of an 86-kg male?

(A) 5 L

(B) 6 L

(C) 5.2 L

(D) 6.8 L

126. How much additional fluid will you administer to a patient undergoing herniorrhaphy?

(A) 4 to 8 mL/kg

(B) 0 to 2 mL/kg

(C) 2 to 4 mL/kg

(D) 10 mL/kg

127. What statement is true regarding colloids?

(A) Inexpensive

(B) Increase plasma volume

(C) Used for initial resuscitation

(D) Used primarily for extracellular expansion

128. While receiving a blood transfusion during general anesthesia tachycardia and hypotension develop. What is the most likely cause?

(A) Delayed hemolytic reaction

(B) Anaphylactic reaction

(C) Urticarial reaction

(D) Acute hemolytic reaction

129. What statement is true regarding a patient who is awake in a supine position?

(A) The blood pressure decreases due to autoregulation.

(B) Venous return decreases.

(C) Blood pressure remains relatively constant.

(D) Sympathetic outflow increases.

130. What effect does the lithotomy position have on arterial pressure?

(A) Lower than supine position

(B) Higher than supine position

(C) Lower than Trendelenburg

(D) Lower than sitting position

131. A patient experiences low vision following a lumbar laminectomy in the prone position. What is the etiology?

(A) Decreased intracranial pressure

(B) Decreased venous pressure

(C) Increased cerebral blood flow

(D) Decreased ocular perfusion pressure

132. Where will you measure the blood pressure for patients undergoing surgery in the lateral decubitus position?

(A) Nondependent arm

(B) Both arms

(C) Dependent arm

(D) Right thigh

133. A sudden decrease in SpO_2, blood pressure, and $ETCO_2$ occur during general anesthesia. A mill-wheel murmur exists. What is the most likely cause?

(A) Venous air embolism

(B) Pneumocephalus

(C) Fat embolism

(D) Cardiovascular accident

134. What nerve injury is most likely when the arm is pronated?

(A) Brachial plexus

(B) Ulnar nerve

(C) Radial nerve

(D) Suprascapular nerve

135. In the supine position, what nerve injury is associated with arm abduction >90 degrees and lateral rotation of the head?

(A) Ulnar nerve

(B) Brachial plexus

(C) Radial nerve

(D) Suprascapular nerve

136. Following surgery in the lithotomy position the patient exhibits foot drop and the inability to extend the toes. What nerves are most likely injured?

(A) Sciatic and common peroneal

(B) Femoral and sciatic

(C) Common peroneal and femoral

(D) Obturator and sciatic

137. Which patient requires a preoperative chest x-ray?

    (A) 55-year-old smoker undergoing a laparoscopic cholecystectomy

    (B) 65-year-old chronic stable bronchitic undergoing a carpal tunnel release

    (C) 60-year-old undergoing a transurethral resection of the prostate

    (D) 50-year-old undergoing a mitral valve replacement

138. What is the average distance from the skin to the epidural space?

    (A) 1 cm

    (B) 1.5 cm

    (C) 5 cm

    (D) 7.5 cm

139. What statement is false regarding the lateral decubitus position?

    (A) Rhabdomyolysis may occur.

    (B) Flex the dependent arm <90 degrees.

    (C) Pad the lateral aspect of the dependent leg.

    (D) Pulmonary blood flow to the dependent lung decreases.

140. In what position is a venous air embolism (VAE) most likely to occur?

    (A) Lateral decubitus

    (B) Sitting

    (C) Prone

    (D) Trendelenburg

141. A T_6 sensory level is identified following administration of a spinal anesthetic. At what level is the sympathetic block?

    (A) T_4

    (B) T_{10}

    (C) T_6

    (D) T_8

142. In which patient is spinal anesthesia contraindicated?

    (A) 30-year-old who takes daily garlic

    (B) 50-year-old taking subcutaneous heparin injections

    (C) 25-year-old taking NSAIDs

    (D) 40-year-old who received thrombolytic therapy

143. What factor least affects the spread of spinal local anesthetic?

    (A) Baricity

    (B) Drug dosage

    (C) Site of injection

    (D) Drug volume

144. How do transient neurologic symptoms (TNS) differ from cauda equina syndrome?

    (A) TNS persists for several weeks following surgery.

    (B) Cauda equina syndrome disappears within 10 days following surgery.

    (C) TNS symptoms spontaneously disappear.

    (D) Cauda equina syndrome symptoms include severe radicular back pain.

145. What local anesthetic is linked to cauda equine syndrome?

    (A) Ropivacaine

    (B) Bupivacaine

    (C) Tetracaine

    (D) Lidocaine

146. Spinal anesthesia using tetracaine 12 mg is given to a patient undergoing a transurethral resection of the prostate. If you add epinephrine what is the longest anticipated duration?

    (A) 0.5 hour

    (B) 1 hour

    (C) 2 hours

    (D) 3 hours

147. Which clotting factor is the first to become inactivated shortly after a patient has begun warfarin therapy?

    (A) IV

    (B) V

    (C) VII

    (D) IX

148. Following administration of 15-mg spinal bupivacaine, the patient's heart rate and blood pressure fall precipitously. What is the cause?

(A) Sympathetic blockade

(B) Motor blockade

(C) Sensory blockade

(D) Sensory and motor blockade

149. A patient states that their feet are numb following administration of an epidural test dose. What is the most likely cause?

(A) Intravascular injection

(B) Local anesthetic toxicity

(C) Intrathecal injection

(D) Normal response to a test dose

150. Twenty-four hours following an epidural anesthesia the patient complains of occipital headache, nausea, vomiting, and double vision. What is the most likely cause?

(A) Neurologic injury

(B) Spinal hematoma

(C) Epidural hematoma

(D) Postdural puncture headache

151. What factor **does not** influence the spread of local anesthetic **placed in the** epidural space?

(A) Concentration

(B) Dose

(C) Site of injection

(D) Age

152. A patient is scheduled for a thoracotomy. A thoracic epidural is placed. What volume of local anesthetic will you use?

(A) 15 mL

(B) 10 mL

(C) 18 mL

(D) 20 mL

153. What is the best approach to avoiding cardiac arrest during spinal anesthesia?

(A) Decrease preload

(B) Give prophylactic ephedrine

(C) Increase preload

(D) Give prophylactic atropine

154. What patient is least likely to experience a postdural puncture headache?

(A) 70-year-old male

(B) 40-year-old male

(C) 20-year-old female

(D) 60-year-old female

155. What ultrasound frequency is used when placing an epidural or spinal?

(A) 2 to 5 MHz

(B) 5 to 10 MHz

(C) 10 to 15 MHz

(D) 20 to 25 MHz

156. Which statement is true regarding ultrasound for peripheral nerve blocks?

(A) Structures that appear white on the ultrasound screen are hypoechoic.

(B) Low frequencies are used for peripheral nerve blocks.

(C) Structures that appear white on the ultrasound screen are hyperechoic.

(D) High-frequency transducers offer a low-resolution picture.

157. What is the innervation of the brachial plexus?

(A) C_5–C_8 and T_1

(B) C_4–C_8

(C) C_4–C_8 and T_1

(D) C_5–C_7 and T_1–T_2

158. What brachial plexus approach is indicated for a patient undergoing shoulder surgery?

(A) Supraclavicular

(B) Infraclavicular

(C) Interscalene

(D) Axillary

159. Which would result from excessive pressure on the sciatic nerve by the piriformis muscle?

(A) Chronic pain in the perineum with voiding difficulty

(B) Anterior thigh pain and weakness upon standing

(C) Gluteal pain with paresthesia in the posterior thigh

(D) Lumbar vertebral pain exacerbated by flexion of the lower back

160. Which of the following is appropriate to use for intravenous regional anesthesia?

(A) 0.5% lidocaine with epinephrine 50 mL

(B) 5.0% lidocaine with epinephrine 40 mL

(C) 0.5% lidocaine 50 mL

(D) 0.5% bupivacaine 50 mL

161. For which medication is regional anesthesia an absolute contraindication?

(A) Clopidogrel

(B) Unfractionated heparin

(C) Low molecular weight heparin

(D) Thrombolytics

162. The patient received a Bier block for hand surgery. The case was completed in 10 minutes. When will you deflate the tourniquet?

(A) 10 minutes after the local anesthetic is injected

(B) 20 minutes after the local anesthetic is injected

(C) 30 minutes after the local anesthetic is injected

(D) 40 minutes after the local anesthetic is injected

163. What statement is true regarding digital nerve blocks?

(A) A small gauge needle is inserted at the distal aspect of the selected digit.

(B) 5 to 7 mL of lidocaine with epinephrine is used.

(C) A small gauge needle is inserted at the medial and lateral borders of the base of the selected digit.

(D) 2 to 3 mL of lidocaine is used.

164. What is the definition of persistent postsurgical pain?

(A) Pain resulting from outpatient surgery sufficient to require inpatient care

(B) Pain for more than 1 to 2 weeks following surgery

(C) Pain for more than 1 to 2 months following surgery

(D) Pain for more than 1 year following surgery

165. Where is local anesthetic injected in a radial block at the wrist?

(A) Medial to the ulnar artery at the wrist

(B) Lateral to the radial artery at the wrist

(C) Medial to the radial artery at the wrist

(D) Lateral to the ulnar artery at the wrist

166. Which nerve provides sensation to the anteromedial foot and medial lower leg?

(A) Deep peroneal

(B) Sural

(C) Superficial peroneal

(D) Saphenous

167. Calculate the Aldrete Score for a patient with the following criteria:

$SpO_2 > 92\%$ (Room Air); Shallow breathing; Blood pressure $+/-20$ mmHg of normal; arousable on calling and moves all extremities.

(A) 4

(B) 6

(C) 8

(D) 10

168. What artery provides most of the blood supply to the anterior, lower two-thirds of the spinal cord?

(A) Posterior spinal artery

(B) Artery of Adamkiewicz

(C) Posterior inferior cerebellar artery

(D) Intercostal arteries

169. After placing a spinal anesthetic the sensory block is assessed at T_8. Where is the most likely level of the motor block?

(A) T_4

(B) T_6

(C) T_{10}

(D) T_2

170. Which of the following characterizes A-*a* nerve fibers?

(A) Diameter 0.5 to 1 micrometer

(B) Heavy myelination with a diameter of 12 to 20 micrometers

(C) Light myelination

(D) Similar to C fibers

171. Following administration of spinal anesthesia the patient becomes hypotensive and bradycardic. What nerve fibers are affected?

    (A) T_1–T_4
    (B) T_5–T_6
    (C) T_7–T_8
    (D) T_{10}–T_{12}

172. Which clotting factor is not synthesized in the liver?

    (A) II
    (B) IV
    (C) VII
    (D) VIII

173. A 70-year-old patient with emphysema is undergoing an open cholecystectomy. What is the best anesthetic choice for this patient?

    (A) Spinal
    (B) Epidural
    (C) General
    (D) MAC

174. Which of the following is an absolute contraindications for regional anesthesia?

    (A) Uncooperative patient
    (B) Preexisting neurological deficits
    (C) Severe aortic stenosis
    (D) Patient refusal

175. A patient who takes ticlopidine requests a spinal anesthetic for a total knee replacement. What is the waiting period for ticlopidine?

    (A) 7 days
    (B) 12 days
    (C) 48 hours
    (D) 8 hours

176. Where is Tuffier's line located?

    (A) L_4
    (B) L_2
    (C) L_1
    (D) L_3

177. What is the correct order of anatomical structure used when placing an epidural needle?

    (A) Skin, subcutaneous tissue, supraspinous ligament, interspinous ligament, ligamentum flavum, epidural space
    (B) Skin, subcutaneous tissue, interspinous ligament, supraspinous ligament, ligamentum flavum, epidural space
    (C) Skin, subcutaneous tissue, interspinous ligament, supraspinous ligament, ligamentum flavum, dura, subarachnoid space
    (D) Skin, subcutaneous tissue, interspinous ligament, supraspinous ligament, ligamentum flavum, dura, epidural space

178. Which statement is true of Aδ fibers?

    (A) Aδ fibers are myelinated, synapse in Rexed laminae I and V, and transmit primarily mechanical or thermal pain.
    (B) Aδ fibers are unmyelinated, synapse in Rexed laminae II and VII, and transmit primarily mechanical or thermal pain.
    (C) Aδ fibers are myelinated, synapse in Rexed laminae III and X, and transmit primarily mechanical or thermal pain.
    (D) Aδ fibers are unmyelinated, synapse in Rexed laminae IV and VI, and transmit primarily mechanical or thermal pain.

179. Which laminae receive input from C fibers?

    (A) III, IV, VI
    (B) I, VI, X
    (C) II, VII, IX
    (D) I, II, V

180. How would postoperative pain localized to the site of skin incision be classified?

    (A) Visceral pain
    (B) Deep somatic pain
    (C) Superficial somatic pain
    (D) Referred pain

181. Referred pain from the diaphragm can be expected in which dermatome?

    (A) C_4
    (B) C_7
    (C) T_4
    (D) T_7

182. What is the surface landmark of the fourth cervical cutaneous dermatome?

    (A) Anterior neck
    (B) Shoulder
    (C) Biceps
    (D) Xiphoid

183. Which act to diminish pain signals?

    (A) Glutamate
    (B) Glycine
    (C) Substance P
    (D) ß-Endorphin

184. What complication is associated with hetastarch?

    (A) Interference with blood typing
    (B) Coagulopathy
    (C) Decreased plasma volume
    (D) Anaphylaxis

185. Which portion of the spinal cord is most associated with transmission of pain signals?

    (A) Dorsal horn
    (B) Central canal
    (C) Ventral horn
    (D) Pia mater

186. Which of these is least likely to relieve pain by decreasing inflammation?

    (A) Acetaminophen
    (B) Ketorolac
    (C) Ibuprofen
    (D) Celecoxib

187. Which is the mechanism of action for gabapentin?

    (A) GABA agonist effect
    (B) Calcium channel activation
    (C) Excitatory neurotransmitter inhibition
    (D) Inhibition of prostaglandin synthesis

188. Which of these analgesic agents is a GABA agonist?

    (A) Baclofen
    (B) Pregabalin
    (C) Dexmedetomidine
    (D) Celecoxib

189. What is the most common level of approach to perform a stellate ganglion block?

    (A) C_3
    (B) C_4
    (C) C_5
    (D) C_6

190. What of the following is a mechanism of action for duloxetine?

    (A) Monoamine oxidase inhibition
    (B) Serotonin reuptake inhibition
    (C) α_2 receptor agonist effect
    (D) Norepinephrine agonist

191. Which is an α_2 agonist?

    (A) Carbamazepine
    (B) Tapentadol
    (C) Phenytoin
    (D) Tizanidine

192. Which route of administration of fentanyl is subject to the hepatic first-pass effect?

    (A) Transdermal patch
    (B) Intravenous injection
    (C) Sublingual spray
    (D) Oral tablet

193. What would be the correct classification of hyperalgesia with sympathetic dysfunction following a traumatic injury that included direct nerve damage persisting beyond the standard healing period in the absence of other conditions that may be responsible for the pain?

    (A) Complex regional pain syndrome type I
    (B) Reflex sympathetic dystrophy
    (C) Complex regional pain syndrome type II
    (D) Persistent allodynia

194. Following placement of a stellate ganglion block the patient becomes hoarse, what has occurred?

    (A) Phrenic nerve block
    (B) Recurrent laryngeal nerve block
    (C) Subdural injection
    (D) Pneumothorax

195. Which are appropriate for inclusion in an epidural steroid injection?

(A) Morphine

(B) Methylprednisolone acetate and saline

(C) Remifentanil

(D) Fentanyl

196. Which steroid has the smallest particulate size?

(A) Methylprednisolone acetate

(B) Triamcinolone diacetate

(C) Dexamethasone sodium phosphate

(D) Betamethasone

197. Which is an indication for a celiac plexus block?

(A) Posttraumatic hypoperfusion of the arm

(B) Lower extremity vascular insufficiency

(C) Intractable lumbar pain

(D) Pain resulting from pancreatic malignancy

198. When selecting a needle for spinal anesthesia, which type is most likely to cause a postdural puncture headache?

(A) 20-g Quincke

(B) 22-g Whitacre

(C) 22-g Sprotte

(D) 22-g Quincke

199. An adult patient with moderate aortic regurgitation receives a spinal anesthetic. Blood pressure decreases to 68/42 and is treated with 100 mcg of phenylephrine. How will this dose impact the patient's underlying disease state?

(A) It will improve the regurgitation.

(B) It will exacerbate the regurgitation.

(C) It will have no impact on the regurgitation.

(D) Phenylephrine is contraindicated in this patient.

200. Which estimated blood volume is correctly paired with its age group?

(A) Preterm neonate: 85 mL/kg

(B) Six-month-old: 90 mL/kg

(C) Adult male: 80 mL/kg

(D) Adult female: 65 mL/kg

201. How will the symptoms of an acute hemolytic transfusion reaction manifest in a patient under general anesthesia?

(A) Fever, unexplained tachycardia, hypotension, and diffuse oozing in surgical field

(B) Nausea, fever, flank pain, unexplained tachycardia, and hypotension

(C) Hemoglobinuria, chest and flank pain, fever, and hypotension

(D) Hypertension, unexplained tachycardia, fever, erythema, and hive

202. 0.5% ropivacaine is injected into the brachial plexus via the interscalene approach. Which of the following is most likely to be spared?

(A) Sensation of the radial side of the forearm

(B) Sensation of the medial upper arm

(C) Sensation of half of the fourth finger and all the fifth finger

(D) Sensation of the palmar surface of the first three fingers

203. How does an opioid inhibit postsynaptic nociceptive signal transmission?

(A) Hyperpolarization and opening potassium channels

(B) Excitation

(C) Opening calcium channels

(D) Opening potassium channels

204. When administering a spinal anesthetic which nerve roots are easily blocked?

(A) Smaller, unmyelinated

(B) Larger, myelinated

(C) Smaller, myelinated

(D) Larger, unmyelinated

205. Which corticosteroid has the most potent glucocorticoid activity?

(A) Hydrocortisone

(B) Prednisone

(C) Methylprednisolone

(D) Dexamethasone

206. Where does the spinal cord end in a 5-year-old?

- (A) L_1
- (B) L_2
- (C) L_3
- (D) L_4

207. When is a type and screen preferable to a type and crossmatch?

- (A) The probability of transfusing blood is low.
- (B) The probability of transfusing blood is high.
- (C) The patient has high risk for alloimmunization.
- (D) The patient has a history of a positive antibody screen.

208. Which of the following is true regarding apneic oxygenation during induction?

- (A) Apneic oxygenation effectively prolongs time to desaturation based on an increased carbon dioxide solubility gradient that allows 100 mL/min of carbon dioxide to diffuse across the alveolar membrane for exhalation.
- (B) Approximately 250 mL/min of oxygen diffuses from the alveoli into the bloodstream during apnea, which allows a prolonged time until desaturation begins from apnea.
- (C) Apneic oxygenation can be achieved by placing a nasal cannula on the patient prior to preoxygenation/denitrogenation and increasing the nasal cannula flows to 5 L/min while keeping a tight-fitting seal on the anesthesia mask.
- (D) Apneic oxygenation is especially beneficial for patients who may decompensate quickly from apnea and morbidly obese patients who have an increased FRC.

209. A patient under general anesthesia's $ETCO_2$ was noted to be 32 mmHg and the ventilator was turned to manual mode to allow the $ETCO_2$ to build enough to breach the apneic threshold. During the first minute of apnea, how much will the $ETCO_2$ rise?

- (A) 6 mmHg
- (B) 3 mmHg
- (C) 0 to 2 mmHg
- (D) 10 mmHg

210. A patient undergoing a right total shoulder arthroplasty has an AICD secondary to heart failure. What is the best practice when developing the anesthesia plan for this patient?

- (A) The generator is on the left side of the patient's chest, no special considerations are needed for this case.
- (B) Monopolar cautery produces less energy than bipolar and thus no grounding pad is needed.
- (C) Communicate with the surgical team that limiting monopolar cautery to <5 seconds is sufficient to prevent device interference.
- (D) Place defibrillator pads on the patient and have the device representative disable the shock feature.

211. Which of the following is not true regarding laryngospasms?

- (A) A history of a viral upper respiratory infection 8 weeks prior to general anesthesia increases the pediatric perioperative risks for laryngospasms.
- (B) ETT and LMA removal should only occur during Guedel's stage I or III of anesthesia.
- (C) Treatment of laryngospasm includes: 100% oxygen, positive pressure ventilation or 1 to 1.5 mg/kg of lidocaine.
- (D) Pharyngeal secretions are a frequent contributing cause of laryngospasms.

212. ENT procedures have unique risks and considerations. Which of the following increased the risk for airway fires?

- (A) For a tracheostomy placement, do not allow the surgeon to use cautery to incise the trachea.
- (B) Regarding laser surgeries, use a laser-resistant tube and inflate the cuff with methylene blue–dyed saline.
- (C) Up to 40% supplemental oxygen can be administered safely without increased risk for an airway fire.
- (D) Manual oxygen flowmeters should only be used with an oxygen analyzer.

213. A 30-year-old Hispanic male with a history of a poorly controlled GERD develops a laryngospasm after extubation. Appropriate measures were taken, and the patient never desaturated during the laryngospasm. Upon arrival at the PACU you note the patient has an oxygen saturation of 89% on 10 L oxygen via face mask and coughs up pink sputum. Which is the best initial response?

(A) Negative pressure pulmonary edema does not present until 1 hour after arrival in the PACU. Continue to observe patient on 10 L oxygen and administer a nebulized albuterol treatment.

(B) The patient is displaying signs of negative pressure pulmonary edema. Provide supplemental oxygen via continuous positive airway pressure (CPAP) with PEEP.

(C) The patient developed negative pressure pulmonary edema. Administer 40 mg of furosemide IVP.

(D) Reintubate the patient in the PACU and perform a bronchoscopy to assess for aspiration.

214. For point-of-care lung ultrasound correctly match the following items.

(A) "Lung point" demonstrated via M mode on ultrasound

(B) A lines

(C) Three or more B lines (or comet tails)

(D) Lung sliding

(E) Shows with interstitial syndrome

(F) Represents a diagnosis of pneumothorax

(G) Hyperechoic horizontal reverberations below the pleura

(H) Presence of this rules out a pneumothorax

215. Which of the following is not a contraindication to TEE placement?

(A) History of alcoholism

(B) Esophageal strictures

(C) Zenker's diverticulum

(D) Esophageal mass

216. Dynamic decision making is one of the key elements to crisis resource management. One major source of poor outcomes is fixation errors. What communication technique is beneficial in preventing or breaking fixation errors?

(A) The use of cognitive aids can help the team leader recognize differential diagnosis.

(B) Anticipating the needs and potential complications of a case assists in preparedness and eliminates the risk of emergencies developing.

(C) Declaring an emergency early rather than late increases the time to gather resources and develop a plan.

(D) Both (A) and (B) are correct.

217. Which is not true about MAC levels regarding volatile anesthetics?

(A) MAC-BAR is the minimum alveolar concentration that blunts an adrenergic response to noxious stimulus. MAC-BAR is 1.9 times the MAC.

(B) MAC awake is the minimum alveolar concentration when patients can open their eyes to command and varies from 0.15 to 0.5 MAC.

(C) MAC values decrease by 6% per decade from ages 40 to 80 years old.

(D) Chronic alcohol abuse, hypernatremia, and hyperthermia all result in increased MAC requirements.

218. A 75-year-old male with a past medical history of coronary artery disease, hypertension, and GERD is scheduled for a right total hip arthroplasty. During the preoperative assessment, the patient disclosed that he needed a blood transfusion when his left hip was replaced. The patient reports he last took his clopidogrel 7 days ago. The patient takes famotidine and garlic daily and took them the morning of surgery. What is the best plan?

(A) Discuss with the surgeon the increased bleeding risks. Consider rescheduling for another day.

(B) Reschedule the surgery for the last case of the day.

(C) Administer 2 units of FFP and 1 g of TXA prior to incision.

(D) Reverse with protamine.

Answers and Explanations: Basic Principles

1. When do symptoms of ischemic optic neuropathy that result in postoperative vision loss typically first occur?

   (A) Immediately postoperatively
   (B) 2 hours postoperatively
   (C) 2 days postoperatively
   (D) 2 weeks postoperatively

   Rationale: Symptoms typically start following emergence from anesthesia but may occur up to 12 days following surgery.
   References: Butterworth JF IV, Mackey DC, Wasnick JD, eds. *Morgan & Mikhail's Clinical Anesthesiology.* 7th ed. New York, NY: McGraw Hill; 2022: Chapter 54.
   Gropper MA. *Miller's Anesthesia.* 9th ed. Philadelphia, PA: Churchill Livingstone Elsevier; 2020: Chapter 34.

2. During a general anesthetic you suspect an episode of MH. What will you do first?

   (A) Call the MHAUS hotline.
   (B) Administer dantrolene.
   (C) Inform the surgeon.
   (D) Turn off inhalational agents.

   Rationale: When suspicion of an episode of malignant hyperthermia exists, each of the responses is in order. However, turning off the inhalational agents is the first priority.
   References: Butterworth JF IV, Mackey DC, Wasnick JD, eds. *Morgan & Mikhail's Clinical Anesthesiology.* 7th ed. New York, NY: McGraw Hill; 2022: Chapter 52.
   Elisha S, Heiner JS, Nagelhout JJ. *Nurse Anesthesia.* 7th ed. St. Louis, MO: Elsevier Saunders; 2023: Chapter 36.
   Gropper MA. *Miller's Anesthesia.* 9th ed. Philadelphia, PA: Churchill Livingstone Elsevier; 2020: Chapter 35.

3. When is body temperature loss the greatest?

   (A) During the preoperative preparation
   (B) During the first hour in the operating room
   (C) During the second and third hour in the operating room
   (D) During the fourth hour in the operating room

   Rationale: The greatest amount of heat loss occurs during the first hour in the operating room (1-2°C). Thereafter temperature decline is gradual and then plateaus.
   References: Butterworth JF IV, Mackey DC, Wasnick JD, eds. *Morgan & Mikhail's Clinical Anesthesiology.* 7th ed. New York, NY: McGraw Hill; 2022: Chapter 52.
   Elisha S, Heiner JS, Nagelhout JJ. *Nurse Anesthesia.* 7th ed. St. Louis, MO: Elsevier Saunders; 2023: Chapter 18.

4. For an awake fiberoptic intubation, anesthesia for the posterior 1/3 of the tongue, vallecula, anterior epiglottis, walls of the pharynx, and tonsils can be performed by injecting local anesthetic into which of the following structures?

   (A) Base of the frenulum
   (B) Palatoglossal arch
   (C) Thyroid membrane
   (D) Cricothyroid membrane

   Rationale: Innervation of the airway related to an awake fiber optic intubation is through two neural pathways: the glossopharyngeal nerve cephalad to the epiglottis and vagal braches (superior laryngeal and recurrent laryngeal nerves) distal to the epiglottis.

   Sensation to the mucosa of the palatine tonsils, soft palate, and sensory branch to the posterior 1/3 of the tongue are provided by the tonsillar nerves (branches of the glossopharyngeal nerve). Blockade of these nerves facilitates intubation by blocking the gag reflex. A submucosal injection can be performed at the cephalad portion of the posterior tonsillar pillars at the palatoglossal arch.
   References: Butterworth JF IV, Mackey DC, Wasnick JD, eds. *Morgan & Mikhail's Clinical Anesthesiology.* 7th ed. New York, NY: McGraw Hill; 2022: Chapter 19.
   Elisha S, Heiner JS, Nagelhout JJ. *Nurse Anesthesia.* 7th ed. St. Louis, MO: Elsevier Saunders; 2023: Chapter 24.

Hagberg CA, Artime CA, Aziz MF, eds. *Hagberg and Benumof's Airway Management.* 4th ed. Philadelphia, PA: Elsevier. 2018: Chapter 12.

5. Which is an example of sensation without stimulus?

    (A) Temporal summation
    (B) Dynamic allodynia
    (C) Paresthesia
    (D) Analgesia

    Rationale: Paresthesia is the spontaneous perception of an abnormal sensation.

    References: Butterworth JF IV, Mackey DC, Wasnick JD, eds. *Morgan & Mikhail's Clinical Anesthesiology.* 7th ed. New York, NY: McGraw Hill; 2022: Chapter 47.

    Elisha S, Heiner JS, Nagelhout JJ. *Nurse Anesthesia.* 7th ed. St. Louis, MO: Elsevier Saunders; 2023: Chapter 56.

6. Which statement about stored blood is correct?

    (A) The amount of extracellular potassium transfused per unit is 10 mEq per unit.
    (B) Stored blood typically has a pH less than 7.45.
    (C) Stored blood contains factors V and VIII.
    (D) Stored blood can contain as much as 150 mEq/L of potassium.

    Rationale: The amount of extracellular potassium transfused per unit is usually less than 4 mEq per unit. Stored blood is acidic due to the citric acid anticoagulant and accumulation of lactic acid. Stored blood does not contain factors V and VIII and stored blood can contain as much as 17 mEq/L of potassium.

    References: Elisha S, Heiner JS, Nagelhout JJ. *Nurse Anesthesia.* 7th ed. St. Louis, MO: Elsevier Saunders; 2023: Chapter 22.

    Butterworth JF IV, Mackey DC, Wasnick JD, eds. *Morgan & Mikhail's Clinical Anesthesiology.* 7th ed. New York, NY: McGraw Hill; 2022: Chapter 51.

7. Which patient is least likely to aspirate?

    (A) Second trimester parturient
    (B) Gastroesophageal reflux
    (C) First trimester parturient
    (D) NPO <6 hours

    Rationale: Patient's at greatest risk for aspiration include the second and third trimester parturient, patients with gastroesophageal reflux disease and those who consumed solid food <6 hours prior to surgery.

    References: Butterworth JF IV, Mackey DC, Wasnick JD, eds. *Morgan & Mikhail's Clinical Anesthesiology.* 7th ed. New York, NY: McGraw Hill; 2022: Chapter 18.

Gropper MA. *Miller's Anesthesia.* 9th ed. Philadelphia, PA: Churchill Livingstone Elsevier; 2020: Chapter 44.

8. What percent of the total body water is extracellular?

    (A) 67%
    (B) 33%
    (C) 25%
    (D) 100%

    Rationale: Extracellular fluid (interstitial and intravascular) contains approximately 30% of the total body water. The intracellular compartment is approximately 67% of the total body water.

TABLE 3-1. Effect of different fluid loads on extracellular and intracellular water contents.[1]

A. Normal

Total body solute = 280 mOsm/kg × 42 kg = 11,760 mOsm
Intracellular solute = 280 mOsm/kg × 25 kg = 7,000 mOsm
Extracellular solute = 280 mOsm/kg × 17 kg = 4,760 mOsm
Extracellular sodium concentration = 280 ÷ 2 = 140 mEq/L

	Intracellular	Extracellular
Osmolality	25	17
Volume (L)	0	0
Net water gain		

B. Isotonic load: 2 L of Isotonic saline (NaCl)

Total body solute = 280 mOsm/kg × 44 kg = 12,320 mOsm
Intracellular solute = 280 mOsm/kg × 25 kg = 7,000 mOsm
Extracellular solute = 280 mOsm/kg × 19 kg = 5,320 mOsm

	Intracellular	Extracellular
Osmolality	280	280
Volume (L)	25	19
Net water gain	0	2

Net effect: Fluid remains in extracellular compartment.

C. Free water (hypotonic) load: 2 L water

New body water = 42 + 2 = 44 kg
New body osmolality = 11,760 mOsm ÷ 44 kg = 267 mOsm/kg
New intracellular volume = 7,000 mOsm ÷ 267 mOsm/kg = 26.2 kg
New extracellular sodium concentration = 267 ÷ 2 = 133 mEq/L

	Intracellular	Extracellular
Osmolality	267.0	267.0
Volume (L)	26.2	17.8
Net water gain	+1.2	+0.8

Net effect: Fluid distributes between both compartments.

D. Hypertonic load: 600 mEq NaCl (no water)

Total body solute = 11,760 + 600 = 12,360 mOsm/kg
New body osmolality = 12,360 mOsm/kg ÷ 42 kg = 294 mOsm
New extracellular solute = 600 + 4760 = 5,360 mOsm
New extracellular volume = 5,360 mOsm ÷ 294 mOsm/kg = 18.2 kg
New intracellular volume = 42 − 18.2 = 23.8 kg
New extracellular sodium concentration = 294 ÷ 2 = 147 mEq/L

	Intracellular	Extracellular
Osmolality	294.0	294.0
Volume (L)	23.8	18.2
Net water gain	−1.2	+1.2

Net effect: An intracellular to extracellular movement of water.

[1]Based on a 70-kg adult man.

(Reproduced with permission from Butterworth JF IV, Mackey DC, Wasnick JD, eds. *Morgan & Mikhail's Clinical Anesthesiology.* 7th ed. New York: McGraw Hill; 2022.)

References: Butterworth JF IV, Mackey DC, Wasnick JD, eds. *Morgan & Mikhail's Clinical Anesthesiology.* 7th ed. New York, NY: McGraw Hill; 2022: Chapter 49.

Elisha S, Heiner JS, Nagelhout JJ. *Nurse Anesthesia.* 7th ed. St. Louis, MO: Elsevier Saunders; 2023: Chapter 21.

9. Which drug is not a trigger for malignant hyperthermia?

   (A) Halothane

   (B) Sevoflurane

   (C) Brevital

   (D) Succinylcholine

   Rationale: All inhalation general anesthetics and depolarizing muscle relaxants trigger malignant hyperthermia. Barbiturates are considered safe anesthetic agents.

   References: Butterworth JF IV, Mackey DC, Wasnick JD, eds. *Morgan & Mikhail's Clinical Anesthesiology.* 7th ed. New York, NY: McGraw Hill; 2022: Chapter 52.

   Gropper MA. *Miller's Anesthesia.* 9th ed. Philadelphia, PA: Churchill Livingstone Elsevier; 2020: Chapter 35.

10. How is the brachial plexus formed?

    (A) Roots, divisions, trunks, cords, branches

    (B) Divisions, trunks, cords, branches

    (C) Cords, divisions, roots, branches

    (D) Trunks, divisions, cords, branches

    Rationale: The brachial plexus arises from the ventral rami of five spinal nerve roots (C_5–C_8 and T_1). As the brachial plexus moves distally, the roots form the trunks, divisions, cords, and terminal branches. Options A, B, and C are in the incorrect order. Even though the *Roots* are missing from "D," the rest of the answer is in order of how the brachial plexus is formed.

    References: Butterworth JF IV, Mackey DC, Wasnick JD, eds. *Morgan & Mikhail's Clinical Anesthesiology.* 7th ed. New York, NY: McGraw Hill; 2022: Chapter 46.

    Elisha S, Heiner JS, Nagelhout JJ. *Nurse Anesthesia.* 7th ed. St. Louis, MO: Elsevier Saunders; 2023: Chapter 50.

    Gropper MA. *Miller's Anesthesia.* 9th ed. Philadelphia, PA: Churchill Livingstone Elsevier; 2020: Chapter 46.

11. Which laboratory test provides the most comprehensive assessment of coagulation in a patient with severe cirrhosis?

    (A) International normalized ratio

    (B) Prothrombin time

    (C) Partial thromboplastin time

    (D) Thromboelastography

Rationale: Thromboelastography allows assessment of the initial clotting process through fibrinolysis which is more comprehensive than an isolated measure of clotting time.

References: Butterworth JF IV, Mackey DC, Wasnick JD, eds. *Morgan & Mikhail's Clinical Anesthesiology.* 7th ed. New York, NY: McGraw Hill; 2022: Chapter 33.

Elisha S, Heiner JS, Nagelhout JJ. *Nurse Anesthesia.* 7th ed. St. Louis, MO: Elsevier Saunders; 2023: Chapter 41.

Gropper MA. *Miller's Anesthesia.* 9th ed. Philadelphia, PA: Churchill Livingstone Elsevier; 2020: Chapter 60.

12. Where does the spinal cord end in adults?

    (A) L_1

    (B) L_2

    (C) L_3

    (D) L_4

    Rationale: In adults the spinal cord ends at L_1 and in some adults to L_2. The spinal cord ends at L_3 in infants.

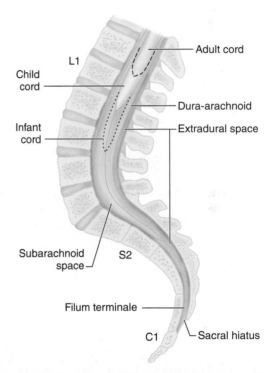

FIG. 3-1. Sagittal view through the lumbar vertebrae and sacrum. Note the end of the spinal cord rises with development from approximately L_3 to L_1. The dural sac normally ends at S_2. (Reproduced with permission from Butterworth JF IV, Mackey DC, Wasnick JD, eds. *Morgan & Mikhail's Clinical Anesthesiology.* 7th ed. New York: McGraw Hill; 2022.)

References: Butterworth JF IV, Mackey DC, Wasnick JD, eds. *Morgan & Mikhail's Clinical Anesthesiology.* 7th ed. New York, NY: McGraw Hill; 2022: Chapter 45.

Gropper MA. *Miller's Anesthesia.* 9th ed. Philadelphia, PA: Churchill Livingstone Elsevier; 2020: Chapter 45.

13. A 25-kg infant has a preoperative hematocrit of 40%. What volume of blood loss will decrease the hematocrit from 36% to 30%?

(A) 250 mL

(B) 360 mL

(C) 400 mL

(D) 450 mL

Rationale: The amount of blood loss that causes the hematocrit to decrease from 35% to 30% in this patient can be calculated as follows:

Step 1: Estimated blood volume = 25 kg × 80 mL/kg = 2,000 mL

Step 2: Estimated initial red blood cell volume = 2,000 mL × 36% = 720 mL

Step 3: Estimated final red blood cell volume = 2,000 mL × 30% = 600 mL

Step 4: Calculate red blood cell loss = 720 mL − 600 mL = 120 mL

Step 5: Multiple red blood cell loss × 3: 120 mL × 3 = 360 mL

References: Butterworth JF IV, Mackey DC, Wasnick JD, eds. *Morgan & Mikhail's Clinical Anesthesiology.* 7th ed. New York, NY: McGraw Hill; 2022: Chapter 51.

Barash PG, Cullen BF, Stoelting RK, et al, eds. *Clinical Anesthesia.* 8th ed. Lippincott Williams & Wilkins; 2017: Chapter 43.

14. Which cranial nerve (CN) provides sensation to the posterior one-third of the tongue?

(A) CN I

(B) CN V

(C) CN IX

(D) CN X

Rationale: CN I (olfactory) provides innervation to the nasal mucosa; the superior and inferior surfaces of the hard and soft palate are innervated by fibers of CN V (trigeminal). CN IX (glossopharyngeal) innervates the posterior one-third of the tongue whereas the lingual nerve provides sensation to the anterior two-thirds of the tongue. Areas of sensation below the epiglottis are innervated by CN X (Vagus).

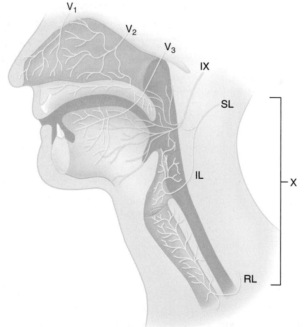

V_1 Ophthalmic division of trigeminal nerve (anterior ethmoidal nerve)

V_2 Maxillary division of trigeminal nerve (sphenopalatine nerves)

V_3 Mandibular division of trigeminal nerve (lingual nerve)

IX Glossopharyngeal nerve

X Vagus nerve
  SL Superior laryngeal nerve
  IL Internal laryngeal nerve
  RL Recurrent laryngeal nerve

FIG. 3-2. Sensory nerve supply of the airway. (Reproduced with permission from Butterworth JF IV, Mackey DC, Wasnick JD, eds. *Morgan & Mikhail's Clinical Anesthesiology.* 7th ed. New York: McGraw Hill; 2022.)

References: Barash PG, Cullen BF, Stoelting RK, et al, eds. *Clinical Anesthesia.* 8th ed. Lippincott Williams & Wilkins; 2017: Chapter 28.

Butterworth JF IV, Mackey DC, Wasnick JD, eds. *Morgan & Mikhail's Clinical Anesthesiology.* 7th ed. New York, NY: McGraw Hill; 2022: Chapter 19.

15. Which patient is more likely to experience complications when using a hypotensive technique?

(A) Uncontrolled glaucoma

(B) Myesthenia gravis

(C) Multiple sclerosis

(D) Osteoarthritis

Rationale: Patients with cerebrovascular, cardiac, hepatic, uncontrolled glaucoma, and renal disease are not the best candidates for hypotensive anesthesia. Hypotensive anesthesia is relatively contraindicated. Complications including blindness, cardiac (myocardial infarction), stroke, and renal dysfunction (acute tubular necrosis) are possible outcomes.

References: Butterworth JF IV, Mackey DC, Wasnick JD, eds. *Morgan & Mikhail's Clinical Anesthesiology.* 7th ed. New York, NY: McGraw Hill; 2022: Chapter 51.

Elisha S, Heiner JS, Nagelhout JJ. *Nurse Anesthesia.* 7th ed. St. Louis, MO: Elsevier Saunders; 2023: Chapter 45.

16. What is the smallest volume of infused ABO-incompatible donor blood that will cause an acute hemolytic reaction?

(A) 40 to 60 mL

(B) 25 to 30 mL

(C) 10 to 15 mL

(D) 1 to 3 mL

Rationale: Acute hemolytic reactions may occur after infusion with as little as 10 mL of ABO-incompatible blood and may result in death for 20 to 60% of patients.

References: Butterworth JF IV, Mackey DC, Wasnick JD, eds. *Morgan & Mikhail's Clinical Anesthesiology.* 7th ed. New York, NY: McGraw Hill; 2022: Chapter 51.

Gropper MA. *Miller's Anesthesia.* 9th ed. Philadelphia, PA: Churchill Livingstone Elsevier; 2020: Chapter 49.

17. Which risk factor does not predispose patients to lower extremity neuropathy?

(A) Hypertension

(B) Surgery <2 hours

(C) Thin body habitus

(D) Cigarette smoking

Rationale: Surgeries longer than 2 hours, positioning that involves the peroneal nerve, extreme lithotomy, hypotension, extremes of weight (low body mass index and obesity), elderly, and vascular diseases are risk factors predisposing patients to lower extremity neuropathy.

References: Butterworth JF IV, Mackey DC, Wasnick JD, eds. *Morgan & Mikhail's Clinical Anesthesiology.* 7th ed. New York, NY: McGraw Hill; 2022: Chapter 54.

Gropper MA. *Miller's Anesthesia.* 9th ed. Philadelphia, PA: Churchill Livingstone Elsevier; 2020: Chapter 34.

18. What is the mechanism of action of a transcutaneous electrical nerve stimulation (TENS) unit?

(A) TENS stimulation of large diameter afferent nerve fibers competitively blocks pain signals from smaller fibers.

(B) TENS stimulation of small diameter afferent nerve fibers competitively blocks pain signals from larger fibers.

(C) TENS stimulation damages the small afferent fibers conducting the pain signals.

(D) TENS stimulation induces a signal conduction interruption in large diameter fibers.

Rationale: TENS is an application of gate theory; stimulation, and activation of large fibers introduces a competing stimulus to counteract pain signals carried along smaller afferent fibers.

References: Butterworth JF IV, Mackey DC, Wasnick JD, eds. *Morgan & Mikhail's Clinical Anesthesiology.* 7th ed. New York, NY: McGraw Hill; 2022: Chapter 47.

Gropper MA. *Miller's Anesthesia.* 9th ed. Philadelphia, PA: Churchill Livingstone Elsevier; 2020: Chapter 57.

19. What are the primary adductors of the vocal cords?

(A) Lateral cricoarytenoid muscles

(B) Recurrent laryngeal nerve

(C) Posterior cricoarytenoid muscles

(D) External laryngeal nerve

Rationale: The primary *abductors* of the vocal cords are the posterior cricoarytenoid muscles. The recurrent laryngeal nerve innervates the muscles of the larynx. The external laryngeal nerve innervates the cricothyroid muscle.

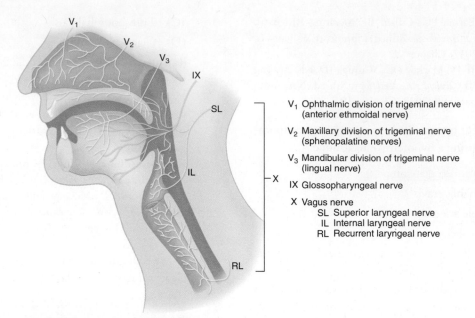

FIG. 3-3. Sensory nerve supply of the airway. (Reproduced with permission from Butterworth JF IV, Mackey DC, Wasnick JD, eds. *Morgan & Mikhail's Clinical Anesthesiology.* 7th ed. New York: McGraw Hill; 2022.)

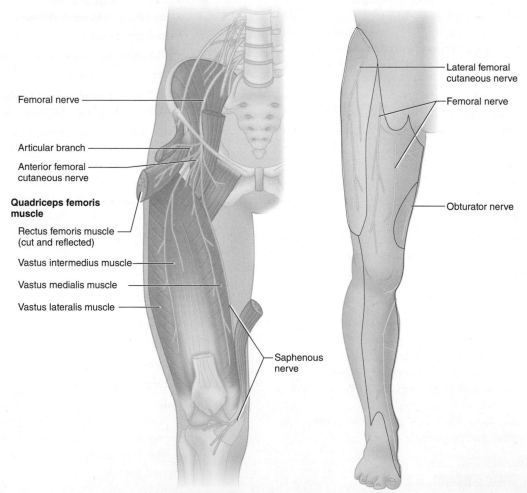

FIG. 3-4. The femoral nerve provides sensory innervation to the hip and thigh, and to the medial leg via its terminal branch, the saphenous nerve. (Reproduced with permission from Butterworth JF IV, Mackey DC, Wasnick JD, eds. *Morgan & Mikhail's Clinical Anesthesiology.* 7th ed. New York: McGraw Hill; 2022.)

References: Elisha S, Heiner JS, Nagelhout JJ. *Nurse Anesthesia.* 7th ed. St. Louis, MO: Elsevier Saunders; 2023: Chapter 24.

Butterworth JF IV, Mackey DC, Wasnick JD, eds. *Morgan & Mikhail's Clinical Anesthesiology.* 7th ed. New York, NY: McGraw Hill; 2022: Chapter 19.

20. Which group lists the vitamin K–dependent clotting factors?

    (A) II, VII, IX, X

    (B) II, IV, IX, XII

    (C) III, VII, X, XI

    (D) I, VII, IX, XI

    Rationale: Vitamin K–dependent factors include factors II, VII, IX, and X. They require vitamin K for completion of their synthesis in the liver. In the absence of vitamin K, these four clotting factors are produced in normal amounts but are nonfunctional.

    References: Butterworth JF IV, Mackey DC, Wasnick JD, eds. *Morgan & Mikhail's Clinical Anesthesiology.* 7th ed. New York, NY: McGraw Hill; 2022: Chapter 33.

    Barash PG, Cullen BF, Stoelting RK, et al, eds. *Clinical Anesthesia.* 8th ed. Lippincott Williams & Wilkins; 2017: Chapter 17.

21. Which of the following chemical mediators is released from peripheral afferent C fibers resulting in dull pain?

    (A) Substance P

    (B) Glutamate

    (C) Histamine

    (D) Serotonin

    Rationale: Glutamate results in fast sharp pain via A-delta and C nerve fibers. Edema and vasodilation result from the release of histamine via Substance P. Platelets release serotonin following tissue injury reacting with multiple receptors.

    References: Barash PG, Cullen BF, Stoelting RK, et al, eds. *Clinical Anesthesia.* 8th ed. Lippincott Williams & Wilkins; 2017: Chapter 55.

    Butterworth JF IV, Mackey DC, Wasnick JD, eds. *Morgan & Mikhail's Clinical Anesthesiology.* 7th ed. New York, NY: McGraw Hill; 2022: Chapter 47.

22. To supplement a brachial plexus block to cover the anterior shoulder, the cervical plexus can be blocked at which of the following locations?

    (A) Anterior to the mastoid process

    (B) The posterior border of the sternocleidomastoid

    (C) At the interscalene groove

    (D) Posterior to the angle of the mandible

    Rationale: Areas of the anterior shoulder are supplied by the superficial cervical plexus, which passes through the platysma at the posterior sternocleidomastoid (SCM) giving off superficial and deep branches. The superficial cervical plexus innervates the skin and the superficial structures of the head, neck, and shoulders. It lies in the plane just behind the SCM and can be blocked with a field block at that location.

    References: Butterworth JF IV, Mackey DC, Wasnick JD, eds. *Morgan & Mikhail's Clinical Anesthesiology.* 7th ed. New York, NY: McGraw Hill; 2022: Chapter 46.

    Hadzic A, ed. *Hadzic's Peripheral Nerve Blocks and Anatomy for Ultrasound-Guided Regional Anesthesia.* 3rd ed. New York, NY: McGraw-Hill; 2022: Chapter 12.

23. Following general endotracheal anesthesia the patient is in respiratory distress and is unable to speak. What nerve(s) may be injured?

    (A) Unilateral recurrent laryngeal nerve

    (B) Bilateral superior laryngeal nerve

    (C) Unilateral superior laryngeal nerve

    (D) Bilateral vagus nerves

    Rationale: Injury to the superior laryngeal nerve may result in vocal fatigue and hoarseness. Unilateral vagal and recurrent laryngeal nerve damage also results in hoarseness. Bilateral vagus (or bilateral recurrent laryngeal) nerve injury results in aphonia.

TABLE 3-2. The effects of laryngeal nerve injury on the voice.

Nerve	Effect of Nerve Injury
Superior laryngeal nerve	
Unilateral	Minimal effects
Bilateral	Hoarseness, tiring of voice
Recurrent laryngeal nerve	
Unilateral	Hoarseness
Bilateral	Stridor, respiratory distress
Acute	Aphonia
Chronic	
Vagus nerve	
Unilateral	Hoarseness
Bilateral	Aphonia

(Reproduced with permission from Butterworth JF IV, Mackey DC, Wasnick JD, eds. *Morgan & Mikhail's Clinical Anesthesiology.* 7th ed. New York: McGraw Hill; 2022.)

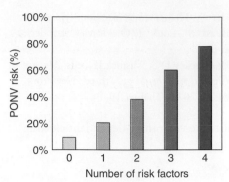

Risk factors	Points
Female gender	1
Nonsmoker	1
History of PONV	1
Postoperative opioids	1
Sum =	0 … 4

FIG. 3-5. Risk score for PONV in adults. Simplified risk score from Apfel et al to predict the patient's risk for PONV. When 0, 1, 2, 3, and 4 of the risk factors are present, the corresponding risk for PONV is about 10%, 20%, 40%, 60%, and 80%, respectively. PONV, postoperative nausea and vomiting. (Reproduced with permission from Gan TJ, Diemunsch P, Habib A, et al. Consensus guidelines for the management of postoperative nausea and vomiting, *Anesth Analg.* 2014;118(1):85-113.)

References: Butterworth JF IV, Mackey DC, Wasnick JD, eds. *Morgan & Mikhail's Clinical Anesthesiology.* 7th ed. New York, NY: McGraw Hill; 2022: Chapter 19.
Elisha S, Heiner JS, Nagelhout JJ. *Nurse Anesthesia.* 7th ed. St. Louis, MO: Elsevier Saunders; 2023: Chapter 24.

24. A patient's serum potassium level is 7.2 mEq/L. In which sequential order will cardiac manifestations of hyperkalemia progress?

    (A) Peaked T waves, loss of P wave, widened QRS complex, sine wave

    (B) Peaked T waves, widened QRS complex, loss of P wave, sine wave

    (C) Loss of R-wave amplitude, peaked T waves, widened QRS complex, sine wave

    (D) Prolonged P-R interval, peaked T waves, widened QRS complex, asystole

Rationale: ECG changes associated with severe hyperkalemia characteristically progress sequentially in the following order: First, peaked T waves, next a widening of the QRS complex, followed by a progression of the P-R interval, then a loss of P wave, then a loss of R wave amplitude, ST-segment depression (sometimes elevation), and finally, a sine wave which will ultimately change into ventricular fibrillation and asystole.
References: Butterworth JF IV, Mackey DC, Wasnick JD, eds. *Morgan & Mikhail's Clinical Anesthesiology.* 7th ed. New York, NY: McGraw Hill; 2022: Chapter 49.
Barash PG, Cullen BF, Stoelting RK, et al, eds. *Clinical Anesthesia.* 8th ed. Lippincott Williams & Wilkins; 2017: Chapter 16.

25. Which of the following is not a physiologic response to pain?

    (A) Increased peripheral vascular resistance

    (B) Decreased tidal volume

    (C) Increased platelet aggregation

    (D) Decreased urinary sphincter tone

Rationale: Pain results in increased urinary sphincter tone.
References: Barash PG, Cullen BF, Stoelting RK, et al, eds. *Clinical Anesthesia.* 8th ed. Lippincott Williams & Wilkins; 2017: Chapter 55.
Elisha S, Heiner JS, Nagelhout JJ. *Nurse Anesthesia.* 7th ed. St. Louis, MO: Elsevier Saunders; 2023: Chapter 56.

26. What is the treatment of choice for hyponatremic patients with decreased total body sodium content?

    (A) 0.9% NS

    (B) D5. ½NS

    (C) 0.5 NS

    (D) 3% NS

Rationale: Isotonic saline is the treatment of choice for hyponatremic patients with decreased total body sodium content. This is sometimes called hypovolemic hypotonic hyponatremia. B is hypertonic; C is hypotonic; and D is hypertonic.
References: Butterworth JF IV, Mackey DC, Wasnick JD, eds. *Morgan & Mikhail's Clinical Anesthesiology.* 7th ed. New York, NY: McGraw Hill; 2022: Chapter 49.
Elisha S, Heiner JS, Nagelhout JJ. *Nurse Anesthesia.* 7th ed. St. Louis, MO: Elsevier Saunders; 2023: Chapter 21.

27. What statement is false regarding nasal airways?

    (A) Nasal airways are 2 to 4 cm shorter than oral airways.

    (B) Thrombocytopenia is a contraindication.

    (C) Nasal airways are 2 to 4 cm longer than oral airways.

    (D) Basilar skull fracture is a contraindication.

Rationale: Any condition leading to nasal bleeding is a relative contraindication to the use of nasal airways. Use of a nasal airway in conditions of the skull including basilar fractures may result in malposition of the airway. Nasal airways are longer than oral airways.

References: Butterworth JF IV, Mackey DC, Wasnick JD, eds. *Morgan & Mikhail's Clinical Anesthesiology.* 7th ed. New York, NY: McGraw Hill; 2022: Chapter 19.

28. A patient-controlled analgesia order is written. What is the lockout interval for morphine?

(A) 8 to 20 minutes

(B) 5 to 10 minutes

(C) 10 to 15 minutes

(D) 15 to 18 minutes

Rationale: The lockout interval for morphine and hydromorphone is 5 to 10 minutes; 8 to 20 minutes for methadone; and 4 to 10 minutes for fentanyl.

References: Elisha S, Heiner JS, Nagelhout JJ. *Nurse Anesthesia.* 7th ed. St. Louis, MO: Elsevier Saunders; 2023: Chapter 56.

Barash PG, Cullen BF, Stoelting RK, et al, eds. *Clinical Anesthesia.* 8th ed. Lippincott Williams & Wilkins; 2017: Chapter 20.

29. A patient taking duloxetine for chronic neuropathic pain is scheduled for a cholecystectomy. How is duloxetine classified?

(A) Tricyclic antidepressant

(B) Selective serotonin reuptake inhibitor

(C) Serotonin-norepinephrine reuptake inhibitor

(D) Non-selective serotonin reuptake inhibitor

Rationale: Selective-norepinephrine reuptake inhibitors commonly used for chronic neuropathic pain include venlafaxine, duloxetine, and milnacipran.

References: Elisha S, Heiner JS, Nagelhout JJ. *Nurse Anesthesia.* 7th ed. St. Louis, MO: Elsevier Saunders; 2023: Chapter 14.

Flood P, Rathmell JP, Urbam RD, eds. *Stoelting's Pharmacology & Physiology in Anesthetic Practice.* 6th ed. Philadelphia, PA: Wolters Kluwer; 2022: Chapter 43.

30. What is the rationale for rapidly freezing plasma for the purpose of making fresh frozen plasma?

(A) Rapid freezing prevents the inactivation of factors VIII and I.

(B) Rapid freezing prevents the inactivation of factors V and VIII.

(C) Rapid freezing prevents the inactivation of all the factors.

(D) Rapid freezing prevents the inactivation of antithrombin III.

Rationale: Plasma is rapidly frozen to help prevent inactivation of the labile coagulation factors, factors V and VIII.

References: Barash PG, Cullen BF, Stoelting RK, et al, eds. *Clinical Anesthesia.* 8th ed. Lippincott Williams & Wilkins; 2017: Chapter 17.

Butterworth JF IV, Mackey DC, Wasnick JD, eds. *Morgan & Mikhail's Clinical Anesthesiology.* 7th ed. New York, NY: McGraw Hill; 2022: Chapter 51.

31. Which of the following is not a risk factor for developing cauda equine syndrome?

(A) 5% Lidocaine spinal anesthesia

(B) Use of glucose to increase baricity of neuraxial anesthetics

(C) Epidural anesthesia

(D) Continuous spinal anesthesia (CSA)

Rationale: Injuries have occurred with CSA most likely because of increased anesthetic doses administered to compensate for an inadequate block. Toxicity can occur with accidental intrathecal injection through what was intended to be an epidural injection.

Most cases of cauda equine syndrome due to local anesthetic neurotoxicity have occurred with the use of 5% lidocaine. Recent cases of cauda equine syndrome have been associated with markedly hyperbaric solutions. Despite this, there is no evidence to suggest that hyperbaric solutions are responsible.

References: Butterworth JF IV, Mackey DC, Wasnick JD, eds. *Morgan & Mikhail's Clinical Anesthesiology.* 7th ed. New York, NY: McGraw Hill; 2022: Chapter 16.

Elisha S, Heiner JS, Nagelhout JJ. *Nurse Anesthesia.* 7th ed. St. Louis, MO: Elsevier Saunders; 2023: Chapter 49.

32. How soon must fresh frozen plasma be transfused once thawed?

(A) Within 4 hours

(B) Within 8 hours

(C) Within 12 hours

(D) Within 24 hours

Rationale: Once fresh frozen plasma has been thawed, it must be given within 24 hours to avoid wastage.

References: Barash PG, Cullen BF, Stoelting RK, et al, eds. *Clinical Anesthesia.* 8th ed. Lippincott Williams & Wilkins; 2017: Chapter 17.

Butterworth JF IV, Mackey DC, Wasnick JD, eds. *Morgan & Mikhail's Clinical Anesthesiology*. 7th ed. New York, NY: McGraw Hill; 2022: Chapter 51.

33. Preoxygenation/denitrogenation results in how many minutes of oxygen reserve?

    (A) 1 to 3 minutes
    (B) 3 to 6 minutes
    (C) 5 to 8 minutes
    (D) >8 minutes

    Rationale: Preoxygenation to an exhaled oxygen content of 90% or greater affords approximately 5 to 8 minutes of oxygen reserve in healthy patients with normal FRC.
    References: Butterworth JF IV, Mackey DC, Wasnick JD, eds. *Morgan & Mikhail's Clinical Anesthesiology*. 7th ed. New York, NY: McGraw Hill; 2022: Chapter 19.
    Elisha S, Heiner JS, Nagelhout JJ. *Nurse Anesthesia*. 7th ed. St. Louis, MO: Elsevier Saunders; 2023: Chapter 24.

34. Which patient should receive a type and crossmatch instead of a type and screen prior to surgery?

    (A) A 48-year-old female scheduled for an endovascular stent of an aortic aneurysm
    (B) An obese 12-year male undergoing an emergency tonsillectomy
    (C) A 22-year-old male with no history of multiple blood transfusions
    (D) A pregnant Rh-positive patient with Rh-negative baby undergoing emergency surgery

    Rationale: Type and cross matches are often performed before the need to transfuse but only when the patient's antibody screen is positive or high risk for a positive screen (C), when the probability of transfusion is high (A), or when the patient is considered at risk for alloimmunization.
    References: Barash PG, Cullen BF, Stoelting RK, et al, eds. *Clinical Anesthesia*. 8th ed. Lippincott Williams & Wilkins; 2017: Chapter 17.
    Butterworth JF IV, Mackey DC, Wasnick JD, eds. *Morgan & Mikhail's Clinical Anesthesiology*. 7th ed. New York, NY: McGraw Hill; 2022: Chapter 51.

35. A 150-kg male patient has a serum sodium concentration of 110 mEq/L. How much sodium would be needed to bring the serum sodium to 125 mEq/L?

    (A) 750 mEq
    (B) 1,350 mEq

    (C) 2,400 mEq
    (D) 3,200 mEq

    Rationale: Using the sodium deficit formula, the answer will be 1,350 mEq. The sodium deficit equation is the following: Sodium deficit (mEq) = ([Na] goal − [Na] plasma) × Total body water; Total body water (TBW) = body weight (in kg) × 60%.
    References: Butterworth JF IV, Mackey DC, Wasnick JD, eds. *Morgan & Mikhail's Clinical Anesthesiology*. 7th ed. New York, NY: McGraw Hill; 2022: Chapter 49.
    Elisha S, Heiner JS, Nagelhout JJ. *Nurse Anesthesia*. 7th ed. St. Louis, MO: Elsevier Saunders; 2023: Chapter 21.

36. How much blood does a fully soaked laparotomy "lap" pad contain?

    (A) 10 to 20 mL
    (B) 25 to 50 mL
    (C) 50 to 100 mL
    (D) 100 to 150 mL

    Rationale: A fully soaked lap pad holds 100 to 150 mL of blood whereas a fully soaked 4 × 4 sponge holds approximately 10 mL.
    References: Butterworth JF IV, Mackey DC, Wasnick JD, eds. *Morgan & Mikhail's Clinical Anesthesiology*. 7th ed. New York, NY: McGraw Hill; 2022: Chapter 51.
    Elisha S, Heiner JS, Nagelhout JJ. *Nurse Anesthesia*. 7th ed. St. Louis, MO: Elsevier Saunders; 2023: Chapter 22.

37. Six hours after a patient received transfusion with 2 units of fresh frozen plasma and 1 unit of platelets, she presents with hypoxia, fever, and noncardiogenic pulmonary edema. What complication do you suspect?

    (A) Post-transfusion purpura
    (B) Transfusion-related acute lung injury
    (C) Delayed hemolytic reaction
    (D) Transfusion-related immunomodulation

    Rationale: Transfusion-related acute lung injury (TRALI) presents as hypoxia, often acute; fever and noncardiogenic pulmonary edema within 6 hours of a blood product transfusion, especially fresh frozen plasma, or platelets. (A) would occur from development of platelet alloantibodies and noted in the precipitous platelet count drop 5 to 10 days after transfusion. Because TRALI is a type of non-hemolytic reaction, (C) is incorrect. (D) would manifest as diminished immune responsiveness and inflammation promotion.
    References: Butterworth JF IV, Mackey DC, Wasnick JD, eds. *Morgan & Mikhail's Clinical Anesthesiology*. 7th ed. New York, NY: McGraw Hill; 2022: Chapter 51.

Elisha S, Heiner JS, Nagelhout JJ. *Nurse Anesthesia.* 7th ed. St. Louis, MO: Elsevier Saunders; 2023: Chapter 22.

38. A 44-year-old 50-kg male received 750 mL of fresh frozen plasma. What percent of normal would you expect his clotting factor concentration to achieve post-transfusion?

(A) 100%

(B) 75%

(C) 60%

(D) 30%

Rationale: The initial therapeutic dose of fresh frozen plasma (FFP) is usually 10 to 15 mL/kg. The final goal of FFP administration is to achieve 30% of the normal coagulation factor concentration.

References: Butterworth JF IV, Mackey DC, Wasnick JD, eds. *Morgan & Mikhail's Clinical Anesthesiology.* 7th ed. New York, NY: McGraw Hill; 2022: Chapter 51.

Elisha S, Heiner JS, Nagelhout JJ. *Nurse Anesthesia.* 7th ed. St. Louis, MO: Elsevier Saunders; 2023: Chapter 22.

Barash PG, Cullen BF, Stoelting RK, et al, eds. *Clinical Anesthesia.* 8th ed. Lippincott Williams & Wilkins; 2017: Chapter 17.

39. For which infectious diseases is donor blood tested after it is collected, typed, and screened?

(A) Hepatitis A, hepatitis B, and hepatitis C

(B) Hepatitis B, hepatitis C, and hepatitis D

(C) Hepatitis C, syphilis, and human immunodeficiency virus

(D) Hepatitis C, cytomegalovirus (CMV), and syphilis

Rationale: Once donor blood is collected, it is typed, screened for antibodies, and tested for hepatitis B, hepatitis C, syphilis, and human immunodeficiency virus.

References: Barash PG, Cullen BF, Stoelting RK, et al, eds. *Clinical Anesthesia.* 8th ed. Lippincott Williams & Wilkins; 2017: Chapter 17.

Butterworth JF IV, Mackey DC, Wasnick JD, eds. *Morgan & Mikhail's Clinical Anesthesiology.* 7th ed. New York, NY: McGraw Hill; 2022: Chapter 51.

40. Which is not an indication for cryoprecipitate administration?

(A) Fibrinogen levels <80 to 100 mg/dL

(B) Factor XIII deficiency

(C) Antithrombin deficiency

(D) Pre-op prophylaxis for patient with von Willebrand disease

Rationale: Cryoprecipitate contains factor VIII, von Willebrand factor (vWF), fibrinogen, fibronectin, and factor XIII. Although factor-specific concentrates can be administered for patients with hemophilia and von Willebrand's disease, it remains an indication for cryoprecipitate administration. Cryoprecipitate is typically administered for documented or suspected fibrinogen levels less than 80 to 100 mg/dL. Antithrombin deficiency is an indication for fresh frozen plasma administration.

References: Barash PG, Cullen BF, Stoelting RK, et al, eds. *Clinical Anesthesia.* 8th ed. Lippincott Williams & Wilkins; 2017: Chapter 17.

Gropper MA. *Miller's Anesthesia.* 9th ed. Philadelphia, PA: Churchill Livingstone Elsevier; 2020: Chapter 49.

41. Which factor is not a complication associated with massive blood transfusion?

(A) Serum K^+ 5.5

(B) Core temperature 35.5°C

(C) Increased 2,3-DPG

(D) Decreased 2,3-DPG

Rationale: Decreased 2,3-DPG is a complication associated with massive transfusion, not increased 2,3-DPG. Hypocalcemia is also associated with massive transfusion. This ionized calcium value is normal. Hyperkalemia (A), hypothermia (B), and decreased 2,3-DPG (D) are all complications of massive blood transfusion.

References: Barash PG, Cullen BF, Stoelting RK, et al, eds. *Clinical Anesthesia.* 8th ed. Lippincott Williams & Wilkins; 2017: Chapter 17.

Butterworth JF IV, Mackey DC, Wasnick JD, eds. *Morgan & Mikhail's Clinical Anesthesiology.* 7th ed. New York, NY: McGraw Hill; 2022: Chapter 51.

Elisha S, Heiner JS, Nagelhout JJ. *Nurse Anesthesia.* 7th ed. St. Louis, MO: Elsevier Saunders; 2023: Chapter 22.

42. What is the approximate half-life of serum albumin?

(A) 12 hours

(B) 6 days

(C) 10 days

(D) 21 days

Rationale: The half-life of serum albumin is approximately 14 to 21 days which is why it is not a reliable indicator of acute liver disease.

References: Barash PG, Cullen BF, Stoelting RK, et al, eds. *Clinical Anesthesia*. 8th ed. Lippincott Williams & Wilkins; 2017: Chapter 46.

Butterworth JF IV, Mackey DC, Wasnick JD, eds. *Morgan & Mikhail's Clinical Anesthesiology*. 7th ed. New York, NY: McGraw Hill; 2022: Chapter 33.

43. Which of the following nerves must be separately blocked during an axillary approach to the brachial plexus?

    (A) Musculocutaneous

    (B) Ulnar

    (C) Medial Brachial Cutaneous

    (D) Median

    Rationale: During the axillary approach to the brachial plexus, the block is performed in the axilla, where large terminal branches have formed. At this point the musculocutaneous nerve (MCN) lies deep within the coracobrachialis, having already left the sheath.

    A separate block is therefore essential to complete forearm and wrist anesthesia. The MCN can be blocked by redirecting the needle, after completing the axillary block, superiorly and posterior to inject within the coracobrachialis.

    References: Butterworth JF IV, Mackey DC, Wasnick JD, eds. *Morgan & Mikhail's Clinical Anesthesiology*. 7th ed. New York, NY: McGraw Hill; 2022: Chapter 46.

    Hadzic, A. (Ed.). *Hadzic's Peripheral Nerve Blocks and Anatomy for Ultrasound-guided Regional Anesthesia* (3rd ed.). McGraw-Hill; 2022: Chapter 17.

44. What is the most effective initial treatment of symptomatic hypercalcemia?

    (A) Hydration with IV normal saline followed by furosemide

    (B) Thiazide followed by IV normal saline hydration

    (C) Hydration with IV normal saline followed by bisphosphonates

    (D) Glucocorticoids followed by IV normal saline hydration

    Rationale: The most effective initial treatment for symptomatic hypercalcemia is hydration with normal saline followed by a loop diuretic to accelerate calcium excretion. Additional therapy would include administering calcitonin or bisphosphonates. Bisphosphonates should only be given once clinical dehydration is treated, or nephrotoxicity may occur secondary to calcium bisphosphonate precipitation. Glucocorticoids would be warranted treatment in the case of vitamin D-induced hypercalemia, but it would not be the most effective initial treatment.

    References: Butterworth JF IV, Mackey DC, Wasnick JD, eds. *Morgan & Mikhail's Clinical Anesthesiology*. 7th ed. New York, NY: McGraw Hill; 2022: Chapter 49.

    Elisha S, Heiner JS, Nagelhout JJ. *Nurse Anesthesia*. 7th ed. St. Louis, MO: Elsevier Saunders; 2023: Chapter 21.

    Gropper MA. *Miller's Anesthesia*. 9th ed. Philadelphia, PA: Churchill Livingstone Elsevier; 2020: Chapter 47.

45. Caudal anesthesia involves needle penetration of the sacrococcygeal ligament covering the sacral hiatus created by which unfused laminae?

    (A) S_1 and S_2

    (B) S_2 and S_3

    (C) S_3 and S_4

    (D) S_4 and S_5

    Rationale: Caudal anesthesia involves needle penetration of the sacrococcygeal ligament covering the sacral hiatus created by unfused S_4 and S_5 laminae.

    References: Barash PG, Cullen BF, Stoelting RK, et al, eds. *Clinical Anesthesia*. 8th ed. Lippincott Williams & Wilkins; 2017: Chapter 42.

    Butterworth JF IV, Mackey DC, Wasnick JD, eds. *Morgan & Mikhail's Clinical Anesthesiology*. 7th ed. New York, NY: McGraw Hill; 2022: Chapter 45.

    Gropper MA. *Miller's Anesthesia*. 9th ed. Philadelphia, PA: Churchill Livingstone Elsevier; 2020: Chapter 76.

46. A 154 lb female has a serum sodium level 120 mEq/L. To correct the sodium level to 128 mEq, how many milliequivalents of sodium are required?

    (A) 280 mEq

    (B) 336 mEq

    (C) 616 mEq

    (D) 739 mEq

    Rationale: Here is the formula: Sodium deficit = TBW × (desired $[Na^+]$ − present $[Na^+]$)
    STEP 1: Convert 154 lbs. to 70 kg by dividing by 2.2.
    STEP 2: Determine that total body water (TBW) for a female is 50%.
    STEP 3: Plug variables into formula: $70 \times 0.50 \times [128 - 120] = 280$ mEq.
    B is derived if TBW was calculated using 60% of body weight for males.
    C is derived if TBW was calculated using 50% of body weight for females but without converting pounds to kg.
    D is derived if TBW was calculated using 60% of body weight for males and without converting pounds to kg.

References: Butterworth JF IV, Mackey DC, Wasnick JD, eds. *Morgan & Mikhail's Clinical Anesthesiology.* 7th ed. New York, NY: McGraw Hill; 2022: Chapter 49.

Elisha S, Heiner JS, Nagelhout JJ. *Nurse Anesthesia.* 7th ed. St. Louis, MO: Elsevier Saunders; 2023: Chapter 21.

47. C fibers transmit what type of sensation?

   (A) Proprioception
   (B) Touch-pressure
   (C) Somatic pain
   (D) Visceral pain

   Rationale: C fibers transmit visceral pain. They are unmyelinated and slow transmitting. Sensation is aching, poorly localized, and usually from a hallow viscus.

References: Butterworth JF IV, Mackey DC, Wasnick JD, eds. *Morgan & Mikhail's Clinical Anesthesiology.* 7th ed. New York, NY: McGraw Hill; 2022: Chapter 47.

Elisha S, Heiner JS, Nagelhout JJ. *Nurse Anesthesia.* 7th ed. St. Louis, MO: Elsevier Saunders; 2023: Chapter 56.

48. Which nerve provides sensory innervation to the lateral thigh?

   (A) Lateral femoral cutaneous
   (B) Saphenous
   (C) Femoral
   (D) Posterior femoral cutaneous

   Rationale: The saphenous nerve provides innervation below the knee. The femoral nerve and its branches innervate the anterior thigh, hip, medial leg, and ankle. The posterior femoral cutaneous nerve innervates the posterior thigh.

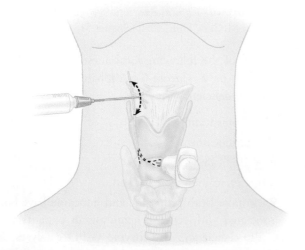

FIG. 3-6. Superior laryngeal nerve block and transtracheal block. (Reproduced with permission from Butterworth JF IV, Mackey DC, Wasnick JD, eds. *Morgan & Mikhail's Clinical Anesthesiology.* 7th ed. New York, NY: McGraw Hill; 2022.)

References: Butterworth JF IV, Mackey DC, Wasnick JD, eds. *Morgan & Mikhail's Clinical Anesthesiology.* 7th ed. New York, NY: McGraw Hill; 2022: Chapter 46.

Elisha S, Heiner JS, Nagelhout JJ. *Nurse Anesthesia.* 7th ed. St. Louis, MO: Elsevier Saunders; 2023: Chapter 50.

49. An axillary block is performed for a surgical procedure on the right forearm and hand. The patient begins to experience pain at the tip of the index finger during the procedure. An effective rescue block would involve injecting local into which of the following sites?

   (A) Antecubital space at the lateral aspect of the biceps tendon
   (B) Antecubital crease medial to the biceps insertion
   (C) One finger breadth proximal to the arcuate ligament
   (D) Immediately lateral to the flexor carpi ulnaris

   Rationale: Sensation for the distal first three fingers is provided by the median nerve. A median nerve rescue block can be performed either at the antecubital crease, medial to the biceps insertion, or at the wrist medial and deep to the palmaris longus tendon.

References: Butterworth JF IV, Mackey DC, Wasnick JD, eds. *Morgan & Mikhail's Clinical Anesthesiology.* 7th ed. New York, NY: McGraw Hill; 2022: Chapter 46.

Hadzic A, ed. *Hadzic's Peripheral Nerve Blocks and Anatomy for Ultrasound-Guided Regional Anesthesia.* 3rd ed. New York, NY: McGraw-Hill; 2022: Chapter 19.

50. Which of the following is associated with slow pain?

   (A) Myelinated A-delta primary efferents
   (B) Action potential 0.5 to 2 m/s
   (C) Myelinated A-delta primary afferents
   (D) Action potential 6 to 30 m/s

   Rationale: Sharp fast pain is characterized by action potentials conducted between 6 and 30 m/s via the myelinated A-delta primary afferent neurons. In contrast, dull, burning, throbbing, or aching pain characterizes slow pain with conduction velocities of 0.5 to 2 m/s via C fibers.

References: Butterworth JF IV, Mackey DC, Wasnick JD, eds. *Morgan & Mikhail's Clinical Anesthesiology.* 7th ed. New York, NY: McGraw Hill; 2022: Chapter 47.

Elisha S, Heiner JS, Nagelhout JJ. *Nurse Anesthesia.* 7th ed. St. Louis, MO: Elsevier Saunders; 2023: Chapter 56.

51. A patient is having pain on the dorsum of the foot and the lateral aspect of the knee. What nerve root is involved?

(A) L_3
(B) L_5
(C) L_4
(D) S_1

Rationale: The dermatome that covers sensation for the dorsum of the foot and the lateral aspect of the knee arises from L_5.

References: Barash PG, Cullen BF, Stoelting RK, et al, eds. *Clinical Anesthesia*. 8th ed. Lippincott Williams & Wilkins; 2017: Chapter 36.

Hadzic A, ed. *Hadzic's Peripheral Nerve Blocks and Anatomy for Ultrasound-Guided Regional Anesthesia*. 3rd ed. New York, NY: McGraw-Hill; 2022: Chapter 21.

52. Which of the following patients are at greatest risk for postdural puncture headaches?

(A) Obese
(B) Elderly
(C) Pregnant
(D) Pediatric

Rationale: Postdural puncture headache is strongly related to young parturients.

References: Barash PG, Cullen BF, Stoelting RK, et al, eds. *Clinical Anesthesia*. 8th ed. Lippincott Williams & Wilkins; 2017: Chapter 35.

Butterworth JF IV, Mackey DC, Wasnick JD, eds. *Morgan & Mikhail's Clinical Anesthesiology*. 7th ed. New York, NY: McGraw Hill; 2022: Chapter 45.

53. While performing an axillary block utilizing the transarterial approach, a paresthesia is elicited after passing through the artery. Which nerve is posterior to the artery?

(A) Ulnar
(B) Radial
(C) Median
(D) Intercostobrachial

Rationale: The radial nerve lies posterior to the axillary artery, and it is anesthetized when injecting posterior to the artery. Ultrasound guided axillary block is now the preferred technique.

References: Butterworth JF IV, Mackey DC, Wasnick JD, eds. *Morgan & Mikhail's Clinical Anesthesiology*. 7th ed. New York, NY: McGraw Hill; 2022: Chapter 46.

Elisha S, Heiner JS, Nagelhout JJ. *Nurse Anesthesia*. 7th ed. St. Louis, MO: Elsevier Saunders; 2023: Chapter 50.

54. A patient receives large volumes of 0.9% normal saline during a case. What is the risk associated with this?

(A) Hypochloremic alkalosis
(B) Hyperchloremic alkalosis
(C) Hypochloremic acidosis
(D) Hyperchloremic acidosis

Rationale: When large volumes of normal saline are given, a dilutional hyperchloremic metabolic acidosis with normal anion gap is produced due to the high sodium and chloride content. As serum chloride concentration increases, plasma bicarbonate concentration decreases.

References: Barash PG, Cullen BF, Stoelting RK, et al, eds. *Clinical Anesthesia*. 8th ed. Lippincott Williams & Wilkins; 2017: Chapter 16.

Butterworth JF IV, Mackey DC, Wasnick JD, eds. *Morgan & Mikhail's Clinical Anesthesiology*. 7th ed. New York, NY: McGraw Hill; 2022: Chapter 51.

55. What causes hypocalcemia?

(A) Hyperparathyroidism
(B) Paget's disease (hypercalcemia)
(C) Fat embolism
(D) Rapid infusion of 1,000 mL normal saline

Rationale: Low PTH levels, fat embolism, and rapid infusion of large volumes of blood preservative with citrate ions (including albumin) cause hypocalcemia.

References: Barash PG, Cullen BF, Stoelting RK, et al, eds. *Clinical Anesthesia*. 8th ed. Lippincott Williams & Wilkins; 2017: Chapter 16.

Butterworth JF IV, Mackey DC, Wasnick JD, eds. *Morgan & Mikhail's Clinical Anesthesiology*. 7th ed. New York, NY: McGraw Hill; 2022: Chapter 51.

56. Which of the following local anesthetics should be avoided in a glucose-6-phosphate dehydrogenase (G_6PD) deficiency?

(A) Ropivacaine
(B) Etidocaine
(C) Prilocaine
(D) Tetracaine

Rationale: Both prilocaine and lidocaine have been associated with red cell hemolysis in patients with G_6PD deficiency. The enzyme G_6PD catalyzes the initial step in the hexose monophosphate shunt which protects red blood cells against oxidative injury by producing NADPH. Hemolysis is triggered when older red blood cells that are deficient in the enzyme are destroyed when exposed to drugs such as prilocaine with high redox potential.

References: Butterworth JF IV, Mackey DC, Wasnick JD, eds. *Morgan & Mikhail's Clinical Anesthesiology*. 7th ed. New York, NY: McGraw Hill; 2022: Chapter 51.

Gropper MA. *Miller's Anesthesia*. 9th ed. Philadelphia, PA: Churchill Livingstone Elsevier; 2020: Chapter 32.

57. You plan to use an intravenous regional technique for hand surgery. What is your greatest concern?

   (A) Duration of the case
   (B) Using the dual tourniquet system
   (C) Tourniquet discomfort
   (D) Tourniquet failure

Rationale: A large volume of local anesthetic from the periphery to the central circulation represents the most serious concern associated with intravenous regional anesthesia. The other variables pose challenges but are readily remedied.

References: Butterworth JF IV, Mackey DC, Wasnick JD, eds. *Morgan & Mikhail's Clinical Anesthesiology*. 7th ed. New York, NY: McGraw Hill; 2022: Chapter 46.

Elisha S, Heiner JS, Nagelhout JJ. *Nurse Anesthesia*. 7th ed. St. Louis, MO: Elsevier Saunders; 2023: Chapter 50.

Gropper MA. *Miller's Anesthesia*. 9th ed. Philadelphia, PA: Churchill Livingstone Elsevier; 2020: Chapter 29.

58. Removal of epidural catheters should be delayed for a minimum of how many hours following the administration of prophylactic low molecular weight heparin (LMWH)?

   (A) 1
   (B) 12
   (C) 3
   (D) 6

Rationale: Due to the risk of spinal hematomas, epidural catheters should be removed at least 12 hours after the last prophylactic dose of LMWH. The next dose of LMWH should not be restarted until 4 hours post epidural catheter was removed. If a patient has been on LMWH more than 4 days, check platelet level prior to removing epidural catheter (based on ASRA guidelines).

References: Elisha S, Heiner JS, Nagelhout JJ. *Nurse Anesthesia*. 7th ed. St. Louis, MO: Elsevier Saunders; 2023: Chapter 38.

Gropper MA. *Miller's Anesthesia*. 9th ed. Philadelphia, PA: Churchill Livingstone Elsevier; 2020: Chapter 45.

59. When performing an ankle block, which of the following nerves is located by identifying the groove formed proximally by the extensor hallucis longus tendon and the extensor digitorum longus tendon?

   (A) Saphenous
   (B) Deep peroneal
   (C) Posterior tibial
   (D) Sural

Rationale: The deep peroneal nerve passes lateral to the anterior tibial artery, extensor hallucis longus and tibialis anterior tendons and medial to the extensor digitorum longus tendon. It is easily accessible as it becomes more superficial to travel with the dorsalis pedis artery. It is located by identifying the groove formed proximally by the extensor hallicus longus tendon and the extensor digitorum longus tendon. This groove can be identified by having the patient extend the great toe, making the extensor hallucis longus tendon more prominent.

References: Barash PG, Cullen BF, Stoelting RK, et al, eds. *Clinical Anesthesia*. 8th ed. Lippincott Williams & Wilkins; 2017: Chapter 36.

Butterworth JF IV, Mackey DC, Wasnick JD, eds. *Morgan & Mikhail's Clinical Anesthesiology*. 7th ed. New York, NY: McGraw Hill; 2022: Chapter 46.

60. Which of the following terms is defined as perception of an ordinary non-noxious stimulus as pain?

   (A) Hyperalgesia
   (B) Allodynia
   (C) Hyperesthesia
   (D) Dysesthesia

Rationale: Allodynia is a perception of an ordinary non-noxious stimulus as pain.

References: Barash PG, Cullen BF, Stoelting RK, et al, eds. *Clinical Anesthesia*. 8th ed. Lippincott Williams & Wilkins; 2017: Chapter 55.

Butterworth JF IV, Mackey DC, Wasnick JD, eds. *Morgan & Mikhail's Clinical Anesthesiology*. 7th ed. New York, NY: McGraw Hill; 2022: Chapter 47.

61. What is your main anesthetic concern when caring for a patient taking anabolic steroids?

   (A) Myocardial infarction
   (B) Hepatotoxicity
   (C) Hypercoagulopathy
   (D) Stroke

Rationale: Each of the responses may be linked to the use of anabolic steroids. Hepatotoxicity poses direct implications for the anesthetic plan specifically regarding medications metabolized by the liver.

References: Butterworth JF IV, Mackey DC, Wasnick JD, eds. *Morgan & Mikhail's Clinical Anesthesiology.* 7th ed. New York, NY: McGraw Hill; 2022: Chapter 47.

Elisha S, Heiner JS, Nagelhout JJ. *Nurse Anesthesia.* 7th ed. St. Louis, MO: Elsevier Saunders; 2023: Chapter 20.

62. Injecting local anesthetic at which site is associated with the greatest risk of systemic absorption?

    (A) Brachial plexus

    (B) Paracervical

    (C) Intercostal

    (D) Caudal

Rationale: Intercostal nerve blocks result in the highest blood levels of any block in the body. In general, more vascular locations result in greater risk of systemic absorption. The risk declines as follows: IV (or intraarterial) > tracheal (transmucosal) > intercostal > caudal epidural space > lumbar epidural space > brachial plexus > sciatic-femoral > subcutaneous.

References: Elisha S, Heiner JS, Nagelhout JJ. *Nurse Anesthesia.* 7th ed. St. Louis, MO: Elsevier Saunders; 2023: Chapter 10.

Gropper MA. *Miller's Anesthesia.* 9th ed. Philadelphia, PA: Churchill Livingstone Elsevier; 2020: Chapter 29.

63. Which topical local anesthetic may cause methemoglobinemia?

    (A) Bupivacaine

    (B) Procaine

    (C) Mepivacaine

    (D) Benzocaine

Rationale: Clinically significant methemoglobinemia may result when using topical prilocaine and benzocaine. Bupivacaine, mepivacaine, and procaine are not topical anesthetics.

References: Butterworth JF IV, Mackey DC, Wasnick JD, eds. *Morgan & Mikhail's Clinical Anesthesiology.* 7th ed. New York, NY: McGraw Hill; 2022: Chapter 16.

Elisha S, Heiner JS, Nagelhout JJ. *Nurse Anesthesia.* 7th ed. St. Louis, MO: Elsevier Saunders; 2023: Chapter 10.

64. Which of the following factors has the greatest effect on the level of spinal anesthesia?

    (A) Age

    (B) Patient height

    (C) Position of patient during injection

    (D) Drug volume

Rationale: The most important factors affecting the level of spinal anesthesia are the solution baricity, drug dose, injection site, and patient position both during and directly after injection. In general, higher levels are obtained with higher doses, higher sites of injection and hypobaric solutions (when in head-up position).

References: Butterworth JF IV, Mackey DC, Wasnick JD, eds. *Morgan & Mikhail's Clinical Anesthesiology.* 7th ed. New York, NY: McGraw Hill; 2022: Chapter 45.

Elisha S, Heiner JS, Nagelhout JJ. *Nurse Anesthesia.* 7th ed. St. Louis, MO: Elsevier Saunders; 2023: Chapter 49.

65. A female patient's preoperative hematocrit is 42%. How much blood could a 90-kg patient lose and still maintain a hematocrit of 30%?

    (A) 702 mL

    (B) 2,106 mL

    (C) 2,457 mL

    (D) 5,850 mL

Rationale: Calculation

Step 1: Calculate EBV for a female: 90 kg × 65 mL/kg = 5,850 mL (D: incorrect)

Step 2: Calculate $RBCV_{42}$: 5,850 × 42% = 2,457 mL (C incorrect)

Step 3: Calculate $RBCS_{30}$: 5,850 × 30% = 1,755 mL

Step 4: Calculate Red cell loss at 30%: 2,457 − 1,755 = 702 mL (A incorrect)

Step 5: Calculate ABL: 702 mL × 2 = 2,106 mL (B is correct)

References: Butterworth JF IV, Mackey DC, Wasnick JD, eds. *Morgan & Mikhail's Clinical Anesthesiology.* 7th ed. New York, NY: McGraw Hill; 2022: Chapter 51.

Elisha S, Heiner JS, Nagelhout JJ. *Nurse Anesthesia.* 7th ed. St. Louis, MO: Elsevier Saunders; 2023: Chapter 22.

66. Interruption of pain impulses can be accomplished through the administration of intrathecal opioids. These opioids act by binding to which of the following sites?

    (A) Periaqueductal gray

    (B) Dorsal root ganglia

    (C) Anterior horn

    (D) Dorsal horn

Rationale: Small quantities of opioids injected within the intrathecal or epidural space produce analgesia segmentally, confined to the sensory nerves entering the dorsal horn of the spinal cord in the vicinity of the area of injection. Presynaptic opioid receptors inhibit primary afferent release of substance P and other neurotransmitters. Postsynaptic opioid receptors decrease spinothalamic tract activity in the dorsal horn.

References: Butterworth JF IV, Mackey DC, Wasnick JD, eds. *Morgan & Mikhail's Clinical Anesthesiology.* 7th ed. New York, NY: McGraw Hill; 2022: Chapter 10.

Elisha S, Heiner JS, Nagelhout JJ. *Nurse Anesthesia.* 7th ed. St. Louis, MO: Elsevier Saunders; 2023: Chapter 11.

67. Epidural morphine was administered for postoperative pain control. What is the duration of action?

(A)   12 to 24 hours

(B)   4 to 6 hours

(C)   24 to 48 hours

(D)   2 to 6 hours

Rationale: The duration of action for epidural narcotics includes morphine 12 to 14 hours; sufentanil 4 to 6 hours; and fentanyl 2 to 6 hours.

References: Butterworth JF IV, Mackey DC, Wasnick JD, eds. *Morgan & Mikhail's Clinical Anesthesiology.* 7th ed. New York, NY: McGraw Hill; 2022: Chapter 41.

Elisha S, Heiner JS, Nagelhout JJ. *Nurse Anesthesia.* 7th ed. St. Louis, MO: Elsevier Saunders; 2023: Chapter 49.

68. A 20-kg child is scheduled for a urology procedure. What is the appropriate dose for a caudal anesthetic?

(A)   10 mL

(B)   5 mL

(C)   3 mL

(D)   25 mL

Rationale: The local anesthetic dose for a caudal block is 0.5 to 1 mL/kg in children.

References: Butterworth JF IV, Mackey DC, Wasnick JD, eds. *Morgan & Mikhail's Clinical Anesthesiology.* 7th ed. New York, NY: McGraw Hill; 2022: Chapter 45.

Elisha S, Heiner JS, Nagelhout JJ. *Nurse Anesthesia.* 7th ed. St. Louis, MO: Elsevier Saunders; 2023: Chapter 49.

69. Which of the following peripheral nerve blocks would provide the most effective analgesia for a total knee arthroplasty?

(A)   Femoral nerve block

(B)   Femoral nerve block and obturator nerve block

(C)   Sciatic nerve block and psoas block

(D)   Sciatic and popliteal block

Rationale: Patients undergoing total knee arthroplasty experience significant postoperative pain. Surgical anesthesia for knee procedures utilizing a tourniquet can be provided through blockade of the femoral, lateral femoral cutaneous, obturator and sciatic nerves.

To provide exclusively regional anesthesia for this procedure, of the listed options, only the sciatic nerve block and the psoas block, also known as the lumbar plexus block (which covers the lateral femoral cutaneous, femoral and obturator nerves) covers the nerves involved.

References: Butterworth JF IV, Mackey DC, Wasnick JD, eds. *Morgan & Mikhail's Clinical Anesthesiology.* 7th ed. New York, NY: McGraw Hill; 2022: Chapter 46.

Elisha S, Heiner JS, Nagelhout JJ. *Nurse Anesthesia.* 7th ed. St. Louis, MO: Elsevier Saunders; 2023: Chapter 50.

70. Which mechanisms of action are common among nonsteroidal anti-inflammatory drugs?

(A)   Inhibition of cyclooxygenase and prostaglandin synthesis

(B)   Promotes release of serotonin

(C)   Inhibition of lipoxygenase

(D)   Inhibition of leukotriene synthesis

Rationale: Nonsteroidal anti-inflammatory drugs inhibit cyclooxygenase and subsequent prostaglandin synthesis.

References: Butterworth JF IV, Mackey DC, Wasnick JD, eds. *Morgan & Mikhail's Clinical Anesthesiology.* 7th ed. New York, NY: McGraw Hill; 2022: Chapter 10.

Hemmings HC Jr, Egan TD, eds. *Pharmacology and Physiology for Anesthesia: Foundations and Clinical Application.* 2nd ed. Philadelphia, PA: Elsevier Saunders; 2019: Chapter 19.

71. What factor is not associated with postoperative pulmonary complications?

(A)   ASA III

(B)   Cigarette smoking

(C)   Aortic aneurysm repair

(D)   Surgery lasting 2 hours

Rationale: Factors that lead to postoperative pulmonary complications include each of the items except surgery last 3 hours. Surgery lasting 4 or more hours is linked to postoperative pulmonary complications.

References: Barash PG, Cullen BF, Stoelting RK, et al, eds. *Clinical Anesthesia.* 8th ed. Lippincott Williams & Wilkins; 2017: Chapter 15.

Butterworth JF IV, Mackey DC, Wasnick JD, eds. *Morgan & Mikhail's Clinical Anesthesiology.* 7th ed. New York, NY: McGraw Hill; 2022: Chapter 24.

72. Which muscle is likely to be unaffected by an axillary brachial plexus block?

(A)   Abductor pollicis brevis

(B)   Interosseous

(C) Brachialis

(D) Pronator teres

Rationale: The axillary block is one of the most common nerve blocks and potential for serious complication is low, however the block is often incomplete. Blockade it at the level of terminal nerves after separation of the musculocutaneous nerve, which requires an additional injection for a complete block. The musculocutaneous nerve enters the coracobrachialis muscle, which it innervates, and goes on to supply the biceps brachii and the brachialis. Sensory innervation is provided to the skin on the radial side of the forearm to the radiocarpal joint.

References: Butterworth JF IV, Mackey DC, Wasnick JD, eds. *Morgan & Mikhail's Clinical Anesthesiology.* 7th ed. New York, NY: McGraw Hill; 2022: Chapter 46.

Elisha S, Heiner JS, Nagelhout JJ. *Nurse Anesthesia.* 7th ed. St. Louis, MO: Elsevier Saunders; 2023: Chapter 50.

73. Which of the following does not define somatic nociceptive pain?

(A) Transduction

(B) Transmission

(C) Thermal

(D) Modulation

Rationale: Transduction, transmission, modulation, and perception are the processes involved with somatic nociceptive pain. Thermal, mechanical, or chemical stimuli result in an action potential via transduction.

References: Butterworth JF IV, Mackey DC, Wasnick JD, eds. *Morgan & Mikhail's Clinical Anesthesiology.* 7th ed. New York, NY: McGraw Hill; 2022: Chapter 47.

Elisha S, Heiner JS, Nagelhout JJ. *Nurse Anesthesia.* 7th ed. St. Louis, MO: Elsevier Saunders; 2023: Chapter 56.

74. During an unremarkable spinal anesthetic a bilateral T_2 level in a healthy parturient results in cardiac arrest. Which of the following is most likely responsible?

(A) Decreased preload

(B) Effect of local anesthetic on the medulla

(C) Blockade of the carotid sinus

(D) Cardiogenic hypertensive chemoreflex

Rationale: Cardiac arrest occurs in approximately 0.07 to 0.15% of spinal anesthetics. Most of these episodes of cardiac arrest are due directly or indirectly to sympathetic blockade. Inhibiting sympathetic efferents decreases venous return with reduction in right atrial pressure by 36% with low spinals and 53% with high spinals. Volume depletion can increase this to 66% on average.

Dramatic reduction in preload initiates three reflexes which can result in bradycardia or sinus arrest: (1) the pacemaker stretch reflex is a result of myocardial pacemaker cells firing in proportion to the degree of stretch. Decreased venous return results in decreased stretch and thus decreased firing. (2) Low pressure barorecptors are stimulated in the right atrium and vena cava which causes bradycardia. (3) The Bezold-Jarisch reflex occurs when intracardiac mechanoreceptors in the left ventricle are stimulated producing bradycardia.

References: Butterworth JF IV, Mackey DC, Wasnick JD, eds. *Morgan & Mikhail's Clinical Anesthesiology.* 7th ed. New York, NY: McGraw Hill; 2022: Chapter 45.

Elisha S, Heiner JS, Nagelhout JJ. *Nurse Anesthesia.* 7th ed. St. Louis, MO: Elsevier Saunders; 2023: Chapter 49.

75. Which medication should be held on the day of surgery?

(A) Beta-adrenergic blockers

(B) Tricyclic antidepressants

(C) Selective serotonin reuptake inhibitors

(D) Beta-adrenergic blocker combinations

Rationale: Stopping tricyclic antidepressants may lead to cholinergic symptoms, cardiac disturbances, and neurological symptoms. There is conflict in the literature regarding holding ACE inhibitors the day of surgery. Miller references to continue ACE inhibitors while Nagelhout and Barash advises to hold the day of surgery. Stopping ACE inhibitors may result in atrial fibrillation and/or congestive heart failure. Severe refractory hypotension may develop in patients who take their ACE inhibitor the day of surgery. Vasopressin is the drug of choice to correct refractory hypotension. If beta-adrenergic blockers are held, cardiac disturbances and withdrawal symptoms may occur. Continued selective serotonin reuptake inhibitors (SSRI) in the perioperative period is associated with increased intraoperative bleeding. However, SSRIs are usually not held the day of surgery (due to side effects from abrupt discontinuation) unless surgical bleeding could result in detrimental outcomes (e.g., intracranial surgery).

References: Elisha S, Heiner JS, Nagelhout JJ. *Nurse Anesthesia.* 7th ed. St. Louis, MO: Elsevier Saunders; 2023: Chapter 25.

Gropper MA. *Miller's Anesthesia.* 9th ed. Philadelphia, PA: Churchill Livingstone Elsevier; 2020: Chapter 31.

76. What nerve injury results most often with the lithotomy position?

(A) Common peroneal

(B) Sciatic

(C) Obturator

(D) Saphenous

Rationale: Each of the nerves may be affected by the lithotomy position. The nerve most likely to be injured in the lithotomy position is the common peroneal.

References: Butterworth JF IV, Mackey DC, Wasnick JD, eds. *Morgan & Mikhail's Clinical Anesthesiology*. 7th ed. New York, NY: McGraw Hill; 2022: Chapter 32.

Elisha S, Heiner JS, Nagelhout JJ. *Nurse Anesthesia*. 7th ed. St. Louis, MO: Elsevier Saunders; 2023: Chapter 23.

77. Which of the following explains the rapid onset of 2-chloroprocaine when used for epidural anesthesia?

(A) It is activated by ester hydrolysis.

(B) It is administered in high concentrations.

(C) It has high potency and lipid solubility.

(D) It has relatively low pKa.

Rationale: 2-Chloroprocaine is a rapidly acting local anesthetic despite its slow onset in isolated nerves. Its high pKa of 9 and large charge would normally result in a slow onset of action. It, however, has a low toxicity and therefore can be administered in high concentrations of 3%. The resultant large number of molecules results in mass diffusion and therefore quick onset.

The onset of local anesthetic in isolated nerves (in vitro) is determined to a large extent by the concentration of lipid soluble (non-ionized) agent administered to the nerve to be anesthetized. The relative concentration of non-ionized to ionized form present in a particular agent is expressed by its pKa, the pH at which these amounts are equal. Agents which have a pKa closer to physiological pH exist in a non-ionized state in larger concentrations, resulting in a faster onset. Reducing the pH of the agent by mixing it with an alkaline solution (sodium bicarbonate) increases the amount of non-ionized free base available and thus increases speed of onset. Other characteristics such as ease of diffusion and concentration affect the clinical onset of action.

References: Barash PG, Cullen BF, Stoelting RK, et al, eds. *Clinical Anesthesia*. 8th ed. Lippincott Williams & Wilkins; 2017: Chapter 42.

Gropper MA. *Miller's Anesthesia*. 9th ed. Philadelphia, PA: Churchill Livingstone Elsevier; 2020: Chapter 29.

78. A patient taking furosemide is scheduled for a total knee arthroscopy. What statement is true?

(A) Continue in patients with chronic renal failure

(B) Discontinue

(C) Continue in patients with diabetes

(D) Discontinue in the elderly

Rationale: Diuretics may be held without concern except for patients with chronic renal failure or congestive heart failure. Patients in chronic renal failure often have hyperkalemia and rely on loop diuretics to increase potassium excretion (kaliuresis).

References: Barash PG, Cullen BF, Stoelting RK, et al, eds. *Clinical Anesthesia*. 8th ed. Lippincott Williams & Wilkins; 2017: Chapter 16.

Gropper MA. *Miller's Anesthesia*. 9th ed. Philadelphia, PA: Churchill Livingstone Elsevier; 2020: Chapter 31.

79. What discontinuation issues may result for patients who take angiotensin converting enzyme (ACE) inhibitors?

(A) Potential clotting abnormalities

(B) Cholinergic symptoms and psychosis

(C) Rebound hypertension

(D) Reduced arterial compliance

Rationale: Discontinuing preoperative medications may result in potential clotting abnormalities with nonsteroidal anti-inflammatories or antiplatelet drugs; cholinergic symptoms with tricyclic antidepressants; psychosis or agitation with selective serotonin reuptake inhibitors (SSRIs) and reduced arterial compliance with ACE inhibitors. Unlike clonidine, abrupt discontinuation of ACE inhibitors does not cause rebound hypertension.

References: Barash PG, Cullen BF, Stoelting RK, et al, eds. *Clinical Anesthesia*. 8th ed. Lippincott Williams & Wilkins; 2017: Chapter 13.

Flood P, Rathmell JP, Urbam RD, eds. *Stoelting's Pharmacology & Physiology in Anesthetic Practice*. 6th ed. Philadelphia, PA: Wolters Kluwer; 2022: Chapter 20.

80. What is the preexisting fluid deficit for a 13-kg patient fasting for 6 hours?

(A) 46 mL/h

(B) 53 mL/h

(C) 138 mL/h

(D) 276 mL/h

Rationale: Calculating the preexisting fluid for this patient is as follows:
Step 1: Using the 4-2-1 rule for a 13-kg patient,
4 mL/kg/h × 10 kg = 40 mL/h
2 mL/kg/h × 3 kg = 6 mL/h
Total maintenance rate: 46 mL/h
Step 2: To calculate the preexisting deficit, 46 mL/hours × 6 hours = 276 mL
References: Barash PG, Cullen BF, Stoelting RK, et al, eds. *Clinical Anesthesia.* 8th ed. Lippincott Williams & Wilkins; 2017: Chapter 16.
Butterworth JF IV, Mackey DC, Wasnick JD, eds. *Morgan & Mikhail's Clinical Anesthesiology.* 7th ed. New York, NY: McGraw Hill; 2022: Chapter 51.

81. Which of the following elements in the postoperative note is not required by the Center for Medicare and Medicaid Services (CMS)?

    (A) Mental status
    (B) Temperature
    (C) Pain
    (D) Urine output

Rationale: In addition to A, B, and C, respiratory and cardiovascular parameters, nausea, vomiting, and hydration are required documentation per CMS.
References: Butterworth JF IV, Mackey DC, Wasnick JD, eds. *Morgan & Mikhail's Clinical Anesthesiology.* 7th ed. New York, NY: McGraw Hill; 2022: Chapter 18.
Gropper MA. *Miller's Anesthesia.* 9th ed. Philadelphia, PA: Churchill Livingstone Elsevier; 2020: Chapter 80.

82. Which nerve is blocked by injection through the thyrohyoid membrane to anesthetize the area between the vocal cords and the epiglottis?

    (A) Hypoglossal
    (B) Recurrent laryngeal
    (C) Superior laryngeal
    (D) Glossopharyngeal

Rationale: Sensory innervation of the airway below the epiglottis is supplied by the vagus nerve. The internal branch of the superior laryngeal nerve provides sensation from the epiglottis to the vocal cords.
References: Barash PG, Cullen BF, Stoelting RK, et al, eds. *Clinical Anesthesia.* 8th ed. Lippincott Williams & Wilkins; 2017: Chapter 28.
Butterworth JF IV, Mackey DC, Wasnick JD, eds. *Morgan & Mikhail's Clinical Anesthesiology.* 7th ed. New York, NY: McGraw Hill; 2022: Chapter 19.

83. Tachycardia, euphoria, delirium, and excitement are noted when conducting the preoperative evaluation in the emergency department. Which of the following is probably not related to the symptoms?

    (A) Narcotics
    (B) Cocaine
    (C) Hallucinogens
    (D) Marijuana

Rationale: Opioids produce respiratory depression, hypotension, and bradycardia. Euphoria may occur as well as pinpoint pupils linked to overdose.
References: Butterworth JF IV, Mackey DC, Wasnick JD, eds. *Morgan & Mikhail's Clinical Anesthesiology.* 7th ed. New York, NY: McGraw Hill; 2022: Chapters 10 and 16.
Flood P, Rathmell JP, Urbam RD, eds. *Stoelting's Pharmacology & Physiology in Anesthetic Practice.* 6th ed. Philadelphia, PA: Wolters Kluwer; 2022: Chapter 7.

84. Which of the following may cause prolonged sedation?

    (A) Echinacea and garlic
    (B) Ephedra and garlic
    (C) Garlic and kava kava
    (D) Kava kava and valerian

Rationale: Anesthetic implications for patients taking echinacea include allergic reactions, liver enzyme induction, and immune system dysfunction. The sympathomimetic effects of ephedra predispose to myocardial infarction and stroke. Garlic increases the possibility of bleeding.
References: Elisha S, Heiner JS, Nagelhout JJ. *Nurse Anesthesia.* 7th ed. St. Louis, MO: Elsevier Saunders; 2023: Chapter 20.
Gropper MA. *Miller's Anesthesia.* 9th ed. Philadelphia, PA: Churchill Livingstone Elsevier; 2020: Chapter 33.

85. Calculate the ideal body weight (BW) for a 6', 90-kg male.

    (A) 80 kg
    (B) 177 kg
    (C) 72 kg
    (D) 145 kg

Rationale: The IBW for males is calculated by the following equation: 105 lb + 6 lb for every inch over 5 feet. For females, add 5 lb for every inch over 5 feet (Nagelhout). Formulas vary by textbook. According to Barash, the formula used is IBW (kg) = height (cm) − x, where x is 100 for adult males and 105 for adult females.

References: Barash PG, Cullen BF, Stoelting RK, et al, eds. *Clinical Anesthesia.* 8th ed. Lippincott Williams & Wilkins; 2017: Chapter 45.

Elisha S, Heiner JS, Nagelhout JJ. *Nurse Anesthesia.* 7th ed. St. Louis, MO: Elsevier Saunders; 2023: Chapter 20.

86. A morbidly obese male patient is scheduled for a bariatric surgery. Which of the following diagnostic tests should be ordered?

    (A) Chest x-ray and coagulation studies

    (B) 12 lead EKG and hCG

    (C) Coagulation studies glucose tolerance test

    (D) hCG

    Rationale: Diagnostic testing for bariatric surgery includes a CBC, complete chemistry, fasting blood glucose, lipid profile, iron, vitamin, and mineral levels. Chest x-ray, 12-lead EKG, and coagulation testing are indicated. The pregnancy test is not indicated.

    References: Barash PG, Cullen BF, Stoelting RK, et al, eds. *Clinical Anesthesia.* 8th ed. Lippincott Williams & Wilkins; 2017: Chapter 45.

    Elisha S, Heiner JS, Nagelhout JJ. *Nurse Anesthesia.* 7th ed. St. Louis, MO: Elsevier Saunders; 2023: Chapter 20.

87. A patient with two peripheral intravenous (PIV) lines is undergoing GETA for an orthopedic procedure. A recent lab value reveals a serum potassium level of 2.9 mEq/L. Which intervention is appropriate for this patient?

    (A) Administer IV replacement K^+ in dextrose solutions

    (B) Maintain $ETCO_2$ levels between 25 and 30 mmHg

    (C) Reduce the rocuronium redose by 25 to 50%

    (D) Administer IV replacement K^+ 20 mEq IV in 0.9% NS over 1 hour

    Rationale: Increased sensitivity to neuromuscular blockers is common in patients with hypokalemia and therefore, dosages should be reduced by 25 to 50%. A is incorrect because dextrose containing solutions will result in hyperglycemia and secondary insulin secretion, thus worsening hypokalemia. B is incorrect because hyperventilation will cause further decreases in plasma K^+. D is incorrect because peripheral replacement of K^+ should not exceed 8 mEq/h. Rapid replacement (i.e., 10 to 20 mEq/L) requires central venous administration.

    References: Butterworth JF IV, Mackey DC, Wasnick JD, eds. *Morgan & Mikhail's Clinical Anesthesiology.* 7th ed. New York, NY: McGraw Hill; 2022: Chapter 49.

Elisha S, Heiner JS, Nagelhout JJ. *Nurse Anesthesia.* 7th ed. St. Louis, MO: Elsevier Saunders; 2023: Chapter 21.

88. What is the primary innervation of the lumbar facet joint?

    (A) The spinal nerve at the level of the joint

    (B) The spinal nerve superior to the joint

    (C) Both the nerve at the joint level and the nerve immediately superior

    (D) Neither the superior nor the inferior spinal nerve

    Rationale: Facet joints are innervated by the spinal nerve at the level of the joint and the immediately superior spinal nerve.

    References: Butterworth JF IV, Mackey DC, Wasnick JD, eds. *Morgan & Mikhail's Clinical Anesthesiology.* 7th ed. New York, NY: McGraw Hill; 2022: Chapter 47.

    Gropper MA. *Miller's Anesthesia.* 9th ed. Philadelphia, PA: Churchill Livingstone Elsevier; 2020: Chapter 51.

89. What is the gold standard diagnostic test for obstructive sleep apnea?

    (A) Polysomnography

    (B) STOP-bang questionnaire

    (C) STOP questionnaire

    (D) Bang questionnaire

    Rationale: The Stop-bank questionnaire is an obstructive sleep apnea screening tool.

    References: Elisha S, Heiner JS, Nagelhout JJ. *Nurse Anesthesia.* 7th ed. St. Louis, MO: Elsevier Saunders; 2023: Chapter 20.

    Barash PG, Cullen BF, Stoelting RK, et al, eds. *Clinical Anesthesia.* 8th ed. Lippincott Williams & Wilkins; 2017: Chapter 45.

90. A patient with rheumatoid arthritis is undergoing a total knee replacement. What is the recommended glucocorticoid dosing regimen?

    (A) Usual corticosteroid dose + hydrocortisone 25 mg

    (B) Usual corticosteroid dose + hydrocortisone 100 mg

    (C) Usual corticosteroid dose + 150 mg

    (D) Usual corticosteroid dose + 50 mg

    Rationale: Steroid coverage is based on the degree of surgical stress. Total join replacements are considered moderate surgical stress. For minor procedures, 25 mg of hydrocortisone is recommended whereas major stress procedures including cardiac and large vascular procedures require 100 to 150 mg every 8 hours for 2 to 3 days (Nagelhout). Conflict exists in the literature regarding treatment with the patient's normal daily dose of steroid either with or without supplementation.

References: Butterworth JF IV, Mackey DC, Wasnick JD, eds. *Morgan & Mikhail's Clinical Anesthesiology*. 7th ed. New York, NY: McGraw Hill; 2022: Chapter 35.
Elisha S, Heiner JS, Nagelhout JJ. *Nurse Anesthesia*. 7th ed. St. Louis, MO: Elsevier Saunders; 2023: Chapter 37.

91. Which diagnostic finding is consistent with intracranial hypertension?

(A) MRI with a 0.5-mm midline brain shift

(B) CT with a 0.5-cm midline brain shift

(C) CT with contrast with a 0.4-cm midline brain shift

(D) MRI with a 0.4-cm midline brain shift

Rationale: A computed tomography (CT) scan or an MRI that evidences a 0.5-cm midline brain shift represents a finding consistent with intracranial hypertension.

References: Butterworth JF IV, Mackey DC, Wasnick JD, eds. *Morgan & Mikhail's Clinical Anesthesiology*. 7th ed. New York, NY: McGraw Hill; 2022: Chapter 27.
Elisha S, Heiner JS, Nagelhout JJ. *Nurse Anesthesia*. 7th ed. St. Louis, MO: Elsevier Saunders; 2023: Chapter 20.

92. Which surgical procedure poses the lowest risk for myocardial infarction within 30 days of surgery?

(A) Liver transplant

(B) Prostatectomy

(C) Liver resection

(D) Cataract

Rationale: Liver transplant and prostatectomy are considered intermediate risk carrying a 1 to 5% likelihood of myocardial infarction following surgery. Vascular and aortic procedures carry the highest risk of infarct (>5%).

References: Barash PG, Cullen BF, Stoelting RK, et al, eds. *Clinical Anesthesia*. 8th ed. Lippincott Williams & Wilkins; 2017: Chapter 23.
Elisha S, Heiner JS, Nagelhout JJ. *Nurse Anesthesia*. 7th ed. St. Louis, MO: Elsevier Saunders; 2023: Chapter 13.

93. What is the most common cause of nonsurgical bleeding following massive blood transfusion?

(A) Dilutional thrombocytopenia

(B) Citrate toxicity

(C) Dilution of factors V and X

(D) Dilution of factors II and VIII

Rationale: Dilutional thrombocytopenia is the most common cause of nonsurgical bleeding following massive blood transfusion. Dilutional coagulopathy is also associated with massive transfusion, specifically dilution of factors V and VIII.

References: Butterworth JF IV, Mackey DC, Wasnick JD, eds. *Morgan & Mikhail's Clinical Anesthesiology*. 7th ed. New York, NY: McGraw Hill; 2022: Chapter 51.
Gropper MA. *Miller's Anesthesia*. 9th ed. Philadelphia, PA: Churchill Livingstone Elsevier; 2020: Chapter 49.

94. The patient weighs 120 kg. The ideal body weight is 60 kg. What is the patient's classification?

(A) Obese

(B) Morbidly obese

(C) Overweight

(D) Moderate obesity

Rationale: Morbid obesity (also called "extreme obesity") is twice the ideal body weight. Obesity reflects 20% over the ideal body weight.

References: Butterworth JF IV, Mackey DC, Wasnick JD, eds. *Morgan & Mikhail's Clinical Anesthesiology*. 7th ed. New York, NY: McGraw Hill; 2022: Chapter 35.
Elisha S, Heiner JS, Nagelhout JJ. *Nurse Anesthesia*. 7th ed. St. Louis, MO: Elsevier Saunders; 2023: Chapter 20.

95. An adult patient's platelet count is 25,000/μL. After transfusing the patient with 2 units of apheresis platelets, what would you expect the platelet count to be?

(A) 30,000 to 35,000/μL

(B) 55,000 to 85,000/μL

(C) 85,000 to 145,000/μL

(D) 145,000 to 165,000/μL

Rationale: One unit of apheresis platelets will increase the platelet count by 30,000 to 60,000/μL. Two units of apheresis platelets will increase the platelet count by 60,000 to 120,000/μL. A single unit of platelets will increase the platelet count by 5,000 to 10,000/μL.

References: Barash PG, Cullen BF, Stoelting RK, et al, eds. *Clinical Anesthesia*. 8th ed. Lippincott Williams & Wilkins; 2017: Chapter 17.
Butterworth JF IV, Mackey DC, Wasnick JD, eds. *Morgan & Mikhail's Clinical Anesthesiology*. 7th ed. New York, NY: McGraw Hill; 2022: Chapter 51.

96. During the preoperative interview the patient shares that they perform light housework, play golf once a week and walk to the grocery store to get the newspaper. What is their metabolic equivalent (METs)?

(A) 1 MET

(B) 2 METs

(C) 3 METs

(D) 4 METs

Rationale: Good functional capacity (4 METs) includes those listed as well as heavy housework, short distance running and climbing a flight of stairs without stopping. Poor functional capacity (1 MET) includes basic activities of daily living and walking one to two blocks (<4 mph).

References: Elisha S, Heiner JS, Nagelhout JJ. *Nurse Anesthesia.* 7th ed. St. Louis, MO: Elsevier Saunders; 2023: Chapter 20.

Gropper MA. *Miller's Anesthesia.* 9th ed. Philadelphia, PA: Churchill Livingstone Elsevier; 2020: Chapter 31.

97. What AANA Standard guides the practice of providing postanesthesia report?

(A) Standard I

(B) Standard III

(C) Standard V

(D) Standard XI

Rationale: Standard XI speaks to the need to "transfer responsibility" for continuity of care.

References: American Association of Nurse Anesthetists (AANA): *AANA Scope and Standards of Nurse Anesthesia Practice:* Standard XI. https://www.aana.com/docs/default-source/practice-aana-com-web-documents-(all)/professional-practice-manual/standards-for-nurse-anesthesia-practice.pdf?sfvrsn=e00049b1_20

Elisha S, Heiner JS, Nagelhout JJ. *Nurse Anesthesia.* 7th ed. St. Louis, MO: Elsevier Saunders; 2023: Chapter 55.

98. Which statement about fresh frozen plasma (FFP) administration is correct?

(A) Each unit of FFP will increase the level of each clotting factor by 2 to 3% in adults.

(B) The initial therapeutic dose is 1 to 5 mL/kg.

(C) It should be ABO-compatible.

(D) It must be Rh-compatible.

Rationale: A unit of FFP will increase the level of each clotting factor by 2 to 3% in adults.

The initial therapeutic dose is generally 10 to 15 mL/kg and should be ABO-compatible. Rh compatibility is not mandatory. The therapeutic goal is to achieve 30% of the normal coagulation factor concentration.

References: Barash PG, Cullen BF, Stoelting RK, et al, eds. *Clinical Anesthesia.* 8th ed. Lippincott Williams & Wilkins; 2017: Chapter 17.

Butterworth JF IV, Mackey DC, Wasnick JD, eds. *Morgan & Mikhail's Clinical Anesthesiology.* 7th ed. New York, NY: McGraw Hill; 2022: Chapter 51.

99. Which of the following are risk factors for postoperative nausea and vomiting?

(A) Male gender

(B) History of motion sickness and opioids

(C) Opioids and laser retinal surgery

(D) Cataract surgery

Rationale: Females are more likely to experience PONV than males. General anesthesia and commonly used opioids, volatile agents, and nitrous oxide contribute to PONV. Patients who are hypotensive postoperatively are at risk for PONV. Certain surgeries are linked to PONV including gynecological and urinary procedures, breast and ear, nose, and throat surgery as well as strabismus surgery.

TABLE 3-3. Risk Factors for PONV.

Evidence	Risk Factors[1]
Positive overall	Female sex (B1) History of PONV or motion sickness (B1) Nonsmoking (B1) Younger age (B1) General versus regional anesthesia (A1) Use of volatile anesthetics and nitrous oxide (A1) Postoperative opioids (A1) Duration of anesthesia (B1) Type of surgery (cholecystectomy, laparoscopic, gynecological) (B1)
Conflicting	ASA physical status (B1) Menstrual cycle (B1) Level of anesthetist's experience (B1) Muscle relaxant antagonists (A2)
Disproven or of limited clinical relevance	BMI (B1) Anxiety (B1) Nasogastric tube (A1) Supplemental oxygen (A1) Perioperative fasting (A2) Migraine (B1)

[1]Risk assessment scoring: A1, randomized trials with supportive meta-analyses; A2, randomized trials but of insufficient number for a meta-analysis; B1, observational studies such as case control or cohort designs.
ASA, American Society of Anesthesiologists; BMI, body mass index; MO, motion sickness; PONV, postoperative nausea and vomiting.
Reproduced with permission from Gan TJ, Diemunsch P, Habib AS, et al. Consensus guidelines for the management of postoperative nausea and vomiting. *Anesth Analg.* 2014;118(1):85-113.

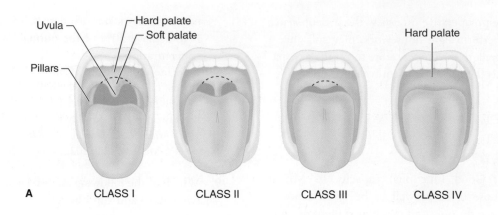

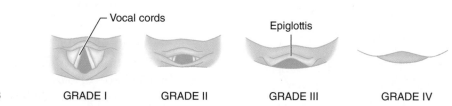

FIG. 3-7. **A**: Mallampati classification of oral opening. **B**: Grading of the laryngeal view. A difficult orotracheal intubation (grade III or IV) may be predicted by the inability to visualize certain pharyngeal structures (class III or IV) during the preoperative examination of a seated patient. Reproduced with permission from Butterworth JF IV, Mackey DC, Wasnick JD, eds. *Morgan & Mikhail's Clinical Anesthesiology.* 7th ed. New York: McGraw Hill; 2022.

References: Butterworth JF IV, Mackey DC, Wasnick JD, eds. *Morgan & Mikhail's Clinical Anesthesiology.* 7th ed. New York, NY: McGraw Hill; 2022: Chapter 17.

Elisha S, Heiner JS, Nagelhout JJ. *Nurse Anesthesia.* 7th ed. St. Louis, MO: Elsevier Saunders; 2023: Chapter 14.

100. Which of the following statements is true regarding airway blocks?

   (A) Topical lidocaine may produce methemoglobinemia.

   (B) 4% lidocaine is injected into the trachea upon inspiration.

   (C) Nerve blocks of the airway pose risk for aspiration.

   (D) Local anesthesia to the mouth and pharynx blocks nerve transmission from the superior laryngeal nerve.

Rationale: Benzocaine is linked to methemoglobinemia. For transtracheal blocks, 2% or 4% local anesthetic is injected into the trachea during end expiration. The trigeminal and glossopharyngeal nerves innervate the airway including the anterior two-thirds of the tongue.

References: Butterworth JF IV, Mackey DC, Wasnick JD, eds. *Morgan & Mikhail's Clinical Anesthesiology.* 7th ed. New York, NY: McGraw Hill; 2022: Chapter 19.

Elisha S, Heiner JS, Nagelhout JJ. *Nurse Anesthesia.* 7th ed. St. Louis, MO: Elsevier Saunders; 2023: Chapter 24.

101. A patient is admitted to the postanesthesia care unit with shallow, rapid respirations, diaphoresis, and tachycardia. What is the most likely cause?

   (A) Delayed awakening

   (B) Hypothermia

   (C) Emergence delirium

   (D) Inadequate oxygenation

Rationale: Common causes of delayed awakening reflect metabolic, neurological, and prolonged action of anesthetic drugs. The patient's presentation is not consistent with delayed awakening. Signs and symptoms of hypothermia reflect depressed metabolism, central nervous system depression, brady- and ventricular arrhythmias. Emergence delirium refers to patients with dysfunctional cognitive signs including agitation, restlessness, fear, lack of orientation, and similar symptoms.

References: Butterworth JF IV, Mackey DC, Wasnick JD, eds. *Morgan & Mikhail's Clinical Anesthesiology.* 7th ed. New York, NY: McGraw Hill; 2022: Chapter 56.

Elisha S, Heiner JS, Nagelhout JJ. *Nurse Anesthesia.* 7th ed. St. Louis, MO: Elsevier Saunders; 2023: Chapter 55.

102. The anesthesia plan includes using topical cocaine for nasal surgery. What is the maximum dose?

    (A) 50 mg
    (B) 200 mg
    (C) 400 mg
    (D) 40 mg

Rationale: To avoid symptoms associated with overdose (arrhythmia, convulsions, respiratory and cardiac arrest) use no more than 200 mg (5 mL 4% solution).

References: Barash PG, Cullen BF, Stoelting RK, et al, eds. *Clinical Anesthesia.* 8th ed. Lippincott Williams & Wilkins; 2017: Chapter 28.

Elisha S, Heiner JS, Nagelhout JJ. *Nurse Anesthesia.* 7th ed. St. Louis, MO: Elsevier Saunders; 2023: Chapter 10.

103. What factors are associated with hypotension in the postanesthesia care unit?

    (A) Hypervolemia
    (B) Nausea
    (C) Shivering
    (D) Pain

Rationale: The main cause of hypotension in the PACU is hypovolemia. Hypertension in the PACU reflects painful stimulation (surgical, intubation, bladder distention) and shivering.

References: Butterworth JF IV, Mackey DC, Wasnick JD, eds. *Morgan & Mikhail's Clinical Anesthesiology.* 7th ed. New York, NY: McGraw Hill; 2022: Chapter 56.

Elisha S, Heiner JS, Nagelhout JJ. *Nurse Anesthesia.* 7th ed. St. Louis, MO: Elsevier Saunders; 2023: Chapter 55.

104. What constitutes the eutectic mixture of local anesthetic?

    (A) Benzocaine and prilocaine
    (B) Prilocaine and tetracaine
    (C) Lidocaine and prilocaine
    (D) Prilocaine and lidocaine

Rationale: EMLA cream is 2.5% lidocaine and 2.5% prilocaine (1:1 mixture).

References: Barash PG, Cullen BF, Stoelting RK, et al, eds. *Clinical Anesthesia.* 8th ed. Lippincott Williams & Wilkins; 2017: Chapter 42.

Butterworth JF IV, Mackey DC, Wasnick JD, eds. *Morgan & Mikhail's Clinical Anesthesiology.* 7th ed. New York, NY: McGraw Hill; 2022: Chapter 16.

Elisha S, Heiner JS, Nagelhout JJ. *Nurse Anesthesia.* 7th ed. St. Louis, MO: Elsevier Saunders; 2023: Chapter 10.

105. During postanesthesia recovery the patient is snoring and use of the accessory muscle for ventilation are noted. What is the most likely cause?

    (A) Airway obstruction
    (B) Hypoventilation
    (C) Hypoxemia
    (D) Bronchospasm

Rationale: Airway obstruction may contribute to hypoventilation. Other signs and symptoms of hypoventilation include decreased respiratory rate or tachypnea with shallow respirations. In the PACU, hypoventilation is the primary cause of hypoxemia resulting in varied signs and symptoms. Airway symptoms including wheezing, secretions, tachypnea, and accessory muscle use are prominent signs.

References: Butterworth JF IV, Mackey DC, Wasnick JD, eds. *Morgan & Mikhail's Clinical Anesthesiology.* 7th ed. New York, NY: McGraw Hill; 2022: Chapter 56.

Elisha S, Heiner JS, Nagelhout JJ. *Nurse Anesthesia.* 7th ed. St. Louis, MO: Elsevier Saunders; 2023: Chapter 55.

106. Gabapentin is most helpful in treating which type of pain?

    (A) Acute somatic pain
    (B) Deep visceral pain
    (C) Neuropathic pain
    (D) Chronic arthritic joint pain

Rationale: Gabapentin and other anticonvulsants are most helpful when used in the treatment neuropathic pain.

References: Butterworth JF IV, Mackey DC, Wasnick JD, eds. *Morgan & Mikhail's Clinical Anesthesiology.* 7th ed. New York, NY: McGraw Hill; 2022: Chapter 47.

Gropper MA. *Miller's Anesthesia.* 9th ed. Philadelphia, PA: Churchill Livingstone Elsevier; 2020: Chapter 51.

107. When using EMLA cream, what is the maximum total dose for children >20 kg?

(A) 20 g

(B) 10 g

(C) 2 g

(D) 1 g

Rationale: The maximum total dose for adults differs from children. Children <3 months and 5 kg (1 g); children 3 to 12 months and more than 5 kg (2 g); and children 1 to 6 years and less than 10 kg (10 g). 20 g is allowed for 7 to 12 years (>20 kg).

References: Butterworth JF IV, Mackey DC, Wasnick JD, eds. *Morgan & Mikhail's Clinical Anesthesiology.* 7th ed. New York, NY: McGraw Hill; 2022: Chapter 16.

Elisha S, Heiner JS, Nagelhout JJ. *Nurse Anesthesia.* 7th ed. St. Louis, MO: Elsevier Saunders; 2023: Chapter 10.

108. Which peripheral nerve block provides complete anesthesia for ankle surgery?

(A) Femoral

(B) Sciatic

(C) Obturator

(D) Popliteal

Rationale: The femoral block is useful for analgesia but not total anesthesia for ankle procedures. For surgical procedures below the knee, the popliteal approach to sciatic nerve block provides complete anesthesia. Surgery above and below the knee and including the knee are anesthetized using other approaches to the sciatic nerve block. The obturator block is useful for knee procedures.

References: Butterworth JF IV, Mackey DC, Wasnick JD, eds. *Morgan & Mikhail's Clinical Anesthesiology.* 7th ed. New York, NY: McGraw Hill; 2022: Chapter 46.

Elisha S, Heiner JS, Nagelhout JJ. *Nurse Anesthesia.* 7th ed. St. Louis, MO: Elsevier Saunders; 2023: Chapter 50.

109. Which nerve block results in the highest blood level of local anesthetic?

(A) Sciatic

(B) Intercostal

(C) Paravertebral

(D) Cervical plexus

Rationale: Along with the highest complication rate of nerve blocks, the intercostal block results in the highest blood level of local anesthetic. The anatomy is a vessel-rich area.

References: Butterworth JF IV, Mackey DC, Wasnick JD, eds. *Morgan & Mikhail's Clinical Anesthesiology.* 7th ed. New York, NY: McGraw Hill; 2022: Chapter 47.

Elisha S, Heiner JS, Nagelhout JJ. *Nurse Anesthesia.* 7th ed. St. Louis, MO: Elsevier Saunders; 2023: Chapter 30.

110. What are the fluid requirements for redistribution and evaporative surgical fluid losses during a bowl resection?

(A) 0 to 2 mL/kg

(B) 2 to 4 mL/kg

(C) 4 to 8 mL/kg

(D) 10 to 14 mL/kg

Rationale: Redistribution and evaporative loss are replaced according to the degree of tissue trauma sustained during surgery: minimal tissue trauma (e.g., herniorrhaphy/short superficial procedure) requires 1 to 2 mL/kg; moderate tissue trauma (e.g., cholecystectomy) requires 2 to 4 mL/kg; and severe tissue trauma (e.g., bowel resection) requires 4 to 6 mL/kg.

References: Butterworth JF IV, Mackey DC, Wasnick JD, eds. *Morgan & Mikhail's Clinical Anesthesiology.* 7th ed. New York, NY: McGraw Hill; 2022: Chapter 51.

Elisha S, Heiner JS, Nagelhout JJ. *Nurse Anesthesia.* 7th ed. St. Louis, MO: Elsevier Saunders; 2023: Chapter 21.

111. Which airway block provides anesthesia below the vocal cords?

(A) Superior laryngeal nerve block and transtracheal block

(B) Tonsillar block

(C) Glossopharyngeal block

(D) Instilling local anesthetic onto the vocal cords

Rationale: A glossopharyngeal nerve block anesthetizes the posterior third of the tongue. Instilling local anesthetic (lidocaine droplet spread) onto the vocal cords provides local anesthesia to the immediate area only.

References: Butterworth JF IV, Mackey DC, Wasnick JD, eds. *Morgan & Mikhail's Clinical Anesthesiology.* 7th ed. New York, NY: McGraw Hill; 2022: Chapter 19.

Elisha S, Heiner JS, Nagelhout JJ. *Nurse Anesthesia.* 7th ed. St. Louis, MO: Elsevier Saunders; 2023: Chapter 24.

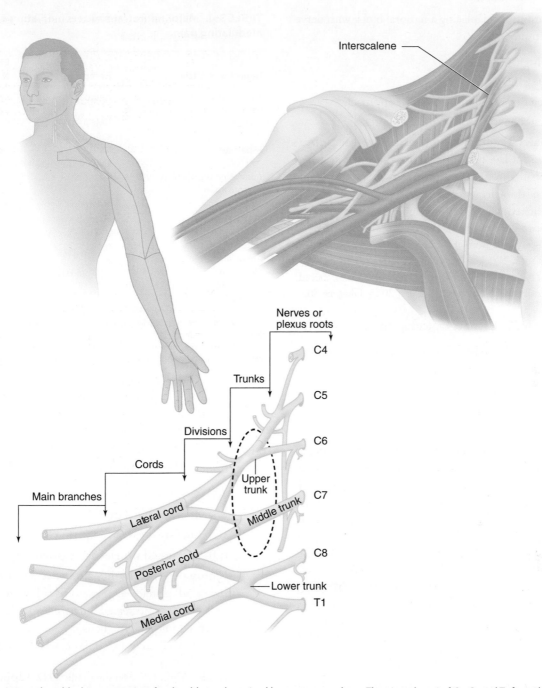

Interscalene

Nerves or
plexus roots

C4

Trunks

C5

C6

Divisions

Upper
trunk

Cords

C7

Lateral cord

Middle trunk

Main branches

C8

Posterior cord

Lower trunk

T1

Medial cord

FIG. 3-8. An interscalene block is appropriate for shoulder and proximal humerus procedures. The ventral rami of C_5–C_8 and T_1 form the brachial plexus. (Reproduced with permission from Butterworth JF IV, Mackey DC, Wasnick JD, eds. *Morgan & Mikhail's Clinical Anesthesiology*. 7th ed. New York: McGraw Hill; 2022.)

112. Which of the following landmarks form the lumbar plexus?

   (A) L1–3 and T-10

   (B) L1–4 and T-10

   (C) L1–4 and T-12

   (D) L1–3 and T-12

Rationale: L1–4 and T-12 ventral rami form the lumbosacral plexus.

References: Butterworth JF IV, Mackey DC, Wasnick JD, eds. *Morgan & Mikhail's Clinical Anesthesiology*. 7th ed. New York, NY: McGraw Hill; 2022: Chapter 46.

Elisha S, Heiner JS, Nagelhout JJ. *Nurse Anesthesia*. 7th ed. St. Louis, MO: Elsevier Saunders; 2023: Chapter 50.

113. What results when placing a femoral block with nerve stimulation?

(A) Thigh adduction

(B) Quadriceps twitch

(C) Sciatic nerve block posterior approach

(D) Sciatic nerve block anterior approach

Rationale: Thigh adduction occurs with an obturator block. The posterior approach to sciatic nerve block results in a gluteal muscle twitch and plantar flexion or dorsiflexion. Foot inversion or plantar flexion is elicited when the anterior approach is used.

References: Butterworth JF IV, Mackey DC, Wasnick JD, eds. *Morgan & Mikhail's Clinical Anesthesiology.* 7th ed. New York, NY: McGraw Hill; 2022: Chapter 46.

Elisha S, Heiner JS, Nagelhout JJ. *Nurse Anesthesia.* 7th ed. St. Louis, MO: Elsevier Saunders; 2023: Chapter 50.

114. Which phrase describes radiculopathy?

(A) Abnormal sensation with or without a stimulus

(B) Pain linked to noxious stimulation

(C) Nerve distribution pain

(D) Abnormal function of nerve roots

Rationale: The unpleasant or abnormal sensation with or without a stimulus is dysesthesia. Hyperalgesia is the increased response to noxious stimulation. Neuralgia describes pain associated with nerve distribution.

References: Barash PG, Cullen BF, Stoelting RK, et al, eds. *Clinical Anesthesia.* 8th ed. Lippincott Williams & Wilkins; 2017: Chapter 56.

Butterworth JF IV, Mackey DC, Wasnick JD, eds. *Morgan & Mikhail's Clinical Anesthesiology.* 7th ed. New York, NY: McGraw Hill; 2022: Chapter 47.

115. Which of the following is not a pain modulating excitatory neurotransmitters?

(A) Glycine

(B) Calcitonin

(C) Adenosine

(D) Asparate

Rationale: Glycine, enkephalin, norepinephrine, GABA, and serotonin are inhibitory neurotransmitters. Other excitatory substances include calcitonin, aspartate, and adenosine triphosphate.

References: Barash PG, Cullen BF, Stoelting RK, et al, eds. *Clinical Anesthesia.* 8th ed. Lippincott Williams & Wilkins; 2017: Chapter 56.

TABLE 3-4. Major neurotransmitters mediating or modulating pain.

Neurotransmitter	Receptor	Effect on Nociception
Substance P	Neurokinin–1	Excitatory
Calcitonin gene-related peptide		Excitatory
Glutamate	NMDA, AMPA, kainate, quisqualate	Excitatory
Aspartate	NMDA, AMPA, kainate, quisqualate	Excitatory
Adenosine triphosphate (ATP)	P_1, P_2	Excitatory
Somatostatin		Inhibitory
Acetylcholine	Muscarinic	Inhibitory
Enkephalins	μ, δ, κ	Inhibitory
β-Endorphin	μ, δ, κ	Inhibitory
Norepinephrine	α_2	Inhibitory
Adenosine	A_1	Inhibitory
Serotonin	5-HT_1 (5-HT_3)	Inhibitory
γ-Aminobutyric acid (GABA)	A, B	Inhibitory
Glycine		Inhibitory

AMPA, 2-(aminomethyl)phenylacetic acid; NMDA, *N*-methyl-D-aspartate; 5-HT, 5-hydroxytryptamine.
(Reproduced with permission from Butterworth JF IV, Mackey DC, Wasnick JD, eds. *Morgan & Mikhail's Clinical Anesthesiology.* 7th ed. New York: McGraw Hill; 2022.)

Butterworth JF IV, Mackey DC, Wasnick JD, eds. *Morgan & Mikhail's Clinical Anesthesiology.* 7th ed. New York, NY: McGraw Hill; 2022: Chapter 47.

116. Which of the following physiological effect results from acute pain stimulation?

(A) Increased myocardial workload

(B) Increasedvital capacity

(C) Increased gastric emptying

(D) Decreased platelet aggregation

Rationale: The physiological effects of pain include increased platelet aggregation leading to thrombosis as well as decreased intestinal motility with the potential for paralytic ileus.

References: Butterworth JF IV, Mackey DC, Wasnick JD, eds. *Morgan & Mikhail's Clinical Anesthesiology.* 7th ed. New York, NY: McGraw Hill; 2022: Chapter 47.

Elisha S, Heiner JS, Nagelhout JJ. *Nurse Anesthesia.* 7th ed. St. Louis, MO: Elsevier Saunders; 2023: Chapter 56.

117. Vocal cord paralysis occurred following intubation. What is the most likely cause?

(A) Recurrent laryngeal nerve damage

(B) Epiglottic damage

(C) Esophageal damage

(D) Superior laryngeal nerve

Rationale: Stridor and respiratory distress result from injury to the superior laryngeal nerve. Unilateral damage to the recurrent laryngeal nerve results in vocal cord paralysis exhibited by hoarseness.

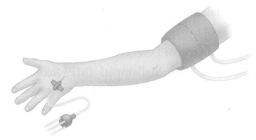

FIG. 3-9. Intravenous regional anesthesia provides surgical anesthesia for procedures of short duration. (Reproduced with permission from Butterworth JF IV, Mackey DC, Wasnick JD, eds. *Morgan & Mikhail's Clinical Anesthesiology.* 7th ed. New York: McGraw Hill; 2022.)

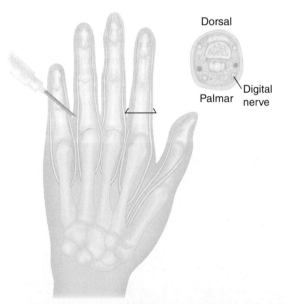

FIG. 3-10. Sensory innervation of the fingers is provided by the digital nerves. (Reproduced with permission from Butterworth JF IV, Mackey DC, Wasnick JD, eds. *Morgan & Mikhail's Clinical Anesthesiology.* 7th ed. New York: McGraw Hill; 2022.)

TABLE 3-5. The effects of laryngeal nerve injury on the voice.

Nerve	Effect of Nerve Injury
Superior laryngeal nerve	
Unilateral	Minimal effects
Bilateral	Hoarseness, tiring of voice
Recurrent laryngeal nerve	
Unilateral	Hoarseness
Bilateral	Stridor, respiratory distress
Acute	Aphonia
Chronic	
Vagus nerve	
Unilateral	Hoarseness
Bilateral	Aphonia

(Reproduced with permission from Butterworth JF IV, Mackey DC, Wasnick JD, eds. *Morgan & Mikhail's Clinical Anesthesiology.* 7th ed. New York: McGraw Hill; 2022.)

References: Butterworth JF IV, Mackey DC, Wasnick JD, eds. *Morgan & Mikhail's Clinical Anesthesiology.* 7th ed. New York, NY: McGraw Hill; 2022: Chapter 19.
Elisha S, Heiner JS, Nagelhout JJ. *Nurse Anesthesia.* 7th ed. St. Louis, MO: Elsevier Saunders; 2023: Chapter 29.

118. A patient with a history of hiatal hernia, diabetes mellitus, and peripheral neuropathy is scheduled for a bowel resection. Which fasting guideline applies?

(A) NPO for 8 hours
(B) Clear fluids up to 2 hours
(C) Light meal up to 6 hours
(D) NPO for 4 hours

Rationale: Even though new ERA's protocols advocate for clear carbohydrate-based liquids 2 hours prior to surgery, the patient's comorbidities and surgery are associated with increased risk for delayed gastric emptying and aspiration. Patients with a history of hiatal hernia commonly have uncontrolled GERD. Fasting guidelines remain conservative for patients at increased risk for aspiration. Relaxed fasting guidelines including a light meal or clear liquids apply only to patients not at risk for delayed gastric emptying.

References: Butterworth JF IV, Mackey DC, Wasnick JD, eds. *Morgan & Mikhail's Clinical Anesthesiology.* 7th ed. New York, NY: McGraw Hill; 2022: Chapter 48.
Gropper MA. *Miller's Anesthesia.* 9th ed. Philadelphia, PA: Churchill Livingstone Elsevier; 2020: Chapter 44.

119. A 40-year-old male with a history of well-controlled hypertension is scheduled for a carpal tunnel release. How will you classify the patient?

(A) ASA-PS IV
(B) ASA-PS III
(C) ASA-PS II
(D) ASA-PS I

Rationale: The American Society of Anesthesiologists (ASA) Physical Status Classification is used to assign patients a physical status prior to anesthesia and surgery. The patient's history of well-controlled hypertension is considered a mild systemic disease.

Rationale: The average blood volume for a male is 70 mL/kg; 65 mL/kg for a female; and 80 mL/kg for a newborn infant.

Reference: Elisha S, Heiner JS, Nagelhout JJ. *Nurse Anesthesia.* 7th ed. St. Louis, MO: Elsevier Saunders; 2023: Chapter 22.

126. How much additional fluid will you administer to a patient undergoing herniorrhaphy?

    (A) 4 to 8 mL/kg
    (B) 0 to 2 mL/kg
    (C) 2 to 4 mL/kg
    (D) 10 mL/kg

Rationale: Surgical procedures with minimal trauma require the least amount of additional fluid replacement. Herniorrhaphy is an example of a minimally invasive procedure with little tissue trauma. Moderate tissue trauma requires 2 to 4 mL/kg and large tissue trauma surgeries require 4 to 8 mL/kg.

TABLE 3-8. Redistribution and evaporative surgical fluid losses.

Degree of Tissue Trauma	Additional Fluid Requirement
Minimal (e.g., herniorrhaphy)	0–2 mL/kg
Moderate (e.g., open cholecystectomy)	2–4 mL/kg
Severe (e.g., open bowel resection)	4–8 mL/kg

(Reproduced with permission from Butterworth JF IV, Mackey DC, Wasnick JD, eds. *Morgan & Mikhail's Clinical Anesthesiology.* 7th ed. New York: McGraw Hill; 2022.)

References: Barash PG, Cullen BF, Stoelting RK, et al, eds. *Clinical Anesthesia.* 8th ed. Lippincott Williams & Wilkins; 2017: Chapter 16.

Butterworth JF IV, Mackey DC, Wasnick JD, eds. *Morgan & Mikhail's Clinical Anesthesiology.* 7th ed. New York, NY: McGraw Hill; 2022: Chapter 51.

127. What statement is true regarding colloids?

    (A) Inexpensive
    (B) Increase plasma volume
    (C) Used for initial resuscitation
    (D) Used primarily for extracellular expansion

Rationale: As compared to crystalloids, colloids are expensive and are useful in increasing plasma volume. Crystalloids are typically used for initial resuscitation and extracellular fluid replacement.

References: Butterworth JF IV, Mackey DC, Wasnick JD, eds. *Morgan & Mikhail's Clinical Anesthesiology.* 7th ed. New York, NY: McGraw Hill; 2022: Chapter 51.

Elisha S, Heiner JS, Nagelhout JJ. *Nurse Anesthesia.* 7th ed. St. Louis, MO: Elsevier Saunders; 2023: Chapter 21.

128. While receiving a blood transfusion during general anesthesia tachycardia and hypotension develop. What is the most likely cause?

    (A) Delayed hemolytic reaction
    (B) Anaphylactic reaction
    (C) Urticarial reaction
    (D) Acute hemolytic reaction

Rationale: When a patient receives incompatible ABO blood, hemolytic reactions result. When patients are awake symptoms include chills, flank pain, nausea, and fever. Patients undergoing general anesthesia exhibit tachycardia hypotension, hemoglobinuria, and oozing. Delayed hemolytic reactions develop 2 to 21 days after the transfusion and are mild compared to the acute hemolytic reaction. Anaphylactic reactions occur in patients with IgA deficiency. Urticarial reactions are linked to plasma proteins.

References: Butterworth JF IV, Mackey DC, Wasnick JD, eds. *Morgan & Mikhail's Clinical Anesthesiology.* 7th ed. New York, NY: McGraw Hill; 2022: Chapter 51.

Elisha S, Heiner JS, Nagelhout JJ. *Nurse Anesthesia.* 7th ed. St. Louis, MO: Elsevier Saunders; 2023: Chapter 22.

129. What statement is true regarding a patient who is awake in a supine position?

    (A) The blood pressure decreases due to autoregulation.
    (B) Venous return decreases.
    (C) Blood pressure remains relatively constant.
    (D) Sympathetic outflow increases.

Rationale: When a patient goes from standing to the supine position, venous return increases. Sympathetic outflow decreases while parasympathetic activity increases due to activation of afferent baroreceptors. Activated atrial and ventricular receptors also decrease sympathetic outflow. These processes along with activation of atrial reflexes result in maintenance of arterial blood pressure.

Reference: Gropper MA. *Miller's Anesthesia.* 9th ed. Philadelphia, PA: Churchill Livingstone Elsevier; 2020: Chapter 34.

130. What effect does the lithotomy position have on arterial pressure?

    (A) Lower than supine position
    (B) Higher than supine position
    (C) Lower than Trendelenburg
    (D) Lower than sitting position

Rationale: The blood pressure in the lithotomy position remains the same as or higher than the supine position. Auto transfusion from the lower extremities occurs in the lithotomy position. The Trendelenburg position typically increases blood pressure whereas the sitting position often results in a lower blood pressure.

References: Butterworth JF IV, Mackey DC, Wasnick JD, eds. *Morgan & Mikhail's Clinical Anesthesiology.* 7th ed. New York, NY: McGraw Hill; 2022: Chapter 32.

Gropper MA. *Miller's Anesthesia.* 9th ed. Philadelphia, PA: Churchill Livingstone Elsevier; 2020: Chapter 34.

131. A patient experiences low vision following a lumbar laminectomy in the prone position. What is the etiology?

   (A) Decreased intracranial pressure
   (B) Decreased venous pressure
   (C) Increased cerebral blood flow
   (D) Decreased ocular perfusion pressure

Rationale: Physiological changes in the prone position include increased intracranial pressure, increased venous pressure, and decreased cerebral blood flow. Postoperative vision loss is due to increased ocular venous pressure as well as decreased ocular perfusion pressure.

References: Butterworth JF IV, Mackey DC, Wasnick JD, eds. *Morgan & Mikhail's Clinical Anesthesiology.* 7th ed. New York, NY: McGraw Hill; 2022: Chapter 54.

Elisha S, Heiner JS, Nagelhout JJ. *Nurse Anesthesia.* 7th ed. St. Louis, MO: Elsevier Saunders; 2023: Chapter 35.

Gropper MA. *Miller's Anesthesia.* 9th ed. Philadelphia, PA: Churchill Livingstone Elsevier; 2020: Chapter 57.

132. Where will you measure the blood pressure for patients undergoing surgery in the lateral decubitus position?

   (A) Nondependent arm
   (B) Both arms
   (C) Dependent arm
   (D) Right thigh

Rationale: In the lateral position, compartment syndrome can develop in either arm. Avoiding compression of the neurovascular bundle in the dependent arm is necessary. To determine perfusion to the extremity, monitor the blood pressure in the dependent arm intermittently. Checking a radial pulse and monitoring for declining pulse oximetry in the dependent arm are additional safety measures.

References: Barash PG, Cullen BF, Stoelting RK, et al, eds. *Clinical Anesthesia.* 8th ed. Lippincott Williams & Wilkins; 2017: Chapter 29.

Elisha S, Heiner JS, Nagelhout JJ. *Nurse Anesthesia.* 7th ed. St. Louis, MO: Elsevier Saunders; 2023: Chapter 23.

Gropper MA. *Miller's Anesthesia.* 9th ed. Philadelphia, PA: Churchill Livingstone Elsevier; 2020: Chapter 34.

133. A sudden decrease in SpO_2, blood pressure, and $ETCO_2$ occur during general anesthesia. A mill-wheel murmur exists. What is the most likely cause?

   (A) Venous air embolism
   (B) Pneumocephalus
   (C) Fat embolism
   (D) Cardiovascular accident

Rationale: Classic signs of a venous air embolism include marked hemodynamic changes, falling end-tidal carbon dioxide, increased nitrogen, arrhythmias, and a mill-wheel murmur.

References: Butterworth JF IV, Mackey DC, Wasnick JD, eds. *Morgan & Mikhail's Clinical Anesthesiology.* 7th ed. New York, NY: McGraw Hill; 2022: Chapter 27.

Elisha S, Heiner JS, Nagelhout JJ. *Nurse Anesthesia.* 7th ed. St. Louis, MO: Elsevier Saunders; 2023: Chapter 23.

134. What nerve injury is most likely when the arm is pronated?

   (A) Brachial plexus
   (B) Ulnar nerve
   (C) Radial nerve
   (D) Suprascapular nerve

Rationale: To avoid injury to the ulnar nerve, the forearm is supinated. An additional measure to avoid injury include the use of elbow padding and flexing elbows <90 degrees.

References: Butterworth JF IV, Mackey DC, Wasnick JD, eds. *Morgan & Mikhail's Clinical Anesthesiology.* 7th ed. New York, NY: McGraw Hill; 2022: Chapter 54.

Elisha S, Heiner JS, Nagelhout JJ. *Nurse Anesthesia.* 7th ed. St. Louis, MO: Elsevier Saunders; 2023: Chapter 23.

135. In the supine position, what nerve injury is associated with arm abduction >90 degrees and lateral rotation of the head?

   (A) Ulnar nerve
   (B) Brachial plexus
   (C) Radial nerve
   (D) Suprascapular nerve

Rationale: Ulnar nerve symptoms may result from injury to the brachial plexus. Keeping the arms abducted <90 degrees as well as proper head alignment minimizes stretching of the brachial plexus.

References: Butterworth JF IV, Mackey DC, Wasnick JD, eds. *Morgan & Mikhail's Clinical Anesthesiology.* 7th ed. New York, NY: McGraw Hill; 2022: Chapter 54.

Elisha S, Heiner JS, Nagelhout JJ. *Nurse Anesthesia.* 7th ed. St. Louis, MO: Elsevier Saunders; 2023: Chapter 23.

136. Following surgery in the lithotomy position the patient exhibits foot drop and the inability to extend the toes. What nerves are most likely injured?

   (A) Sciatic and common peroneal
   (B) Femoral and sciatic
   (C) Common peroneal and femoral
   (D) Obturator and sciatic

   Rationale: Foot drop and the inability to extend the toes are seen with sciatic and common peroneal nerve injury. These nerves are the most injured when placed in the lithotomy position. Injury to the obturator and femoral nerves results in femoral neuropathy demonstrated by decreased hip flexion, inability to extend the knee, and/or sensory loss (superior thigh and anteromedial or medial leg).

TABLE 3-9. Complications associated with patient positioning.

Complication	Position	Prevention
Venous air embolism	Sitting, prone, reverse Trendelenburg	Maintain adequate venous pressure; ligate "open" veins
Alopecia	Supine, lithotomy, Trendelenburg	Avoid prolonged hypotension, padding, and occasional head turning
Backache	Any	Lumbar support, padding, and slight hip flexion
Extremity compartment syndromes	Especially lithotomy	Maintain perfusion pressure and avoid external compression
Corneal abrasion	Any, but especially prone	Taping or lubricating eye
Digit amputation	Any	Check for protruding digits before changing table configuration
Nerve palsies		
Brachial plexus	Any	Avoid stretching or direct compression at neck, shoulder, or axilla
Common peroneal	Lithotomy, lateral decubitus	Avoid sustained pressure on lateral aspect of upper fibula
Radial	Any	Avoid compression of lateral humerus
Ulnar	Any	Avoid sustained pressure on ulnar groove
Retinal ischemia	Prone, sitting	Avoid pressure on globe
Skin necrosis	Any	Avoid sustained pressure over bony prominences

(Reproduced with permission from Butterworth JF IV, Mackey DC, Wasnick JD, eds. *Morgan & Mikhail's Clinical Anesthesiology.* 7th ed. New York: McGraw Hill; 2022.)

References: Butterworth JF IV, Mackey DC, Wasnick JD, eds. *Morgan & Mikhail's Clinical Anesthesiology.* 7th ed. New York, NY: McGraw Hill; 2022: Chapter 54.

Elisha S, Heiner JS, Nagelhout JJ. *Nurse Anesthesia.* 7th ed. St. Louis, MO: Elsevier Saunders; 2023: Chapter 23.

137. Which patient requires a preoperative chest x-ray?

   (A) 55-year-old smoker undergoing a laparoscopic cholecystectomy
   (B) 65-year-old chronic stable bronchitic undergoing a carpal tunnel release
   (C) 60-year-old undergoing a transurethral resection of the prostate
   (D) 50-year-old undergoing a mitral valve replacement

   Rationale: Preoperative chest x-rays are indicated for patients with acute or chronic symptomatic pulmonary dysfunction, cardiac conditions, or malignancies of the chest.

   References: Elisha S, Heiner JS, Nagelhout JJ. *Nurse Anesthesia.* 7th ed. St. Louis, MO: Elsevier Saunders; 2023: Chapter 20.

   Gropper MA. *Miller's Anesthesia.* 9th ed. Philadelphia, PA: Churchill Livingstone Elsevier; 2020: Chapter 31.

138. What is the average distance from the skin to the epidural space?

   (A) 1 cm
   (B) 1.5 cm
   (C) 5 cm
   (D) 7.5 cm

   Rationale: The distance from the skin to the epidural space ranges from 2.5 to 8 cm with an average of 5 cm.

   References: Elisha S, Heiner JS, Nagelhout JJ. *Nurse Anesthesia.* 7th ed. St. Louis, MO: Elsevier Saunders; 2023: Chapter 49.

   Gropper MA. *Miller's Anesthesia.* 9th ed. Philadelphia, PA: Churchill Livingstone Elsevier; 2020: Chapter 45.

139. What statement is false regarding the lateral decubitus position?

   (A) Rhabdomyolysis may occur.
   (B) Flex the dependent arm <90 degrees.
   (C) Pad the lateral aspect of the dependent leg.
   (D) Pulmonary blood flow to the dependent lung decreases.

   Rationale: In the lateral decubitus position, blood flow to the dependent lung is increased.

References: Butterworth JF IV, Mackey DC, Wasnick JD, eds. *Morgan & Mikhail's Clinical Anesthesiology.* 7th ed. New York, NY: McGraw Hill; 2022: Chapter 25.

Elisha S, Heiner JS, Nagelhout JJ. *Nurse Anesthesia.* 7th ed. St. Louis, MO: Elsevier Saunders; 2023: Chapter 23.

140. In what position is a venous air embolism (VAE) most likely to occur?

    (A) Lateral decubitus

    (B) Sitting

    (C) Prone

    (D) Trendelenburg

    Rationale: In surgeries above the level of the heart, the risk of VAE exists. Approximately 20 to 40% of open craniotomies develop a VAE. Usually, these are small. Any position where the surgery is above the level of the heart predisposes the patient to VAE. Open sinuses allow for the entrainment of air.

    References: Butterworth JF IV, Mackey DC, Wasnick JD, eds. *Morgan & Mikhail's Clinical Anesthesiology.* 7th ed. New York, NY: McGraw Hill; 2022: Chapter 27.

    Gropper MA. *Miller's Anesthesia.* 9th ed. Philadelphia, PA: Churchill Livingstone Elsevier; 2020: Chapter 34.

141. A T_6 sensory level is identified following administration of a spinal anesthetic. At what level is the sympathetic block?

    (A) T_4

    (B) T_{10}

    (C) T_6

    (D) T_8

    Rationale: Differential blockade exists following administration of a spinal anesthetic. The sympathetic block is two or more (may even extend up to six) segments higher than the sensory block which is two segments higher than a motor block.

    References: Butterworth JF IV, Mackey DC, Wasnick JD, eds. *Morgan & Mikhail's Clinical Anesthesiology.* 7th ed. New York, NY: McGraw Hill; 2022: Chapter 45.

    Gropper MA. *Miller's Anesthesia.* 9th ed. Philadelphia, PA: Churchill Livingstone Elsevier; 2020: Chapter 45.

    Elisha S, Heiner JS, Nagelhout JJ. *Nurse Anesthesia.* 7th ed. St. Louis, MO: Elsevier Saunders; 2023: Chapter 49.

142. In which patient is spinal anesthesia contraindicated?

    (A) 30-year-old who takes daily garlic

    (B) 50-year-old taking subcutaneous heparin injections

    (C) 25-year-old taking NSAIDs

    (D) 40-year-old who received thrombolytic therapy

    Rationale: Herbal remedies including garlic, ginkgo, and ginseng increase the risk of bleeding, but are not contraindicated for regional anesthesia. No contraindication exists for patients taking aspirin, NSAIDs, or subcutaneous heparin. Low-dose heparin recommendations: wait 4 to 6 hours or confirm normal coagulation. Thrombolytic therapy is an absolute contraindication for regional anesthesia.

    References: Butterworth JF IV, Mackey DC, Wasnick JD, eds. *Morgan & Mikhail's Clinical Anesthesiology.* 7th ed. New York, NY: McGraw Hill; 2022: Chapter 45.

    Gropper MA. *Miller's Anesthesia.* 9th ed. Philadelphia, PA: Churchill Livingstone Elsevier; 2020: Chapter 45.

143. What factor least affects the spread of spinal local anesthetic?

    (A) Baricity

    (B) Drug dosage

    (C) Site of injection

    (D) Drug volume

    Rationale: While each of the factors affects the spread of local anesthetic in the CSF, drug volume least affects the spread. Other factors influencing the spread of spinal local anesthetic include the patient's age, curvature of the spine, intraabdominal pressure, needle direction, patient height, and pregnancy.

TABLE 3-10. Factors affecting the dermatomal spread of spinal anesthesia.

Most important factors
- Baricity of anesthetic solution
- Position of the patient
  - During injection
  - Immediately after injection
- Drug dosage
- Site of injection

Other factors
- Age
- Cerebrospinal fluid
- Curvature of the spine
- Drug volume
- Intraabdominal pressure
- Needle direction
- Patient height
- Pregnancy

(Reproduced with permission from Butterworth JF IV, Mackey DC, Wasnick JD, eds. *Morgan & Mikhail's Clinical Anesthesiology.* 7th ed. New York: McGraw Hill; 2022.)

References: Butterworth JF IV, Mackey DC, Wasnick JD, eds. *Morgan & Mikhail's Clinical Anesthesiology.* 7th ed. New York, NY: McGraw Hill; 2022: Chapter 45.

Gropper MA. *Miller's Anesthesia.* 9th ed. Philadelphia, PA: Churchill Livingstone Elsevier; 2020: Chapter 45.

144. How do transient neurologic symptoms (TNS) differ from cauda equina syndrome?

(A) TNS persists for several weeks following surgery.

(B) Cauda equina syndrome disappears within 10 days following surgery.

(C) TNS symptoms spontaneously disappear.

(D) Cauda equina syndrome symptoms include severe radicular back pain.

Rationale: Cauda equine syndrome is a persistent condition that results in lower extremity weakness, bowel, and bladder dysfunction. TNS occurs within 24 hours of surgery. Mild to severe radicular back pain results, but symptoms spontaneously disappear.

References: Butterworth JF IV, Mackey DC, Wasnick JD, eds. *Morgan & Mikhail's Clinical Anesthesiology.* 7th ed. New York, NY: McGraw Hill; 2022: Chapter 45.

Elisha S, Heiner JS, Nagelhout JJ. *Nurse Anesthesia.* 7th ed. St. Louis, MO: Elsevier Saunders; 2023: Chapter 45.

Gropper MA. *Miller's Anesthesia.* 9th ed. Philadelphia, PA: Churchill Livingstone Elsevier; 2020: Chapter 45.

145. What local anesthetic is linked to cauda equine syndrome?

(A) Ropivacaine

(B) Bupivacaine

(C) Tetracaine

(D) Lidocaine

Rationale: Administration of spinal lidocaine and epidural 2-chloroprocaine (inadvertent dural puncture) has been implicated in cauda equina syndrome as well as transient neurological symptoms.

References: Butterworth JF IV, Mackey DC, Wasnick JD, eds. *Morgan & Mikhail's Clinical Anesthesiology.* 7th ed. New York, NY: McGraw Hill; 2022: Chapter 45.

Elisha S, Heiner JS, Nagelhout JJ. *Nurse Anesthesia.* 7th ed. St. Louis, MO: Elsevier Saunders; 2023: Chapter 10.

Gropper MA. *Miller's Anesthesia.* 9th ed. Philadelphia, PA: Churchill Livingstone Elsevier; 2020: Chapter 45.

146. Spinal anesthesia using Tetracaine 12 mg is given to a patient undergoing a transurethral resection of the prostate. If you add epinephrine what is the longest anticipated duration?

(A) 0.5 hour

(B) 1 hour

(C) 2 hours

(D) 3 hours

Rationale: Addition of epinephrine to tetracaine extends the duration of action from 2 to 4 hours.

References: Butterworth JF IV, Mackey DC, Wasnick JD, eds. *Morgan & Mikhail's Clinical Anesthesiology.* 7th ed. New York, NY: McGraw Hill; 2022: Chapter 45.

Elisha S, Heiner JS, Nagelhout JJ. *Nurse Anesthesia.* 7th ed. St. Louis, MO: Elsevier Saunders; 2023: Chapter 49.

147. Which clotting factor is the first to become inactivated shortly after a patient has begun warfarin therapy?

(A) IV

(B) V

(C) VII

(D) IX

Rationale: Because factor VII has the shortest half-life (4-6 hours), it is the first factor to become inactivated after a patient begins treatment with warfarin.

References: Butterworth JF IV, Mackey DC, Wasnick JD, eds. *Morgan & Mikhail's Clinical Anesthesiology.* 7th ed. New York, NY: McGraw Hill; 2022: Chapter 33.

Gropper MA. *Miller's Anesthesia.* 9th ed. Philadelphia, PA: Churchill Livingstone Elsevier; 2020: Chapter 16.

148. Following administration of 15-mg spinal bupivacaine, the patient's heart rate and blood pressure fall precipitously. What is the cause?

(A) Sympathetic blockade

(B) Motor blockade

(C) Sensory blockade

(D) Sensory and motor blockade

Rationale: Administration of a spinal anesthetic may cause blocking the cardiac accelerators (T_1–T_4) and decreasing venous return with resultant bradycardia. Venous return, cardiac output, and systemic vascular resistance decrease in response to sympathetic nervous system blockade.

References: Butterworth JF IV, Mackey DC, Wasnick JD, eds. *Morgan & Mikhail's Clinical Anesthesiology.* 7th ed. New York, NY: McGraw Hill; 2022: Chapter 45.

Elisha S, Heiner JS, Nagelhout JJ. *Nurse Anesthesia.* 7th ed. St. Louis, MO: Elsevier Saunders; 2023: Chapter 49.

149. A patient states that their feet are numb following administration of an epidural test dose. What is the most likely cause?

(A) Intravascular injection

(B) Local anesthetic toxicity

(C) Intrathecal injection

(D) Normal response to a test dose

Rationale: The test dose determines correct epidural needle placement. Inadvertent injection of an epidural test dose into the intrathecal space results in signs and symptoms consistent with a spinal anesthetic (typically within 3 minutes of injection). In laboring women, suspicion for an intrathecal placement is warranted if the patient suddenly reports rapid onset of analgesia. Intravascular injection is demonstrated by tachycardia.

References: Barash PG, Cullen BF, Stoelting RK, et al, eds. *Clinical Anesthesia.* 8th ed. Lippincott Williams & Wilkins; 2017: Chapter 35.

Butterworth JF IV, Mackey DC, Wasnick JD, eds. *Morgan & Mikhail's Clinical Anesthesiology.* 7th ed. New York, NY: McGraw Hill; 2022: Chapter 45.

Gropper MA. *Miller's Anesthesia.* 9th ed. Philadelphia, PA: Churchill Livingstone Elsevier; 2020: Chapter 62.

150. Twenty-four hours following an epidural anesthesia the patient complains of occipital headache, nausea, vomiting, and double vision. What is the most likely cause?

(A) Neurologic injury

(B) Spinal hematoma

(C) Epidural hematoma

(D) Postdural puncture headache

Rationale: Signs and symptoms are consistent with a postdural puncture headache. Specifically, a headache associated with changes in position, i.e., sitting or standing worsens the pain. Sharp back and leg pain with accompanying motor weakness are symptoms of spinal or epidural hematoma.

References: Butterworth JF IV, Mackey DC, Wasnick JD, eds. *Morgan & Mikhail's Clinical Anesthesiology.* 7th ed. New York, NY: McGraw Hill; 2022: Chapter 45.

Elisha S, Heiner JS, Nagelhout JJ. *Nurse Anesthesia.* 7th ed. St. Louis, MO: Elsevier Saunders; 2023: Chapter 49.

151. What factor does not influence the spread of local anesthetic placed in the epidural space?

(A) Concentration

(B) Dose

(C) Site of injection

(D) Age

Rationale: The dose and site of injection influence the spread of local anesthetic. The density of the block is influenced by the concentration of local anesthetic.

With advanced age, the dose of local anesthetic decreases due to anatomical changes. Additional factors that influence the spread of local anesthetic in the epidural space are pregnancy, weight, height, rate of injection, and patient position. However, *volume* is the most important drug-related factor that affects block height.

References: Butterworth JF IV, Mackey DC, Wasnick JD, eds. *Morgan & Mikhail's Clinical Anesthesiology.* 7th ed. New York, NY: McGraw Hill; 2022: Chapter 45.

Elisha S, Heiner JS, Nagelhout JJ. *Nurse Anesthesia.* 7th ed. St. Louis, MO: Elsevier Saunders; 2023: Chapter 49.

Gropper MA. *Miller's Anesthesia.* 9th ed. Philadelphia, PA: Churchill Livingstone Elsevier; 2020: Chapter 45.

152. A patient is scheduled for a thoracotomy. A thoracic epidural is placed. What volume of local anesthetic will you use?

(A) 15 mL

(B) 10 mL

(C) 18 mL

(D) 20 mL

Rationale: Epidural placement is T_4–T_5 for thoracic surgery. Cervical and thoracic epidural volume is calculated based upon 0.7 to 1.0 mL/segment. 1 to 2 mL/segment volume is administered for lumbar epidural anesthesia.

References: Butterworth JF IV, Mackey DC, Wasnick JD, eds. *Morgan & Mikhail's Clinical Anesthesiology.* 7th ed. New York, NY: McGraw Hill; 2022: Chapter 45.

Elisha S, Heiner JS, Nagelhout JJ. *Nurse Anesthesia.* 7th ed. St. Louis, MO: Elsevier Saunders; 2023: Chapter 49.

153. What is the best approach to avoiding cardiac arrest during spinal anesthesia?

(A) Decrease preload

(B) Give prophylactic ephedrine

(C) Increase preload

(D) Give prophylactic atropine

Rationale: Preload is essential when administering spinal and epidural anesthesia. Giving a fluid bolus improves preload in anticipation of sympathetic blockade. When significant bradycardia occurs following administration of local anesthetic, give ephedrine and atropine in sequence. These measures will help to avoid cardiac arrest.

References: Butterworth JF IV, Mackey DC, Wasnick JD, eds. *Morgan & Mikhail's Clinical Anesthesiology.* 7th ed. New York, NY: McGraw Hill; 2022: Chapter 45.

Elisha S, Heiner JS, Nagelhout JJ. *Nurse Anesthesia.* 7th ed. St. Louis, MO: Elsevier Saunders; 2023: Chapter 49.

154. What patient is least likely to experience a postdural puncture headache?

    (A) 70-year-old male
    (B) 40-year-old male
    (C) 20-year-old female
    (D) 60-year-old female

Rationale: Risk factors linked to postdural puncture headache include age, gender, needle size, and pregnancy. Young females represent the highest risk population. The incidence of PDPH in females is greater than males. The incidence of PDPH is greater in younger versus older populations.

References: Butterworth JF IV, Mackey DC, Wasnick JD, eds. *Morgan & Mikhail's Clinical Anesthesiology.* 7th ed. New York, NY: McGraw Hill; 2022: Chapter 45.

Elisha S, Heiner JS, Nagelhout JJ. *Nurse Anesthesia.* 7th ed. St. Louis, MO: Elsevier Saunders; 2023: Chapter 51.

155. What ultrasound frequency is used when placing an epidural or spinal?

    (A) 2 to 5 MHz
    (B) 5 to 10 MHz
    (C) 10 to 15 MHz
    (D) 20 to 25 MHz

Rationale: The ultrasound probe for peripheral nerve blocks utilizes high frequency. Lower frequency ultrasound probes are used for spinal and epidural placement.

References: Barash PG, Cullen BF, Stoelting RK, et al, eds. *Clinical Anesthesia.* 8th ed. Lippincott Williams & Wilkins; 2017: Chapter 35.

Elisha S, Heiner JS, Nagelhout JJ. *Nurse Anesthesia.* 7th ed. St. Louis, MO: Elsevier Saunders; 2023: Chapter 49.

156. Which statement is true regarding ultrasound for peripheral nerve blocks?

    (A) Structures that appear white on the ultrasound screen are hypoechoic.
    (B) Low frequencies are used for peripheral nerve blocks.
    (C) Structures that appear white on the ultrasound screen are hyperechoic.
    (D) High-frequency transducers offer a low-resolution picture.

Rationale: Hypoechoic refers to dark structures on the ultrasound screen. Higher frequencies are used for peripheral nerve blocks whereas lower frequencies are used for spinal and epidural anesthesia when ultrasound technology is employed. High-frequency transducers provide high resolution pictures but poor tissue penetration. Low-frequency transducers allow for deeper tissue penetration.

References: Butterworth JF IV, Mackey DC, Wasnick JD, eds. *Morgan & Mikhail's Clinical Anesthesiology.* 7th ed. New York, NY: McGraw Hill; 2022: Chapter 46.

Elisha S, Heiner JS, Nagelhout JJ. *Nurse Anesthesia.* 7th ed. St. Louis, MO: Elsevier Saunders; 2023: Chapter 50.

157. What is the innervation of the brachial plexus?

    (A) C_5–C_8 and T_1
    (B) C_4–C_8
    (C) C_4–C_8 and T_1
    (D) C_5–C_7 and T_1–T_2

Rationale: The C_4 and T_2 innervation is minimal or absent.

References: Butterworth JF IV, Mackey DC, Wasnick JD, eds. *Morgan & Mikhail's Clinical Anesthesiology.* 7th ed. New York, NY: McGraw Hill; 2022: Chapter 46.

Elisha S, Heiner JS, Nagelhout JJ. *Nurse Anesthesia.* 7th ed. St. Louis, MO: Elsevier Saunders; 2023: Chapter 50.

158. What brachial plexus approach is indicated for a patient undergoing shoulder surgery?

    (A) Supraclavicular
    (B) Infraclavicular
    (C) Interscalene
    (D) Axillary

Rationale: Surgeries distal to the mid-humerus employ supraclavicular, infraclavicular, and axillary blocks. The interscalene block is used for surgeries proximal to the humerus including the shoulder.

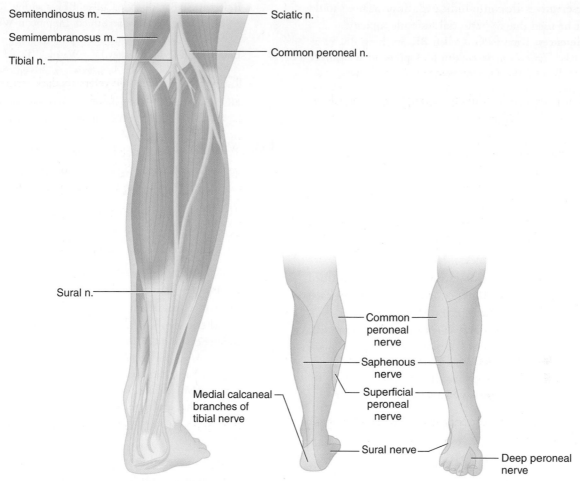

FIG. 3-12. The sciatic nerve divides into tibial and peroneal branches just proximal to the popliteal fossa and provides sensory innervation to much of the lower leg. (Reproduced with permission from Butterworth JF IV, Mackey DC, Wasnick JD, eds. *Morgan & Mikhail's Clinical Anesthesiology.* 7th ed. New York: McGraw Hill; 2022.)

References: Butterworth JF IV, Mackey DC, Wasnick JD, eds. *Morgan & Mikhail's Clinical Anesthesiology.* 7th ed. New York, NY: McGraw Hill; 2022: Chapter 46.

Elisha S, Heiner JS, Nagelhout JJ. *Nurse Anesthesia.* 7th ed. St. Louis, MO: Elsevier Saunders; 2023: Chapter 50.

159. Which would result from excessive pressure on the sciatic nerve by the piriformis muscle?

(A) Chronic pain in the perineum with voiding difficulty

(B) Anterior thigh pain and weakness upon standing

(C) Gluteal pain with paresthesia in the posterior thigh

(D) Lumbar vertebral pain exacerbated by flexion of the lower back

Rationale: The sciatic nerve emerges from the greater sciatic foramen immediately approximate to the piriformis muscle. Nerve compression by this muscle results in gluteal pain and posterior paresthesia.

References: Barash PG, Cullen BF, Stoelting RK, et al, eds. *Clinical Anesthesia.* 8th ed. Lippincott Williams & Wilkins; 2017: Chapter 56.

Butterworth JF IV, Mackey DC, Wasnick JD, eds. *Morgan & Mikhail's Clinical Anesthesiology.* 7th ed. New York, NY: McGraw Hill; 2022: Chapter 47.

160. Which of the following is appropriate to use for intravenous regional anesthesia?

(A) 0.5% lidocaine with epinephrine 50 mL

(B) 5.0% lidocaine with epinephrine 40 mL

(C) 0.5% lidocaine 50 mL

(D) 0.5% bupivacaine 50 mL

Rationale: Vasoconstrictors are contraindicated in regional blocks involving extremities. Low versus high local anesthetic concentration is used. In addition, preservatives are contraindicated. Bupivacaine should not be used due to potential systemic toxicity.

References: Barash PG, Cullen BF, Stoelting RK, et al, eds. *Clinical Anesthesia*. 8th ed. Lippincott Williams & Wilkins; 2017: Chapter 36.

Butterworth JF IV, Mackey DC, Wasnick JD, eds. *Morgan & Mikhail's Clinical Anesthesiology*. 7th ed. New York, NY: McGraw Hill; 2022: Chapter 46.

161. For which medication is regional anesthesia an absolute contraindication?

(A) Clopidogrel

(B) Unfractionated heparin

(C) Low molecular weight heparin

(D) Thrombolytics

Rationale: Regional anesthesia may be performed safely when the waiting period is adhered to for each of the medications except thrombolytics.

References: Butterworth JF IV, Mackey DC, Wasnick JD, eds. *Morgan & Mikhail's Clinical Anesthesiology*. 7th ed. New York, NY: McGraw Hill; 2022: Chapter 45.

Elisha S, Heiner JS, Nagelhout JJ. *Nurse Anesthesia*. 7th ed. St. Louis, MO: Elsevier Saunders; 2023: Chapter 49.

162. The patient received a Bier block for hand surgery. The case was completed in 10 minutes. When will you deflate the tourniquet?

(A) 10 minutes after the local anesthetic is injected

(B) 20 minutes after the local anesthetic is injected

(C) 30 minutes after the local anesthetic is injected

(D) 40 minutes after the local anesthetic is injected

Rationale: The tourniquet should remain inflated for a minimum of 20 minutes after the local anesthetic is injected to avoid local anesthetic toxicity.

References: Barash PG, Cullen BF, Stoelting RK, et al, eds. *Clinical Anesthesia*. 8th ed. Lippincott Williams & Wilkins; 2017: Chapter 36.

Butterworth JF IV, Mackey DC, Wasnick JD, eds. *Morgan & Mikhail's Clinical Anesthesiology*. 7th ed. New York, NY: McGraw Hill; 2022: Chapter 46.

Elisha S, Heiner JS, Nagelhout JJ. *Nurse Anesthesia*. 7th ed. St. Louis, MO: Elsevier Saunders; 2023: Chapter 50.

163. What statement is true regarding digital nerve blocks?

(A) A small gauge needle is inserted at the distal aspect of the selected digit.

(B) 5 to 7 mL of lidocaine with epinephrine is used.

(C) A small gauge needle is inserted at the medial and lateral borders of the base of the selected digit.

(D) 2 to 3 mL of lidocaine is used.

Rationale: The digital block is performed by injecting 2 to 3 mL of a non-epinephrine containing local anesthetic solution at the base of the selected digit.

References: Butterworth JF IV, Mackey DC, Wasnick JD, eds. *Morgan & Mikhail's Clinical Anesthesiology*. 7th ed. New York, NY: McGraw Hill; 2022: Chapter 46.

Gropper MA. *Miller's Anesthesia*. 9th ed. Philadelphia, PA: Churchill Livingstone Elsevier; 2020: Chapter 76.

164. What is the definition of persistent postsurgical pain?

(A) Pain resulting from outpatient surgery sufficient to require inpatient care

(B) Pain for more than 1 to 2 weeks following surgery

(C) Pain for more than 1 to 2 months following surgery

(D) Pain for more than 1 year following surgery

Rationale: Chronic pain persisting beyond 4 to 8 weeks following surgery defines persistent postsurgical pain.

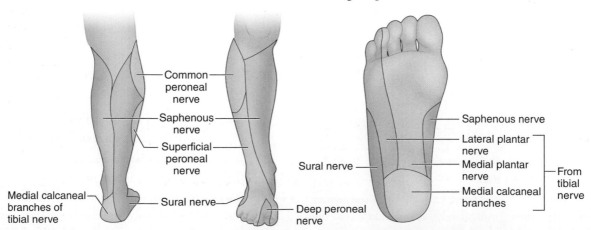

FIG. 3-13. Cutaneous innervation of the foot. (Reproduced with permission from Butterworth JF IV, Mackey DC, Wasnick JD, eds. *Morgan & Mikhail's Clinical Anesthesiology*. 7th ed. New York: McGraw Hill; 2022.)

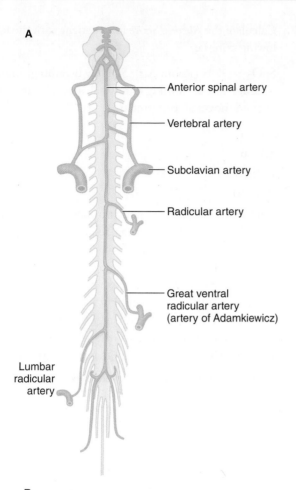

A

Anterior spinal artery

Vertebral artery

Subclavian artery

Radicular artery

Great ventral radicular artery (artery of Adamkiewicz)

Lumbar radicular artery

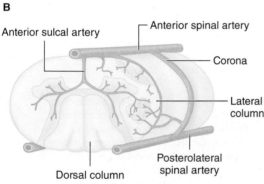

B

Anterior sulcal artery

Anterior spinal artery

Corona

Lateral column

Posterolateral spinal artery

Dorsal column

FIG. 3-14. Arterial supply to the spinal cord. **A:** Anterior view showing principal sources of blood supply. **B:** Cross-sectional view through the spinal cord showing paired posterior spinal arteries and a single anterior spinal artery. (Reproduced with permission from Waxman SG. *Correlative Neuroanatomy.* 24th ed. New York: McGraw Hill; 2000.)

References: Butterworth JF IV, Mackey DC, Wasnick JD, eds. *Morgan & Mikhail's Clinical Anesthesiology.* 7th ed. New York, NY: McGraw Hill; 2022: Chapter 47.
Elisha S, Heiner JS, Nagelhout JJ. *Nurse Anesthesia.* 7th ed. St. Louis, MO: Elsevier Saunders; 2023: Chapter 57.

165. Where is local anesthetic injected in a radial block at the wrist?

(A) Medial to the ulnar artery at the wrist

(B) Lateral to the radial artery at the wrist

(C) Medial to the radial artery at the wrist

(D) Lateral to the ulnar artery at the wrist

Rationale: The radial nerve block at the wrist requires injecting 3 to 5 mL of local anesthetic lateral to the radial artery. The ulnar nerve block requires injecting local anesthetic medial to the ulnar artery at the wrist.

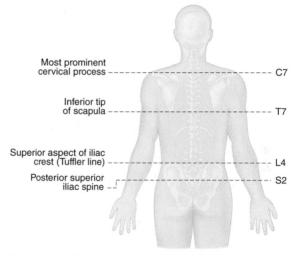

Most prominent cervical process — C7

Inferior tip of scapula — T7

Superior aspect of iliac crest (Tuffler line) — L4

Posterior superior iliac spine — S2

FIG. 3-15. Surface landmarks for identifying spinal levels. (Reproduced with permission from Butterworth JF IV, Mackey DC, Wasnick JD, eds. *Morgan & Mikhail's Clinical Anesthesiology.* 7th ed. New York: McGraw Hill; 2022.)

References: Butterworth JF IV, Mackey DC, Wasnick JD, eds. *Morgan & Mikhail's Clinical Anesthesiology.* 7th ed. New York, NY: McGraw Hill; 2022: Chapter 46.
Hadzic A, ed. *Hadzic's Peripheral Nerve Blocks and Anatomy for Ultrasound-Guided Regional Anesthesia.* 3rd ed. New York, NY: McGraw-Hill; 2022: Chapter 20.

166. Which nerve provides sensation to the anteromedial foot and medial lower leg?

(A) Deep peroneal

(B) Sural

(C) Superficial peroneal

(D) Saphenous

Rationale: The deep peroneal nerve provides sensation to webbing between the first and second digits. The superficial peroneal nerve supplies sensation to the dorsum of the foot and toes. The sural nerve provides sensation to the lateral foot.

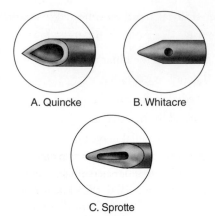

A. Quincke   B. Whitacre

C. Sprotte

FIG. 3-16. Spinal needles. (Reproduced with permission from Butterworth JF IV, Mackey DC, Wasnick JD, eds. *Morgan & Mikhail's Clinical Anesthesiology*. 7th ed. New York: McGraw Hill; 2022.)

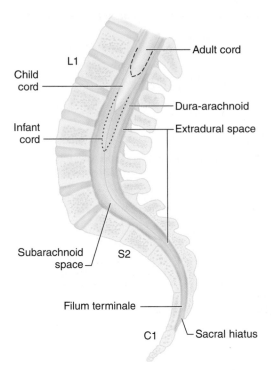

FIG. 3-17. Sagittal view through the lumbar vertebrae and sacrum. Note the end of the spinal cord rises with development from approximately L_3 to L_1. The dural sac normally ends at S_2. (Reproduced with permission from Butterworth JF IV, Mackey DC, Wasnick JD, eds. *Morgan & Mikhail's Clinical Anesthesiology*. 7th ed. New York: McGraw Hill; 2022.)

References: Barash PG, Cullen BF, Stoelting RK, et al, eds. *Clinical Anesthesia*. 8th ed. Lippincott Williams & Wilkins; 2017: Chapter 36.

Butterworth JF IV, Mackey DC, Wasnick JD, eds. *Morgan & Mikhail's Clinical Anesthesiology*. 7th ed. New York, NY: McGraw Hill; 2022: Chapter 46.

167. Calculate the Aldrete Score for a patient with the following criteria:

$SpO_2 > 92\%$ (Room Air); Shallow breathing; Blood pressure $+/-20$ mmHg of normal; arousable on calling and moves all extremities.

(A) 4
(B) 6
(C) 8
(D) 10

Rationale: The Aldrete Score provides discharge criteria. Each criterion (oxygenation, respiration, circulation, consciousness, and activity) earns 2 points maximum. Full deep breathing and coughing receive 2 points as compared to shallow or limited breathing (1 point). Blood pressure $+/-20$ mmHg of normal receives 2 points. A fully awake patient receives 2 points as compared to a patient who arouses on calling (1 point). Lastly, moving all four extremities receives 2 points.

TABLE 3-11. Postanesthetic Aldrete recovery score.[1]

Original Criteria	Modified Criteria	Point Value
Color	**Oxygenation**	
Pink	$SpO_2 > 92\%$ on room air	2
Pale or dusky	$SpO_2 > 90\%$ on oxygen	1
Cyanotic	$SpO_2 < 90\%$ on oxygen	0
Respiration		
Can breathe deeply and cough	Breathes deeply and coughs freely	2
Shallow but adequate exchange	Dyspneic, shallow, or limited breathing	1
Apnea or obstruction	Apnea	0
Circulation		
Blood pressure within 20% of normal	Blood pressure ± 20 mmHg of normal	2
Blood pressure within 20% to 50% of normal	Blood pressure ± 20-50 mmHg of normal	1
Blood pressure deviating >50% from normal	Blood pressure more than ± 50 mmHg of normal	0
Consciousness		
Awake, alert, and oriented	Fully awake	2
Arousable but readily drifts back to sleep	Arousable on calling	1
No response	Not responsive	0
Activity		
Moves all extremities	Same	2
Moves two extremities	Same	1
No movement	Same	0

[1]Ideally, the patient should be discharged when the total score is 10, but a minimum of 9 is required.
(Data from Aldrete JA, Kronlik D. A postanesthetic recovery score. *Anesth Analg.* 1970;49:924; and Aldrete JA. The postanesthesia recovery score revisited. *J Clin Anesth.* 1995;7(1):89.)

References: Butterworth JF IV, Mackey DC, Wasnick JD, eds. *Morgan & Mikhail's Clinical Anesthesiology.* 7th ed. New York, NY: McGraw Hill; 2022: Chapter 56.

Elisha S, Heiner JS, Nagelhout JJ. *Nurse Anesthesia.* 7th ed. St. Louis, MO: Elsevier Saunders; 2023: Chapter 55.

168. What artery provides most of the blood supply to the anterior, lower two-thirds of the spinal cord?

(A) Posterior spinal artery

(B) Artery of Adamkiewicz

(C) Posterior inferior cerebellar artery

(D) Intercostal arteries

Rationale: Blood flow to the posterior one-third of the spinal cord is provided by the posterior spinal artery. The posterior inferior cerebellar artery feeds the posterior spinal arteries. The intercostal arteries provide blood flow to the anterior and posterior spinal arteries. The largest of the arteries supplying the spinal cord is the arteria radicularis magna (Artery of Adamkiewicz).

References: Butterworth JF IV, Mackey DC, Wasnick JD, eds. *Morgan & Mikhail's Clinical Anesthesiology.* 7th ed. New York, NY: McGraw Hill; 2022: Chapter 45.

Gropper MA. *Miller's Anesthesia.* 9th ed. Philadelphia, PA: Churchill Livingstone Elsevier; 2020: Chapter 45.

169. After placing a spinal anesthetic the sensory block is assessed at T_8. Where is the most likely level of the motor block?

(A) T_4

(B) T_6

(C) T_{10}

(D) T_2

Rationale: A motor block is typically two or more segments below the sensory block.

References: Butterworth JF IV, Mackey DC, Wasnick JD, eds. *Morgan & Mikhail's Clinical Anesthesiology.* 7th ed. New York, NY: McGraw Hill; 2022: Chapter 45.

Flood P, Rathmell JP, Urbam RD, eds. *Stoelting's Pharmacology & Physiology in Anesthetic Practice.* 6th ed. Philadelphia, PA: Wolters Kluwer; 2022: Chapter 10.

170. Which of the following characterizes A-*a* nerve fibers?

(A) Diameter 0.5 to 1 micrometer

(B) Heavy myelination with a diameter of 12 to 20 micrometers

(C) Light myelination

(D) Similar to C fibers

Rationale: B fibers are lightly myelinated, 1 to 4 micrometers in diameter possessing preganglionic and autonomic function. C fibers are not myelinated, 0.5 to 1 micrometer in diameter and are responsible for touch and temperature sensation.

TABLE 3-12. Nerve fiber classification.[1]

Fiber Type	Modality Served	Diameter (mm)	Conduction (m/s)	Myelinated?
Aα	Motor efferent	12-20	70-120	Yes
Aα	Proprioception	12-20	70-120	Yes
Aβ	Touch, pressure	5-12	30-70	Yes
Aγ	Motor efferent (muscle spindle)	3-6	15-30	Yes
Aδ	Pain	2-5	12-30	Yes
	Temperature			
	Touch			
B	Preganglionic autonomic fibers	<3	3-14	Some
C	Pain	0.4-1.2	0.5-2	No
Dorsal root	Temperature			
C	Postganglionic sympathetic fibers	0.3-1.3	0.7-2.3	No
Sympathetic				

[1]An alternative numerical system is sometimes used to classify sensory fibers.

(Reproduced with permission from Butterworth JF IV, Mackey DC, Wasnick JD, eds. *Morgan & Mikhail's Clinical Anesthesiology.* 7th ed. New York: McGraw Hill; 2022.)

References: Butterworth JF IV, Mackey DC, Wasnick JD, eds. *Morgan & Mikhail's Clinical Anesthesiology.* 7th ed. New York, NY: McGraw Hill; 2022: Chapter 16.

Elisha S, Heiner JS, Nagelhout JJ. *Nurse Anesthesia.* 7th ed. St. Louis, MO: Elsevier Saunders; 2023: Chapter 49.

171. Following administration of spinal anesthesia the patient becomes hypotensive and bradycardic. What nerve fibers are affected?

    (A) T_1–T_4
    (B) T_5–T_6
    (C) T_7–T_8
    (D) T_{10}–T_{12}

    Rationale: Blocking the cardiac accelerator fibers leaves vagal tone unopposed and results in bradycardia and hypotension.

    References: Butterworth JF IV, Mackey DC, Wasnick JD, eds. *Morgan & Mikhail's Clinical Anesthesiology.* 7th ed. New York, NY: McGraw Hill; 2022: Chapter 45.

    Elisha S, Heiner JS, Nagelhout JJ. *Nurse Anesthesia.* 7th ed. St. Louis, MO: Elsevier Saunders; 2023: Chapter 49.

172. Which clotting factor is not synthesized in the liver?

    (A) II
    (B) IV
    (C) VII
    (D) VIII

    Rationale: Most clotting factors are synthesized in the liver except factor VIII, i.e., von Willebrand factor, which is synthesized by vascular endothelial cells.

    References: Barash PG, Cullen BF, Stoelting RK, et al, eds. *Clinical Anesthesia.* 8th ed. Lippincott Williams & Wilkins; 2017: Chapter 17.

    Elisha S, Heiner JS, Nagelhout JJ. *Nurse Anesthesia.* 7th ed. St. Louis, MO: Elsevier Saunders; 2023: Chapter 20.

173. A 70-year-old patient with emphysema is undergoing an open cholecystectomy. What is the best anesthetic choice for this patient?

    (A) Spinal
    (B) Epidural
    (C) General
    (D) MAC

    Rationale: Regional anesthesia is used with caution for patients with pulmonary disease, specifically for surgical procedures above the umbilicus. The patient would benefit however from epidural analgesia.

TABLE 3-13. Contraindications to neuraxial blockade.

Absolute
Infection at the site of injection
Lack of consent
Coagulopathy or other bleeding diathesis
Severe hypovolemia
Increased intracranial pressure
Relative
Sepsis
Uncooperative patient
Preexisting neurological deficits
Demyelinating lesions
Stenotic valvular heart lesions
Left ventricular outflow obstruction (hypertrophic obstructive cardiomyopathy)
Severe spinal deformity
Controversial
Prior back surgery at the site of injection
Complicated surgery
Prolonged operation
Major blood loss
Maneuvers that compromise respiration

(Reproduced with permission from Butterworth JF IV, Mackey DC, Wasnick JD, eds. *Morgan & Mikhail's Clinical Anesthesiology.* 7th ed. New York: McGraw Hill; 2022.)

References: Butterworth JF IV, Mackey DC, Wasnick JD, eds. *Morgan & Mikhail's Clinical Anesthesiology.* 7th ed. New York, NY: McGraw Hill; 2022: Chapter 45.

Elisha S, Heiner JS, Nagelhout JJ. *Nurse Anesthesia.* 7th ed. St. Louis, MO: Elsevier Saunders; 2023: Chapter 29.

174. Which of the following is an absolute contraindication for regional anesthesia?

    (A) Uncooperative patient
    (B) Preexisting neurological deficits
    (C) Severe aortic stenosis
    (D) Patient refusal

    Rationale: Absolute contraindications for regional anesthesia include patient refusal, infection at the injection site, and increased intracranial pressure (neuraxial technique). Extreme caution is used when considering regional anesthesia for patients with coagulopathies, stenotic valves, and significant hypovolemia. The risks and benefits must be weighed.

    References: Butterworth JF IV, Mackey DC, Wasnick JD, eds. *Morgan & Mikhail's Clinical Anesthesiology.* 7th ed. New York, NY: McGraw Hill; 2022: Chapter 45.

    Elisha S, Heiner JS, Nagelhout JJ. *Nurse Anesthesia.* 7th ed. St. Louis, MO: Elsevier Saunders; 2023: Chapter 49.

    Gropper MA. *Miller's Anesthesia.* 9th ed. Philadelphia, PA: Churchill Livingstone Elsevier; 2020: Chapter 45.

175. A patient who takes ticlopidine requests a spinal anesthetic for a total knee replacement. What is the waiting period for ticlopidine?

(A) 7 days

(B) 12 days

(C) 48 hours

(D) 8 hours

Rationale: The waiting period to provide regional anesthesia for patients taking antiplatelet drugs varies. The waiting period for clopidogrel is 5 to 7 days; abciximab is 48 hours; and eptifibatide is 8 hours. The waiting period for rivaroxaban and apixaban is 72 hours.

References: Elisha S, Heiner JS, Nagelhout JJ. *Nurse Anesthesia.* 7th ed. St. Louis, MO: Elsevier Saunders; 2023: Chapter 38.

Gropper MA. *Miller's Anesthesia.* 9th ed. Philadelphia, PA: Churchill Livingstone Elsevier; 2020: Chapters 31 and 45.

176. Where is Tuffier's line located?

(A) L₄

(B) L₂

(C) L₁

(D) L₃

Rationale: Tuffier's line is located just above the iliac crests crossing the L₄–L₅ vertebrae.

References: Butterworth JF IV, Mackey DC, Wasnick JD, eds. *Morgan & Mikhail's Clinical Anesthesiology.* 7th ed. New York, NY: McGraw Hill; 2022: Chapter 45.

Elisha S, Heiner JS, Nagelhout JJ. *Nurse Anesthesia.* 7th ed. St. Louis, MO: Elsevier Saunders; 2023: Chapter 50.

177. What is the correct order of anatomical structure used when placing an epidural needle?

(A) Skin, subcutaneous tissue, supraspinous ligament, interspinous ligament, ligamentum flavum, epidural space

(B) Skin, subcutaneous tissue, interspinous ligament, supraspinous ligament, ligamentum flavum, epidural space

(C) Skin, subcutaneous tissue, interspinous ligament, supraspinous ligament, ligamentum flavum, dura, subarachnoid space

(D) Skin, subcutaneous tissue, interspinous ligament, supraspinous ligament, ligamentum flavum, dura, epidural space

Rationale: Once the needle reaches the epidural space, further advancement penetrates the dura

reaching the subarachnoid space and presence of cerebral spinal fluid.

References: Butterworth JF IV, Mackey DC, Wasnick JD, eds. *Morgan & Mikhail's Clinical Anesthesiology.* 7th ed. New York, NY: McGraw Hill; 2022: Chapter 45.

Elisha S, Heiner JS, Nagelhout JJ. *Nurse Anesthesia.* 7th ed. St. Louis, MO: Elsevier Saunders; 2023: Chapter 49.

Gropper MA. *Miller's Anesthesia.* 9th ed. Philadelphia, PA: Churchill Livingstone Elsevier; 2020: Chapter 45.

178. Which statement is true of Aδ fibers?

(A) Aδ fibers are myelinated, synapse in Rexed laminae I and V, and transmit primarily mechanical or thermal pain.

(B) Aδ fibers are unmyelinated, synapse in Rexed laminae II and VII, and transmit primarily mechanical or thermal pain.

(C) Aδ fibers are myelinated, synapse in Rexed laminae III and X, and transmit primarily mechanical or thermal pain.

(D) Aδ fibers are unmyelinated, synapse in Rexed laminae IV and VI, and transmit primarily mechanical or thermal pain.

Rationale: Aδ fibers are myelinated, terminate in laminae I and V, and respond to mechanical and thermal stimuli.

References: Butterworth JF IV, Mackey DC, Wasnick JD, eds. *Morgan & Mikhail's Clinical Anesthesiology.* 7th ed. New York, NY: McGraw Hill; 2022: Chapter 47.

Elisha S, Heiner JS, Nagelhout JJ. *Nurse Anesthesia.* 7th ed. St. Louis, MO: Elsevier Saunders; 2023: Chapter 10.

179. Which laminae receive input from C fibers?

(A) III, IV, VI

(B) I, VI, X

(C) II, VII, IX

(D) I, II, V

Rationale: Signals from C fibers travel to laminae I, II, and V.

References: Barash PG, Cullen BF, Stoelting RK, et al, eds. *Clinical Anesthesia.* 8th ed. Lippincott Williams & Wilkins; 2017: Chapter 56.

Butterworth JF IV, Mackey DC, Wasnick JD, eds. *Morgan & Mikhail's Clinical Anesthesiology.* 7th ed. New York, NY: McGraw Hill; 2022: Chapter 47.

180. How would postoperative pain localized to the site of skin incision be classified?

(A) Visceral pain

(B) Deep somatic pain

(C)   Superficial somatic pain

(D)   Referred pain

Rationale: This is an example of acute superficial somatic pain.

References: Butterworth JF IV, Mackey DC, Wasnick JD, eds. *Morgan & Mikhail's Clinical Anesthesiology*. 7th ed. New York, NY: McGraw Hill; 2022: Chapter 47.
Elisha S, Heiner JS, Nagelhout JJ. *Nurse Anesthesia*. 7th ed. St. Louis, MO: Elsevier Saunders; 2023: Chapter 56.

181.   Referred pain from the diaphragm can be expected in which dermatome?

(A) C_4

(B) C_7

(C) T_4

(D) T_7

Rationale: Diaphragmatic innervation originates in cervical levels 3, 4, and 5.

TABLE 3-14. Patterns of referred pain.

Location	Cutaneous Dermatome
Central diaphragm	C_4
Lungs	T_2–T_6
Aorta	T_1–L_2
Heart	T_1–T_4
Esophagus	T_3–T_8
Pancreas and spleen	T_5–T_{10}
Stomach, liver, and gallbladder	T_6–T_9
Adrenals	T_8–L_1
Small intestine	T_9–T_{11}
Colon	T_{10}–L_1
Kidney, ovaries, and testes	T_{10}–L_1
Ureters	T_{10}–T_{12}
Uterus	T_{11}–L_2
Bladder and prostate	S_2–S_4
Urethra and rectum	S_2–S_4

(Reproduced with permission from Butterworth JF IV, Mackey DC, Wasnick JD, eds. *Morgan & Mikhail's Clinical Anesthesiology*. 7th ed. New York: McGraw Hill; 2022.)

References: Butterworth JF IV, Mackey DC, Wasnick JD, eds. *Morgan & Mikhail's Clinical Anesthesiology*. 7th ed. New York, NY: McGraw Hill; 2022: Chapter 47.
Elisha S, Heiner JS, Nagelhout JJ. *Nurse Anesthesia*. 7th ed. St. Louis, MO: Elsevier Saunders; 2023: Chapter 29.

182.   What is the surface landmark of the fourth cervical cutaneous dermatome?

(A)   Anterior neck

(B)   Shoulder

(C)   Biceps

(D)   Xiphoid

Rationale: Referred diaphragm pain occurs in the shoulder due to innervation at C_3–C_5.

References: Butterworth JF IV, Mackey DC, Wasnick JD, eds. *Morgan & Mikhail's Clinical Anesthesiology*. 7th ed. New York, NY: McGraw Hill; 2022: Chapter 47.
Elisha S, Heiner JS, Nagelhout JJ. *Nurse Anesthesia*. 7th ed. St. Louis, MO: Elsevier Saunders; 2023: Chapter 49.

183.   Which act to diminish pain signals?

(A)   Glutamate

(B)   Glycine

(C)   Substance P

(D)   ß-Endorphin

Rationale: Endogenous opioids modulate pain by decreasing severity.

TABLE 3-15. Major neurotransmitters mediating or modulating pain.

Neurotransmitter	Receptor	Effect on Nociception
Substance P	Neurokinin–1	Excitatory
Calcitonin gene-related peptide		Excitatory
Glutamate	NMDA, AMPA, kainate, quisqualate	Excitatory
Aspartate	NMDA, AMPA, kainate, quisqualate	Excitatory
Adenosine triphosphate (ATP)	P_1, P_2	Excitatory
Somatostatin		Inhibitory
Acetylcholine	Muscarinic	Inhibitory
Enkephalins	μ, δ, κ	Inhibitory
β-Endorphin	μ, δ, κ	Inhibitory
Norepinephrine	α_2	Inhibitory
Adenosine	A_1	Inhibitory
Serotonin	5-HT$_1$ (5-HT$_3$)	Inhibitory
γ-Aminobutyric acid (GABA)	A, B	Inhibitory
Glycine		Inhibitory

AMPA, 2-(aminomethyl)phenylacetic acid; NMDA, *N*-methyl-D-aspartate; 5-HT, 5-hydroxytryptamine.
(Reproduced with permission from Butterworth JF IV, Mackey DC, Wasnick JD, eds. *Morgan & Mikhail's Clinical Anesthesiology*. 7th ed. New York: McGraw Hill; 2022.)

References: Butterworth JF IV, Mackey DC, Wasnick JD, eds. *Morgan & Mikhail's Clinical Anesthesiology*. 7th ed. New York, NY: McGraw Hill; 2022: Chapter 47.
Elisha S, Heiner JS, Nagelhout JJ. *Nurse Anesthesia*. 7th ed. St. Louis, MO: Elsevier Saunders; 2023: Chapter 11.

184.   What complication is associated with hetastarch?

(A)   Interference with blood typing

(B)   Coagulopathy

(C)   Decreased plasma volume

(D)   Anaphylaxis

Rationale: The size of the starch molecule is responsible for the therapeutic effects and side effects of hetastarch. Larger molecules can increase plasma volume by up to 80%. Complications associated with hetastarch include coagulopathy, accumulation (which may persist for several years), and renal failure (even with smaller starches). Perioperative use of hetastarch remains controversial. Dextran is associated with interference with blood typing and kidney failure. Unlike dextran, which is antigenic and known to cause anaphylaxis, hetastarch is nonantigenic.

References: Butterworth JF IV, Mackey DC, Wasnick JD, eds. *Morgan & Mikhail's Clinical Anesthesiology.* 7th ed. New York, NY: McGraw Hill; 2022: Chapter 51.

Elisha S, Heiner JS, Nagelhout JJ. *Nurse Anesthesia.* 7th ed. St. Louis, MO: Elsevier Saunders; 2023: Chapter 21.

Gropper MA. *Miller's Anesthesia.* 9th ed. Philadelphia, PA: Churchill Livingstone Elsevier; 2020: Chapter 47.

185. Which portion of the spinal cord is most associated with transmission of pain signals?

(A) Dorsal horn

(B) Central canal

(C) Ventral horn

(D) Pia mater

Rationale: The proximal portion of pain receptors terminate in the dorsal horn.

References: Butterworth JF IV, Mackey DC, Wasnick JD, eds. *Morgan & Mikhail's Clinical Anesthesiology.* 7th ed. New York, NY: McGraw Hill; 2022: Chapter 47.

Elisha S, Heiner JS, Nagelhout JJ. *Nurse Anesthesia.* 7th ed. St. Louis, MO: Elsevier Saunders; 2023: Chapter 56.

186. Which of these is least likely to relieve pain by decreasing inflammation?

(A) Acetaminophen

(B) Ketorolac

(C) Ibuprofen

(D) Celecoxib

Rationale: The exact MOA of acetaminophen is unclear. Acetaminophen inhibits COX in the brain, but not peripherally. The primary effect of acetaminophen is analgesia and as an antipyretic. It has a minimal anti-inflammatory effect.

References: Butterworth JF IV, Mackey DC, Wasnick JD, eds. *Morgan & Mikhail's Clinical Anesthesiology.* 7th ed. New York, NY: McGraw Hill; 2022: Chapter 17.

Elisha S, Heiner JS, Nagelhout JJ. *Nurse Anesthesia.* 7th ed. St. Louis, MO: Elsevier Saunders; 2023: Chapter 56.

187. Which is the mechanism of action for gabapentin?

(A) GABA agonist effect

(B) Calcium channel activation

(C) Excitatory neurotransmitter inhibition

(D) Inhibition of prostaglandin synthesis

Rationale: Possible mechanisms include blocking the alpha 2 delta ($\alpha 2\delta$) subunit of the presynaptic voltage-gated calcium channels in the CNS, thus inhibiting the release of the excitatory neurotransmitter, glutamate.

References: Butterworth JF IV, Mackey DC, Wasnick JD, eds. *Morgan & Mikhail's Clinical Anesthesiology.* 7th ed. New York, NY: McGraw Hill; 2022: Chapter 17.

Elisha S, Heiner JS, Nagelhout JJ. *Nurse Anesthesia.* 7th ed. St. Louis, MO: Elsevier Saunders; 2023: Chapter 56.

188. Which of these analgesic agents is a GABA agonist?

(A) Baclofen

(B) Pregabalin

(C) Dexmedetomidine

(D) Celecoxib

Rationale: Baclofen is a GABA agonist. Baclofen activates GABA-B receptors pre- and postsynaptically.

References: Butterworth JF IV, Mackey DC, Wasnick JD, eds. *Morgan & Mikhail's Clinical Anesthesiology.* 7th ed. New York, NY: McGraw Hill; 2022: Chapter 47.

Gropper MA. *Miller's Anesthesia.* 9th ed. Philadelphia, PA: Churchill Livingstone Elsevier; 2020: Chapter 51.

189. What is the most common level of approach to perform a stellate ganglion block?

(A) C_3

(B) C_4

(C) C_5

(D) C_6

Rationale: Both the landmark, paratracheal technique, and ultrasound utilize Chassaignac's tubercle which is the transverse process of C_6. However, real time ultrasound use reduces the risk for complications. After visualizing the relevant structures (carotid artery, internal jugular vein, longus colli muscle, and the transverse process of C_6), the needle is inserted until it pierces the prevertebral fascial layer of the longus colli muscle. After a negative aspiration, 1 mL of test dose is administered. Total volume: 4 to 5 mL.

References: Butterworth JF IV, Mackey DC, Wasnick JD, eds. *Morgan & Mikhail's Clinical Anesthesiology.* 7th ed. New York, NY: McGraw Hill; 2022: Chapter 47.

Murray MJ, Harrison BA, Mueller JT, et al, eds. *Faust's Anesthesiology Review.* 4th ed. Elsevier; 2015: Chapter 218.

190. Which of the following is a mechanism of action for duloxetine?

(A) Monoamine oxidase inhibition

(B) Serotonin reuptake inhibition

(C) α_2 receptor agonist effect

(D) Norepinephrine agonist

Rationale: This drug inhibits serotonin and norepinephrine reuptake.

References: Butterworth JF IV, Mackey DC, Wasnick JD, eds. *Morgan & Mikhail's Clinical Anesthesiology.* 7th ed. New York, NY: McGraw Hill; 2022: Chapter 47.

Elisha S, Heiner JS, Nagelhout JJ. *Nurse Anesthesia.* 7th ed. St. Louis, MO: Elsevier Saunders; 2023: Chapter 14.

191. Which is an α_2 agonist?

(A) Carbamazepine

(B) Tapentadol

(C) Phenytoin

(D) Tizanidine

Rationale: Tizanidine is a centrally acting α_2 agonist sometimes useful in spastic pain.

References: Butterworth JF IV, Mackey DC, Wasnick JD, eds. *Morgan & Mikhail's Clinical Anesthesiology.* 7th ed. New York, NY: McGraw Hill; 2022: Chapter 47.

Flood P, Rathmell JP, Urbam RD, eds. *Stoelting's Pharmacology & Physiology in Anesthetic Practice.* 6th ed. Philadelphia, PA: Wolters Kluwer; 2022: Chapter 13.

192. Which route of administration of fentanyl is subject to the hepatic first-pass effect?

(A) Transdermal patch

(B) Intravenous injection

(C) Sublingual spray

(D) Oral tablet

Rationale: Gastrointestinal absorption is subject to hepatic first-pass effect. IV injection is subject to an estimated 75% first-pass pulmonary uptake.

References: Flood P, Rathmell JP, Urbam RD, eds. *Stoelting's Pharmacology & Physiology in Anesthetic Practice.* 6th ed. Philadelphia, PA: Wolters Kluwer; 2022: Chapter 7.

Elisha S, Heiner JS, Nagelhout JJ. *Nurse Anesthesia.* 7th ed. St. Louis, MO: Elsevier Saunders; 2023: Chapter 11.

193. What would be the correct classification of hyperalgesia with sympathetic dysfunction following a traumatic injury that included direct nerve damage persisting

beyond the standard healing period in the absence of other conditions that may be responsible for the pain?

(A) Complex regional pain syndrome type I

(B) Reflex sympathetic dystrophy

(C) Complex regional pain syndrome type II

(D) Persistent allodynia

Rationale: Precipitating injury to the nerve itself identifies complex regional pain syndrome type II. Type I does not include distinct injury to the nerve. Reflex sympathetic dystrophy is a synonym for type I.

References: Barash PG, Cullen BF, Stoelting RK, et al, eds. *Clinical Anesthesia.* 8th ed. Lippincott Williams & Wilkins; 2017: Chapter 56.

Butterworth JF IV, Mackey DC, Wasnick JD, eds. *Morgan & Mikhail's Clinical Anesthesiology.* 7th ed. New York, NY: McGraw Hill; 2022: Chapter 47.

194. Following placement of a stellate ganglion block the patient becomes hoarse, what has occurred?

(A) Phrenic nerve block

(B) Recurrent laryngeal nerve block

(C) Subdural injection

(D) Pneumothorax

Rationale: Unilateral recurrent laryngeal nerve block results in hoarseness.

References: Butterworth JF IV, Mackey DC, Wasnick JD, eds. *Morgan & Mikhail's Clinical Anesthesiology.* 7th ed. New York, NY: McGraw Hill; 2022: Chapter 47.

Elisha S, Heiner JS, Nagelhout JJ. *Nurse Anesthesia.* 7th ed. St. Louis, MO: Elsevier Saunders; 2023: Chapter 50.

195. Which are appropriate for inclusion in an epidural steroid injection?

(A) Morphine

(B) Methylprednisolone acetate and saline

(C) Remifentanil

(D) Fentanyl

Rationale: Opioids are not indicated.

References: Butterworth JF IV, Mackey DC, Wasnick JD, eds. *Morgan & Mikhail's Clinical Anesthesiology.* 7th ed. New York, NY: McGraw Hill; 2022: Chapter 47.

Elisha S, Heiner JS, Nagelhout JJ. *Nurse Anesthesia.* 7th ed. St. Louis, MO: Elsevier Saunders; 2023: Chapter 56.

196. Which steroid has the smallest particulate size?

(A) Methylprednisolone acetate

(B) Triamcinolone diacetate

(C) Dexamethasone sodium phosphate

(D) Betamethasone

Rationale: Dexamethasone is a nonparticulate corticosteroid which minimizes the risk of vasoocclusive complications if inadvertently injected into a vessel during an epidural steroid injection.

References: Butterworth JF IV, Mackey DC, Wasnick JD, eds. *Morgan & Mikhail's Clinical Anesthesiology.* 7th ed. New York, NY: McGraw Hill; 2022: Chapter 47.

Elisha S, Heiner JS, Nagelhout JJ. *Nurse Anesthesia.* 7th ed. St. Louis, MO: Elsevier Saunders; 2023: Chapter 57.

197. Which is an indication for a celiac plexus block?

(A) Posttraumatic hypoperfusion of the arm

(B) Lower extremity vascular insufficiency

(C) Intractable lumbar pain

(D) Pain resulting from pancreatic malignancy

Rationale: Pain associated with an intraabdominal malignancy is a primary indication for this intervention.

References: Butterworth JF IV, Mackey DC, Wasnick JD, eds. *Morgan & Mikhail's Clinical Anesthesiology.* 7th ed. New York, NY: McGraw Hill; 2022: Chapter 47.

Gropper MA. *Miller's Anesthesia.* 9th ed. Philadelphia, PA: Churchill Livingstone Elsevier; 2020: Chapter 15.

198. When selecting a needle for spinal anesthesia, which type is most likely to cause a postdural puncture headache?

(A) 20-g Quincke

(B) 22-g Whitacre

(C) 22-g Sprotte

(D) 22-g Quincke

Rationale: Cutting needles (Quincke) are more likely to cause postdural puncture headaches as compared to pencil point needles. Larger gauge needles are also more likely to cause postdural puncture headaches.

References: Butterworth JF IV, Mackey DC, Wasnick JD, eds. *Morgan & Mikhail's Clinical Anesthesiology.* 7th ed. New York, NY: McGraw Hill; 2022: Chapter 45.

Elisha S, Heiner JS, Nagelhout JJ. *Nurse Anesthesia.* 7th ed. St. Louis, MO: Elsevier Saunders; 2023: Chapter 49.

Gropper MA. *Miller's Anesthesia.* 9th ed. Philadelphia, PA: Churchill Livingstone Elsevier; 2020: Chapter 45.

199. An adult patient with moderate aortic regurgitation receives a spinal anesthetic. Blood pressure decreases to 68/42 and is treated with 100 mcg of phenylephrine. How will this dose impact the patient's underlying disease state?

(A) It will improve the regurgitation.

(B) It will exacerbate the regurgitation.

(C) It will have no impact on the regurgitation.

(D) Phenylephrine is contraindicated in this patient.

Rationale: Phenylephrine can be used to treat anesthetic-induced hypotension in a patient with aortic regurgitation, but the doses should be small and incremental, i.e., 25 to 50 mcg. Larger doses such as 100 mcg will increase the systemic vascular resistance and exacerbate the regurgitation.

References: Butterworth JF IV, Mackey DC, Wasnick JD, eds. *Morgan & Mikhail's Clinical Anesthesiology.* 7th ed. New York, NY: McGraw Hill; 2022: Chapter 21.

Elisha S, Heiner JS, Nagelhout JJ. *Nurse Anesthesia.* 7th ed. St. Louis, MO: Elsevier Saunders; 2023: Chapter 25.

Gropper MA. *Miller's Anesthesia.* 9th ed. Philadelphia, PA: Churchill Livingstone Elsevier; 2020: Chapter 54.

200. Which estimated blood volume is correctly paired with its age group?

(A) Preterm neonate: 85 mL/kg

(B) Six-month-old: 90 mL/kg

(C) Adult male: 80 mL/kg

(D) Adult female: 65 mL/kg

Rationale: The estimated blood volume for an adult female is 65 mL/kg. The estimated blood volume for a preterm neonate ranges from 95 to 100 mL/kg; for an infant, 80 mL/kg; and for an adult male, 80 mL/kg.

References: Butterworth JF IV, Mackey DC, Wasnick JD, eds. *Morgan & Mikhail's Clinical Anesthesiology.* 7th ed. New York, NY: McGraw Hill; 2022: Chapter 51.

Elisha S, Heiner JS, Nagelhout JJ. *Nurse Anesthesia.* 7th ed. St. Louis, MO: Elsevier Saunders; 2023: Chapter 22.

201. How will the symptoms of an acute hemolytic transfusion reaction manifest in a patient under general anesthesia?

(A) Fever, unexplained tachycardia, hypotension, and diffuse oozing in surgical field

(B) Nausea, fever, flank pain, unexplained tachycardia, and hypotension

(C) Hemoglobinuria, chest and flank pain, fever, and hypotension

(D) Hypertension, unexplained tachycardia, fever, erythema, and hive

Rationale: Unlike the symptoms of acute hemolytic reaction in awake patients (chills, nausea, fever, chest pain and flank pain); in anesthetized patients, these symptoms are masked. Symptoms include fever, unexplained tachycardia, hypotension, hemoglobinuria, and diffuse oozing in the surgical field.

References: Barash PG, Cullen BF, Stoelting RK, et al, eds. *Clinical Anesthesia*. 8th ed. Lippincott Williams & Wilkins; 2017: Chapter 17.

Butterworth JF IV, Mackey DC, Wasnick JD, eds. *Morgan & Mikhail's Clinical Anesthesiology*. 7th ed. New York, NY: McGraw Hill; 2022: Chapter 51.

202. 0.5% ropivacaine is injected into the brachial plexus via the interscalene approach. Which of the following is most likely to be spared?

    (A) Sensation of the radial side of the forearm

    (B) Sensation of the medial upper arm

    (C) Sensation of half of the fourth finger and all the fifth finger

    (D) Sensation of the palmar surface of the first three fingers

    Rationale: The interscalene block of the brachial plexus is the most proximal approach to the brachial plexus and ideal for shoulder surgery with advantages of clear landmarks and a low risk of pneumothorax because of the distance to the dome of the pleura.

    This approach can be used for forearm and hand surgery; however, blockade of the inferior trunk is typically incomplete. The inferior trunk provides innervation to C_8 and T_1. Supplementation at the site of the ulnar nerve can assist with providing coverage for that distribution.

    References: Barash PG, Cullen BF, Stoelting RK, et al, eds. *Clinical Anesthesia*. 8th ed. Lippincott Williams & Wilkins; 2017: Chapter 36.

    Butterworth JF IV, Mackey DC, Wasnick JD, eds. *Morgan & Mikhail's Clinical Anesthesiology*. 7th ed. New York, NY: McGraw Hill; 2022: Chapter 46.

203. How does an opioid inhibit postsynaptic nociceptive signal transmission?

    (A) Hyperpolarization and opening potassium channels

    (B) Excitation

    (C) Opening calcium channels

    (D) Opening potassium channels

    Rationale: Opioids impede postsynaptic signal transmission by opening potassium channels resulting in hyperpolarization.

    References: Butterworth JF IV, Mackey DC, Wasnick JD, eds. *Morgan & Mikhail's Clinical Anesthesiology*. 7th ed. New York, NY: McGraw Hill; 2022: Chapter 10.

    Elisha S, Heiner JS, Nagelhout JJ. *Nurse Anesthesia*. 7th ed. St. Louis, MO: Elsevier Saunders; 2023: Chapter 11.

204. When administering a spinal anesthetic which nerve roots are easily blocked?

    (A) Smaller, unmyelinated

    (B) Larger, myelinated

    (C) Smaller, myelinated

    (D) Larger, unmyelinated

    Rationale: Smaller unmyelinated nerves are blocked easier than larger, myelinated nerve roots.

    References: Butterworth JF IV, Mackey DC, Wasnick JD, eds. *Morgan & Mikhail's Clinical Anesthesiology*. 7th ed. New York, NY: McGraw Hill; 2022: Chapter 45.

    Gropper MA. *Miller's Anesthesia*. 9th ed. Philadelphia, PA: Churchill Livingstone Elsevier; 2020: Chapter 45.

205. Which corticosteroid has the most potent glucocorticoid activity?

    (A) Hydrocortisone

    (B) Prednisone

    (C) Methylprednisolone

    (D) Dexamethasone

    Rationale: The relative glucocorticoid potency of dexamethasone is roughly 25 times that of hydrocortisone.

TABLE 3-16. Selected corticosteroids.

Drug	Routes Given	Glucocorticoid Activity	Mineralocorticoid Activity	Equivalent Dose (mg)	Half-Life (h)
Hydrocortisone	O, I, T	1	1	20	8-12
Prednisone	O	4	0.8	5	12-36
Prednisolone	O, I	4	0.8	5	12-36
Methylprednisolone (Depo-Medrol, Solu-Medrol)	O, I, T	5	0.5	4	12-36
Triamcinolone (Aristocort)	O, I, T	5	0.5	4	12-36
Betamethasone (Celestone)	O, I, T	25	0	0.75	36-72
Dexamethasone (Decadron)	O, I, T	25	0	0.75	36-72

O, oral; I, injectable; T, topical.
(Reproduced with permission from Goodman LS, Gilman AG. *The Pharmacologic Basis of Therapeutics*. 8th ed. New York: McGraw Hill, 1990.)

References: Butterworth JF IV, Mackey DC, Wasnick JD, eds. *Morgan & Mikhail's Clinical Anesthesiology.* 7th ed. New York, NY: McGraw Hill; 2022: Chapter 47.

Elisha S, Heiner JS, Nagelhout JJ. *Nurse Anesthesia.* 7th ed. St. Louis, MO: Elsevier Saunders; 2023: Chapter 37.

Gropper MA. *Miller's Anesthesia.* 9th ed. Philadelphia, PA: Churchill Livingstone Elsevier; 2020: Chapter 32.

206. Where does the spinal cord end in a 5-year-old?

    (A) L_1

    (B) L_2

    (C) L_3

    (D) L_4

    Rationale: The spinal cord ends at L_1 in adults and L_3 in children.

    References: Butterworth JF IV, Mackey DC, Wasnick JD, eds. *Morgan & Mikhail's Clinical Anesthesiology.* 7th ed. New York, NY: McGraw Hill; 2022: Chapter 45.

    Gropper MA. *Miller's Anesthesia.* 9th ed. Philadelphia, PA: Churchill Livingstone Elsevier; 2020: Chapter 45.

207. When is a type and screen preferable to a type and crossmatch?

    (A) The probability of transfusing blood is low.

    (B) The probability of transfusing blood is high.

    (C) The patient has high risk for alloimmunization.

    (D) The patient has a history of a positive antibody screen.

    Rationale: A type and screen is preferable when the probability of transfusing blood is low. A type and cross is preferable when the probability of transfusing blood is high.

    References: Butterworth JF IV, Mackey DC, Wasnick JD, eds. *Morgan & Mikhail's Clinical Anesthesiology.* 7th ed. New York, NY: McGraw Hill; 2022: Chapter 51.

    Gropper MA. *Miller's Anesthesia.* 9th ed. Philadelphia, PA: Churchill Livingstone Elsevier; 2020: Chapter 49.

208. Which of the following are true regarding apneic oxygenation during induction?

    (A) Apneic oxygenation effectively prolongs time to desaturation based on an increased carbon dioxide solubility gradient that allows 100 mL/min of carbon dioxide to diffuse across the alveolar membrane for exhalation.

    (B) Approximately 250 mL/min of oxygen diffuses from the alveoli into the bloodstream during apnea, which allows a prolonged time until desaturation begins from apnea.

    (C) Apneic oxygenation can be achieved by placing a nasal cannula on the patient prior to preoxygenation/denitrogenation and increasing the nasal cannula flows to 5 L/min while keeping a tight-fitting seal on the anesthesia mask.

    (D) Apneic oxygenation is especially beneficial for patients who may decompensate quickly from apnea and morbidly obese patients who have an increased FRC.

    Rationale: The solubility of carbon dioxide allows only 8 to 20 mL/min of CO_2 to diffuse across the alveolar membrane. Five minutes of preoxygenation/denitrogenation with a tight-fitting mask increases the time until desaturation during apnea by up to 8 minutes. However, adding a nasal cannula at 15 L/min under a tight-fitting face mask will significantly increase the time until desaturation during apnea. The patient must have an unobstructed oral/pharyngeal airway to build an oxygen reservoir. Both Fick's Law of Diffusion and hemoglobin's affinity for oxygen encourages oxygen to move down the concentration gradient into the bloodstream at a rate of 250 mL/min.

    References: Elisha S, Heiner JS, Nagelhout JJ. *Nurse Anesthesia.* 7th ed. St. Louis, MO: Elsevier Saunders; 2023: Chapter 24.

    Gropper MA. *Miller's Anesthesia.* 9th ed. Philadelphia, PA: Churchill Livingstone Elsevier; 2020: Chapter 44.

209. A patient under general anesthesia's $ETCO_2$ was noted to be 32 mmHg and the ventilator was turned to manual mode to allow the $ETCO_2$ to build enough to breach the apneic threshold. During the first minute of apnea, how much will the $ETCO_2$ rise?

    (A) 6 mmHg

    (B) 3 mmHg

    (C) 0 to 2 mmHg

    (D) 10 mmHg

    Rationale: The apneic threshold is the highest amount of $PaCO_2$ at which the patient remains apneic. Breaching the apneic threshold is required to stimulate spontaneous ventilation. The first minute of apnea will raise carbon dioxide by 6 mmHg. Each subsequent minute results in a 3 mmHg increase in $ETCO_2$.

    References: Barash PG, Cullen BF, Stoelting RK, et al, eds. *Clinical Anesthesia.* 8th ed. Lippincott Williams & Wilkins; 2017: Chapter 38.

    Butterworth JF IV, Mackey DC, Wasnick JD, eds. *Morgan & Mikhail's Clinical Anesthesiology.* 7th ed. New York, NY: McGraw Hill; 2022: Chapters 8 and 25.

210. A patient undergoing a right total shoulder arthroplasty has an AICD secondary to heart failure. What is the best practice when developing the anesthesia plan for this patient?

(A) The generator is on the left side of the patient's chest, no special considerations are needed for this case.

(B) Monopolar cautery produces less energy than bipolar and thus no grounding pad is needed.

(C) Communicate with the surgical team that limiting monopolar cautery to <5 seconds is sufficient to prevent device interference.

(D) Place defibrillator pads on the patient and have the device representative disable the shock feature.

Rationale: Electronic magnetic interference (EMI) is greatest in patients with implantable cardiac devices when surgery is above the umbilicus and electrocautery is used. Monopolar cautery produces more energy than bipolar cautery and a grounding pad is required. The grounding pad should be placed close to the surgical site and further away from the AICD. While limiting cautery to <5 seconds may help prevent electronic magnetic interference (EMI) best practice is to have the shock feature disabled for the case.

References: Barash PG, Cullen BF, Stoelting RK, et al, eds. *Clinical Anesthesia*. 8th ed. Lippincott Williams & Wilkins; 2017: Appendix 3.

Elisha S, Heiner JS, Nagelhout JJ. *Nurse Anesthesia*. 7th ed. St. Louis, MO: Elsevier Saunders; 2023: Chapter 27.

211. Which of the following is not true regarding laryngospasms?

(A) A history of a viral upper respiratory infection 8 weeks prior to general anesthesia increases the pediatric perioperative risks for laryngospasms.

(B) ETT and LMA removal should only occur during Guedel's stage I or III of anesthesia.

(C) Treatment of laryngospasm includes: 100% oxygen, positive pressure ventilation or 1 to 1.5 mg/kg of lidocaine.

(D) Pharyngeal secretions are a frequent contributing cause of laryngospasms.

Rationale: A viral infection up to 6 weeks before general anesthesia increases the risk for laryngospasm in pediatric patients; especially in patients younger than 1 year old.

References: Butterworth JF IV, Mackey DC, Wasnick JD, eds. *Morgan & Mikhail's Clinical Anesthesiology*. 7th ed. New York, NY: McGraw Hill; 2022: Chapter 19.

Elisha S, Heiner JS, Nagelhout JJ. *Nurse Anesthesia*. 7th ed. St. Louis, MO: Elsevier Saunders; 2023: Chapter 20.

212. ENT procedures have unique risks and considerations. Which of the following increased the risk for airway fires?

(A) For a tracheostomy placement, do not allow the surgeon to use cautery to incise the trachea.

(B) Regarding laser surgeries, use a laser-resistant tube and inflate the cuff with methylene blue–dyed saline.

(C) Up to 40% supplemental oxygen can be administered safely without increased risk for an airway fire.

(D) Manual oxygen flowmeters should only be used with an oxygen analyzer.

Rationale: Inspired FiO_2 should be as low as possible (ideally 21%). Avoid nitrous oxide. If supplemental oxygen is needed, an oxygen concentration <30% decreases the chances of an airway fire developing. When airway fires occur, it is frequently because of the laser penetrating the ETT, hence a laser resistant tube *and* methylene blue–dyed saline in the cuff will allow quicker identification of a cuff perforation.

References: Butterworth JF IV, Mackey DC, Wasnick JD, eds. *Morgan & Mikhail's Clinical Anesthesiology*. 7th ed. New York, NY: McGraw Hill; 2022: Chapter 37.

Elisha S, Heiner JS, Nagelhout JJ. *Nurse Anesthesia*. 7th ed. St. Louis, MO: Elsevier Saunders; 2023: Chapter 47.

213. A 30-year-old Hispanic male with a history of a poorly controlled GERD develops a laryngospasm after extubation. Appropriate measures were taken, and the patient never desaturated during the laryngospasm. Upon arrival at the PACU you note the patient has an oxygen saturation of 89% on 10 L oxygen via face mask and coughs up pink sputum with a respiratory rate of 24 breaths per minute. Which is the best initial response?

(A) Negative pressure pulmonary edema does not present until 1 hour after arrival in the PACU. Continue to observe patient on 10 L oxygen and administer a nebulized albuterol treatment.

(B) The patient is displaying signs of negative pressure pulmonary edema. Provide supplemental oxygen via continuous positive airway pressure (CPAP) with PEEP.

(C) The patient developed negative pressure pulmonary edema. Administer 40 mg of furosemide IVP.

(D) Reintubate the patient in the PACU and perform a bronchoscopy to assess for aspiration.

Rationale: Negative pressure pulmonary edema develops rapidly after attempting inspiration against a closed glottis. The best initial response is to provide oxygen via CPAP with PEEP. Patients who display severe respiratory distress may require reintubation, steroids, and diuretics.

References: Barash PG, Cullen BF, Stoelting RK, et al, eds. *Clinical Anesthesia*. 8th ed. Lippincott Williams & Wilkins; 2017: Chapter 28.

Elisha S, Heiner JS, Nagelhout JJ. *Nurse Anesthesia*. 7th ed. St. Louis, MO: Elsevier Saunders; 2023: Chapter 29.

214. For point-of-care lung ultrasound correctly match the following items.

(A) "Lung point" demonstrated via M mode on ultrasound

(B) A lines

(C) Three or more B lines (or comet tails)

(D) Lung sliding

(E) Shows with interstitial syndrome

(F) Represents a diagnosis of pneumothorax

(G) Hyperechoic horizontal reverberations below the pleura

(H) Presence of this rules out a pneumothorax

Matching answers: A → F, B → G, C → E, D → H

Rationale: The lung point is the specific area during the M mode where the image on the ultrasound transitions from moving pleura to the absence of lung sliding. The lung point is seen only during M mode (where the seashore and barcode signs meet) and is indicative of a pneumothorax. Arterial lines are normal reverberations deep to the pleura. Three or more B lines (in a longitudinal plane at one intercostal level) is an abnormal finding and indicates interstitial-alveolar syndrome (cardiogenic pulmonary edema). Lung sliding is normal and would be absent at the level of a pneumothorax.

References: Gropper MA. *Miller's Anesthesia*. 9th ed. Philadelphia, PA: Churchill Livingstone Elsevier; 2020: Chapter 41.

Soni NJ, Arntfield R, Kory P, eds. *Point-of-Care Ultrasound*. 2nd ed. Philadelphia, PA: Elsevier; 2020: Chapters 8 and 9.

215. Which of the following is not a contraindication to TEE placement?

(A) History of alcoholism

(B) Esophageal strictures

(C) Zenker's diverticulum

(D) Esophageal mass

Rationale: A history of alcoholism is not a contraindication to TEE; however, recent or active bleeding esophageal varices is a contraindication. A patient who recently had gastric bypass should not receive a TEE. Esophageal or gastric perforation are the two most-feared complications.

References: Barash PG, Cullen BF, Stoelting RK, et al, eds. *Clinical Anesthesia*. 8th ed. Lippincott Williams & Wilkins; 2017: Chapter 27.

Gropper MA. *Miller's Anesthesia*. 9th ed. Philadelphia, PA: Churchill Livingstone Elsevier; 2020: Chapter 37.

216. Dynamic decision making is one of the key elements to crisis resource management. One major source of poor outcomes is fixation errors. What technique is beneficial in preventing or breaking fixation errors?

(A) The use of cognitive aids can help the team leader recognize differential diagnosis.

(B) Anticipating the needs and potential complications of a case assists in preparedness and eliminates the risk of emergencies developing.

(C) Declaring an emergency early rather than late increases the time to gather resources and develop a plan.

(D) Both (A) and (B) are correct.

Rationale: Cognitive aids have a proven value in improving outcomes from anesthesia emergencies. Preprinting cognitive aids with an order of steps and rule out differential diagnosis helps to prevent fixation errors such as "It can be this and only this." No amount of preplanning can guarantee an intraoperative emergency does not develop.

References: Barash PG, Cullen BF, Stoelting RK, et al, eds. *Clinical Anesthesia*. 8th ed. Lippincott Williams & Wilkins; 2017: Chapter 2.

Elisha S, Heiner JS, Nagelhout JJ. *Nurse Anesthesia*. 7th ed. St. Louis, MO: Elsevier Saunders; 2023: Chapter 60.

Gaba DM, Fish KJ, Howard SK, Burden AR, eds. *Crisis Management in Anesthesiology*. 2nd ed. Philadelphia, PA: Saunders. 2015: Chapter 2.

217. Which is not true about MAC levels regarding volatile anesthetics?

(A) MAC-BAR is the minimum alveolar concentration that blunts an adrenergic response to noxious stimulus. MAC-BAR is 1.9 times the MAC.

(B) MAC awake is the minimum alveolar concentration when patients can open their eyes to command and varies from 0.15 to 0.5 MAC.

(C) MAC values decrease by 6% per decade from ages 40 to 80 years old.

(D) Chronic alcohol abuse, hypernatremia, and hyperthermia all result in increased MAC requirements.

Rationale: MAC-BAR is 1.6 times higher than a MAC level for any given volatile anesthetic. MAC awake is variable. It takes about 0.5 MAC for patients to lose consciousness; however, MAC awake on emergence is as low as 0.15 MAC.

References: Barash PG, Cullen BF, Stoelting RK, et al, eds. *Clinical Anesthesia*. 8th ed. Lippincott Williams & Wilkins; 2017: Chapter 18.

Elisha S, Heiner JS, Nagelhout JJ. *Nurse Anesthesia*. 7th ed. St. Louis, MO: Elsevier Saunders; 2023: Chapter 8.

218. A 75-year-old male with a past medical history of coronary artery disease, hypertension, and GERD is scheduled for a right total hip arthroplasty. During the preoperative assessment, the patient disclosed that he needed a blood transfusion when his left hip was replaced. The patient reports he last took his clopidogrel 7 days ago. The patient takes famotidine and garlic daily and took them the morning of surgery. What is the best plan?

(A) Discuss with the surgeon the increased bleeding risks. Consider rescheduling for another day.

(B) Reschedule the surgery for the last case of the day.

(C) Administer 2 units of FFP and 1 g of TXA prior to incision.

(D) Reverse with protamine.

(E) Continue with surgery as planned.

Rationale: Garlic is useful as an antihypertensive and inhibits platelet aggregation. Considering the patient needed a blood transfusion with his previous hip replacement, it is prudent to discuss with the surgeon rescheduling the case when the patient can appropriately hold the garlic.

References: Barash PG, Cullen BF, Stoelting RK, et al, eds. *Clinical Anesthesia*. 8th ed. Lippincott Williams & Wilkins; 2017: Appendix 7.

Elisha S, Heiner JS, Nagelhout JJ. *Nurse Anesthesia*. 7th ed. St. Louis, MO: Elsevier Saunders; 2023: Chapter 20.

CHAPTER 4

Advanced Principles
Questions

1. During induction of general anesthesia the pregnant patient quickly desaturates. Which factors most likely caused the desaturation?

   (A) Increased functional residual capacity and increased oxygen consumption

   (B) Decreased residual volume and increased expiratory reserve volume

   (C) Decreased functional residual capacity and increased oxygen consumption

   (D) Increased residual volume and decreased expiratory reserve volume

2. Which cardiac variable leads to heart failure due to obesity?

   (A) Decreased preload

   (B) Left ventricular systolic dysfunction

   (C) Decreased afterload

   (D) Hypotension

3. What is the average weight of a 6-year-old?

   (A) 15 kg

   (B) 18 kg

   (C) 21 kg

   (D) 24 kg

4. Which of the following is not a symptom of fat embolism associated with a long bone fracture?

   (A) Dyspnea

   (B) Confusion

   (C) Petechiae

   (D) Decreased free fatty acids

5. An 80-year-old female with moderate aortic stenosis is undergoing an emergent open reduction and internal fixation of her left hip. Preoperative vital signs include a blood pressure of 175/95 mmHg and a heart rate in sinus rhythm of 65 beats/min. Shortly after induction with propofol and general anesthesia maintained with sevoflurane, the patient's heart rate increases to an irregular 133 beats/min. The blood pressure decreases to 69/55 mmHg. What would be the most effective action to restore a stable hemodynamic profile?

   (A) Administer 100 mcg of phenylephrine intravenously.

   (B) Request that the surgery begin immediately in order that a painful stimulus may increase blood pressure.

   (C) Cardiovert the patient with a synchronized transthoracic shock of 170 joules.

   (D) Administer a 500 mL bolus of lactated ringers.

6. What finding may be identified during preoperative examination of an awake and alert patient with a posterior cerebral artery aneurysm?

   (A) Brown-Séquard syndrome

   (B) Abnormal gaze or pupil response

   (C) Decorticate posturing

   (D) Hypertensive crisis

7. What is the uterine blood flow at term?

   (A) 200 to 300 mL/min

   (B) 300 to 400 mL/min

   (C) 400 to 500 mL/min

   (D) 600 to 700 mL/min

8. What is resting cerebral oxygen consumption?

    (A) 3.5 mL/100 g/min

    (B) 5 mL/100 g/min

    (C) 100 mL/min

    (D) 250 mL/min

9. What dose of protamine sulfate would be appropriate to reverse 5,000 units of heparin?

    (A) 500 mcg

    (B) 5 mg

    (C) 50 mg

    (D) 5 mcg

10. Which of the following is not harmful when in proximity to the magnetic resonance imaging (MRI) machine?

    (A) Implanted medication pumps

    (B) Pacing wires

    (C) Cardiac pacemakers

    (D) Pulse oximeter

11. A patient is scheduled for bariatric surgery. What is the recommended induction dose for propofol?

    (A) Dose based on ideal body weight

    (B) Dose based on body mass index

    (C) Dose based on obesity scale

    (D) Dose based on morbid obesity

12. What is an indication of significant venous air embolism during a seated craniotomy?

    (A) Increased end-tidal carbon dioxide

    (B) Unchanged end-tidal carbon dioxide

    (C) Decreased end-tidal carbon dioxide

    (D) Hypertension

13. Which of the following is not associated with pulseless electrical activity?

    (A) Hypovolemia

    (B) Hypoxia

    (C) Hyperkalemia

    (D) Hyperthermia

14. A patient with dysmenorrhea is scheduled for dilation and curettage (D&C). What preoperative testing is required?

    (A) CBC

    (B) Electrolyte panel

    (C) Chest x-ray

    (D) HCG

15. The addition of an intravenous inotrope will move the Frank-Starling curve in which direction?

    (A) Up

    (B) Down

    (C) Left

    (D) Right

16. During an uncomplicated vaginal delivery, what is the expected blood loss?

    (A) 250 mL

    (B) 400 mL

    (C) 750 mL

    (D) 800 mL

17. What should the activated clotting time be prior to initiation of cardiopulmonary bypass (CPB)?

    (A) <150 seconds

    (B) >200 seconds but <350 seconds

    (C) >350 seconds but <450 seconds

    (D) >400 seconds

18. What level of neural blockade is needed for analgesia during the first stage of labor?

    (A) T_{10}-L_1 motor level

    (B) T_{10}-S_4 sensory level

    (C) T_{10}-L_1 sensory level

    (D) T_{10}-S_4 motor level

19. How is cardiac index calculated?

   (A) $\dfrac{Cardiac\ Output}{Stroke\ Volume}$

   (B) $\dfrac{Cardiac\ Output}{Systemic\ Vascular\ Resistance}$

   (C) $\dfrac{Cardiac\ Output}{Body\ Surface\ Area}$

   (D) $\dfrac{Cardiac\ Output}{Heart\ Rate}$

20. What is the goal of hemodynamic management for patients with mitral stenosis?

   (A) Avoiding bradycardia
   (B) Maintenance of sinus rhythm
   (C) Aggressive volume resuscitation
   (D) Inotropic support with phosphodiesterase inhibitors

21. A peribulbar block was performed. There was notable resistance during the injection. The patient becomes agitated and complains of pain. What do you suspect?

   (A) Retrobulbar hemorrhage
   (B) Globe puncture
   (C) Extraocular muscle palsy
   (D) Intravascular injection

22. Which sign is associated with placenta previa?

   (A) Painless vaginal bleeding
   (B) Uterine irritability
   (C) Painful vaginal bleeding
   (D) Coagulopathy

23. What sign is not an effect of hyperparathyroidism?

   (A) Hypertension
   (B) Ventricular arrhythmias
   (C) Muscle weakness
   (D) Hypochloremic metabolic acidosis

24. Which factor does not contribute to respiratory fatigue in neonates and infants?

   (A) Weaker intercostal muscles
   (B) More horizontal ribs

   (C) Sunken abdomen
   (D) Decreased chest wall compliance

25. Which valvular disorder leads to largest left ventricular volume?

   (A) Mitral stenosis
   (B) Aortic stenosis
   (C) Mitral regurgitation
   (D) Aortic regurgitation

26. Which narcotic analgesic is not used for patient-controlled analgesia (PCA)?

   (A) Meperidine
   (B) Morphine
   (C) Fentanyl
   (D) Hydromorphone

27. With which patient would the anesthetist most want to maintain spontaneous ventilation while under general anesthesia?

   (A) Severe aortic stenosis
   (B) Severe mitral regurgitation
   (C) Acute pulmonary edema
   (D) Mitral valve prolapse

28. The a-wave on the central venous pressure tracing corresponds to which what on the EKG tracing?

   (A) P wave
   (B) QRS wave
   (C) QT interval
   (D) T wave

29. What do you anticipate during laparoscopic cholecystectomy for an obese patient?

   (A) Increased functional residual capacity
   (B) Increased closing capacity
   (C) Decreased functional residual capacity
   (D) Decreased peak inspiratory pressure

30. Which of the following symptoms is consistent with cardiac tamponade?

    (A) Hypotension, tachycardia, tachypnea, muffled heart sounds, and pulsus paradoxus

    (B) Hypertension, tachycardia, tachypnea, and widened pulse pressure

    (C) Jugular venous distension, muffled heart sounds, and bradycardia

    (D) Hypotension, widened pulse pressure, and tachycardia

31. Which of the following is an absolute contraindication for electroconvulsive therapy (ECT)?

    (A) Myocardial infarction <6 weeks

    (B) Intercranial mass

    (C) Glaucoma

    (D) Pregnancy

32. What is the most common cause of acute epiglottitis?

    (A) *Streptococcus pneumoniae*

    (B) Allergic reaction

    (C) *Haemophilus influenza B*

    (D) COVID-19 infection

33. The patient is scheduled for a thyroidectomy. Which of the following is not a primary anesthetic concern?

    (A) Arrhythmias

    (B) Tachycardia

    (C) Body temperature

    (D) Hypotension

34. What is the lowest recommended $PaCO_2$ if hyperventilation is used during intracranial tumor resection?

    (A) 35 mmHg

    (B) 30 mmHg

    (C) 25 mmHg

    (D) 20 mmHg

35. How is coronary perfusion pressure defined?

    (A) Difference between mean arterial pressure and central venous pressure

    (B) Difference between aortic diastolic pressure and left-ventricular end-diastolic pressure

    (C) Difference between aortic systolic pressure and left-ventricular end-diastolic pressure

    (D) Difference between systolic pressure and central venous pressure

36. What results when a limb tourniquet is released?

    (A) Hypokalemia

    (B) Metabolic acidosis

    (C) Metabolic alkalosis

    (D) Bradycardia

37. Which patient faces the greatest risk of complete cardiovascular collapse?

    (A) 75-year-old female with bilateral carotid artery disease with an aortic valve area of 1.1 cm^2 undergoing left carotid endarterectomy

    (B) 82-year-old male with severe mitral regurgitation and severe tricuspid regurgitation with atrial fibrillation undergoing bowel resection for colon cancer

    (C) 67-year-old male with aortic valve area of 0.7 cm^2 undergoing left carotid endarterectomy

    (D) 59-year-old male with aortic valve area of 0.7 cm^2 undergoing colon resection for ischemic colon

38. What risk factor places patients at greater risk of perioperative vision loss (POVL)?

    (A) Low estimated blood loss

    (B) Prolonged surgery in the head down position

    (C) Controlled hypertension

    (D) Thin stature

39. While observing the fetal heart monitor during labor you note a decreased fetal heart rate. What is the probable cause?

    (A) Epidural opioids

    (B) Terbutaline

    (C) Ritodrine

    (D) Atropine

40. Estimate the total difference in cerebral blood flow if $PaCO_2$ is decreased from 40 mmHg to 34 mmHg. Assume total brain weight is 1,400 g.

   (A) 0 to 50 mL/min
   (B) 30 to 60 mL/min
   (C) 60 to 120 mL/min
   (D) 90 to 180 mL/min

41. Which of the following rate control agents should be avoided in a patient undergoing general anesthesia with acute onset wide-complex supraventricular tachycardia (SVT)?

   (A) Digitalis
   (B) Adenosine
   (C) Esmolol
   (D) Amiodarone

42. Which factor contributes to the rapid development of hypoxia seen during apnea in neonates?

   (A) High functional residual capacity
   (B) Low basal metabolic rate
   (C) High oxygen reserve
   (D) High oxygen demand

43. What is cerebral metabolic rate?

   (A) 3.5 mL/100 g/min
   (B) 5 mL/100 g/min
   (C) 100 mL/min
   (D) 250 mL/min

44. A 100-kg patient is administered 40,000 units of heparin. Five minutes later the ACT was measured to be 182 seconds. What is the next step?

   (A) Proceed with cardiopulmonary bypass.
   (B) Wait 5 more minutes and recheck ACT.
   (C) Administer an additional 40,000 units of heparin.
   (D) Administer two units of fresh frozen plasma.

45. Because you are concerned with factors contributing to cerebral ischemia during mediastinoscopy, where will you place the blood pressure cuff and arterial line?

   (A) Blood pressure cuff on right arm, arterial line in left hand
   (B) Blood pressure cuff on right arm, pulse oximeter on right hand
   (C) Blood pressure cuff on left arm, arterial line in right hand
   (D) Blood pressure cuff on left arm, pulse oximeter on left hand

46. Which symptom is not present in advanced aortic stenosis?

   (A) Angina
   (B) Dyspnea on exertion
   (C) Orthostatic syncope
   (D) Dyspnea at rest

47. Which nerve is at greatest risk for injury during thyroid surgery?

   (A) Recurrent laryngeal nerve
   (B) Superior laryngeal nerve
   (C) Facial nerve
   (D) Glossopharyngeal nerve

48. Which statement is true regarding gastrointestinal changes during pregnancy?

   (A) Pregnant patients are not considered a "full stomach."
   (B) Gastric acid increases.
   (C) Gastric volume increases.
   (D) Lower esophageal sphincter relaxation occurs due to progesterone and estrogen.

49. What is the cervical level of the larynx in a child?

   (A) C_1–C_3
   (B) C_2–C_4
   (C) C_3–C_5
   (D) C_4–C_7

50. How does general anesthesia affect the functional residual capacity (FRC)?

    (A) Increases FRC by 50%
    (B) Decreases FRC by 20%
    (C) Increases FRC by 20%
    (D) Decreases FRC by 50%

51. Which is least adaptive in an infant as compared to an adult?

    (A) Heart rate
    (B) Cardiac output
    (C) Stroke volume
    (D) Chest wall

52. A spinal anesthetic is planned for an obese patient. How will you adjust the dose of local anesthetic?

    (A) Decrease by 20%
    (B) Increase by 20%
    (C) Decrease by 10%
    (D) Increase by 10%

53. What is the primary determinant of cerebral perfusion?

    (A) Position
    (B) Mean arterial pressure
    (C) Intracranial pressure
    (D) Central venous pressure

54. What is the efferent limb of the oculocardiac reflex?

    (A) Cranial nerve V
    (B) Cranial nerve X
    (C) Cranial nerve I
    (D) Cranial nerve III

55. What factor is increased in a neonate as compared to an adult?

    (A) Surface area to weight ratio
    (B) Systolic blood pressure
    (C) Plasma protein concentration
    (D) Lung compliance

56. When calculating medication doses for obese patients, what is the best weight parameter to use?

    (A) Total body weight
    (B) Ideal body weight
    (C) Lean body weight
    (D) Total body mass index

57. Which is true regarding morbidity and mortality in pediatric anesthesia?

    (A) Anesthetic risk is directly related to patient age.
    (B) Anesthetic risk is greatest in patients younger than 1 year.
    (C) Anesthetic risk is greater now than in the past.
    (D) Anesthetic risk is similar throughout childhood.

58. With which of the following preoperative EKG findings will the anesthetist be particularly careful to avoid bradycardia?

    (A) Sinus rhythm with prolonged QT interval
    (B) Sinus rhythm with left bundle branch block
    (C) Sinus rhythm with premature ventricular complexes
    (D) Atrial fibrillation

59. A patient is scheduled for a total knee arthroscopy under general anesthesia. The patient's history includes retina surgery using sulfur hexafluoride 2 weeks ago. What will you avoid?

    (A) Nitrous oxide
    (B) Rocuronium
    (C) Sevoflurane
    (D) Fentanyl

60. What is the maintenance intravenous fluid replacement rate for a toddler weighing 12 kg?

    (A) 48 mL/h
    (B) 44 mL/h
    (C) 40 mL/h
    (D) 36 mL/h

61. How much intravenous replacement should be given in the first hour of the anesthetic for a child weighing 16 kg who last had anything by mouth at 0400 if the current time is 0700?

   (A) 52 mL
   (B) 104 mL
   (C) 208 mL
   (D) 130 mL

62. Which feature of a pediatric endotracheal tube will have greatest influence on the work of breathing?

   (A) External diameter
   (B) Length
   (C) Internal diameter
   (D) Curvature

63. During laparoscopic bariatric surgery, you add positive end expiratory pressure (PEEP). What is the recommended upper limit?

   (A) 5 cm H_2O
   (B) 10 cm H_2O
   (C) 15 cm H_2O
   (D) 20 cm H_2O

64. Which of the following agents will cause the greatest decrease on afterload?

   (A) Verapamil
   (B) Nicardipine
   (C) Metoprolol
   (D) Nitroglycerine

65. What is the correct depth for an endotracheal tube placed in a 4-year-old?

   (A) Internal diameter 3.5 mm
   (B) Internal diameter 5.0 cm
   (C) Internal diameter of 4.5 mm
   (D) Internal diameter of 5.0 mm

66. You are planning to add fentanyl to the epidural for labor. How much will you add to the local anesthetic solution?

   (A) 5 mg
   (B) 10 μg
   (C) 50 to 150 mcg
   (D) 0.5 mg

67. A patient with ischemic cardiomyopathy, with a preoperative ejection fraction of 15%, presents for a general anesthetic. After induction of general anesthesia, the vital signs include a blood pressure of 79/61 mmHg and a heart rate of 54 beats/min. What intravenous drip is best?

   (A) Epinephrine
   (B) Vasopressin
   (C) Phenylephrine
   (D) Milrinone

68. Which solution is appropriate for replacement of calculated fluid deficits, blood loss, or third-space loss in the pediatric patient?

   (A) Lactated Ringer's
   (B) 5% dextrose in water
   (C) 5% dextrose in 0.45% normal saline
   (D) 25% albumin

69. Which estimation of blood volume per kilogram is correct for a 2-week-old?

   (A) 65 mL
   (B) 75 mL
   (C) 85 mL
   (D) 95 mL

70. Which patient requires the highest minimum alveolar concentration (MAC)?

   (A) Newborn of 35 weeks gestation
   (B) A 4-month-old
   (C) An 18-month-old
   (D) A 3-year-old

71. If intramuscular succinylcholine were indicated, what would be the correct dose for a 1-year-old child?

    (A) 0.5 mg/kg
    (B) 4.5 mg/kg
    (C) 5 mg/kg
    (D) 4 mg/kg

72. Why does an infant require an increased induction dose (mg/kg) of propofol than an adult?

    (A) Enzyme induction
    (B) Increased central volume of distribution
    (C) Immature renal function
    (D) Decreased adipose for redistribution

73. What is the best means to avoid lung overdistension for obese ventilated patients?

    (A) Tidal volume 10 to 15 mL/kg
    (B) Tidal volume 12 to 15 mL/kg
    (C) Tidal volume 6 to 10 mL/kg
    (D) Tidal volume 4 to 8 mL/kg

74. Which patient is at greatest risk of central apnea following anesthesia?

    (A) A 3-month-old born at 40 weeks gestation
    (B) A 9-week-old born at 39 weeks gestation
    (C) A 4-month-old born at 30 weeks gestation
    (D) An 8-month-old born at 28 weeks gestation

75. Following administration of intrathecal anesthesia for cesarean section the patient is unable to speak, loses consciousness, and is hypotensive. What is the most likely cause?

    (A) High spinal
    (B) Use of ropivacaine
    (C) Spinal hematoma
    (D) Use of bupivacaine

76. What is the best position for optimizing airway patency during pediatric airway management?

    (A) Small pad placed under the shoulders
    (B) Small pad placed behind the head
    (C) The "sniffing position"
    (D) "Ramp" of towels behind the back

77. What is the best indication for a caudal block in a pediatric patient?

    (A) Anesthesia or analgesia for procedures below the xyphoid process
    (B) Analgesia for the first stage of labor
    (C) Anesthesia or analgesia for procedures below the umbilicus
    (D) Significant deformity of the sacral region

78. Which valve disorder most likely predisposes a patient to coronary ischemia with hypotension?

    (A) Mitral stenosis
    (B) Mitral regurgitation
    (C) Aortic stenosis
    (D) Aortic regurgitation

79. What is the hallmark laboratory finding associated with pyloric stenosis?

    (A) Hypokalemic hypochloremic metabolic acidosis
    (B) Hypokalemic hyperchloremic metabolic alkalosis
    (C) Hyperkalemic hypochloremic metabolic acidosis
    (D) Hypokalemic hypochloremic metabolic alkalosis

80. Which of the following is true regarding a patient with septal defects?

    (A) An increase in SVR relative to PVR will increase cyanosis.
    (B) An increase in PVR relative to SVR favors right to left shunting.
    (C) An increase in PVR relative to SVR will decrease risk of paradoxical air embolism.
    (D) Eisenmenger syndrome is most often due to left ventricular hypertrophy.

81. What is the most common site of herniation in congenital diaphragmatic hernia?

    (A) Right foramen of Bochdalek
    (B) Foramen of Morgagni
    (C) Left foramen of Bochdalek
    (D) Foramen of Luschka

82. Which is the most common type of tracheoesophageal fistula?

    (A) Type IIIb, esophageal atresia with a fistula between the distal esophagus and trachea

    (B) Type I, proximal tracheoesophageal fistula without distal fistula between stomach and trachea

    (C) Type IIIc, fistula between the trachea and both the upper and lower esophageal sections

    (D) Type II, esophageal atresia without communication with the trachea

83. Which statement is true regarding omphalocele and gastroschisis?

    (A) Gastroschisis is less common and presents with a peritoneal covering.

    (B) Omphalocele is less common and presents without peritoneal covering.

    (C) Gastroschisis is more common and presents without peritoneal covering.

    (D) Omphalocele is more common and presents with a peritoneal covering.

84. Which congenital cardiac malformation is most associated with Trisomy 21 (Down syndrome)?

    (A) Transposition of the great vessels

    (B) Coarctation of the aorta

    (C) Endocardial cushion defect

    (D) Aortic stenosis

85. Which of the following is an anatomic characteristic of the pediatric airway that distinguishes it from the adult patient?

    (A) The rima glottis is the narrowest point of the airway until the age of 5.

    (B) The tongue is proportionately smaller.

    (C) The larynx is located at the level of C4.

    (D) The epiglottis is flat and flexible.

86. Which type of surgical procedure will result in the greatest increase in afterload accompanied by acute hypertension during aortic cross-clamping?

    (A) Stanford Type A dissection of the ascending aorta

    (B) Suprarenal descending aortic aneurysm

    (C) Infrarenal descending aortic aneurysm

    (D) Stanford Type B dissection

87. At what gestational age does surfactant production begin?

    (A) 30 weeks

    (B) 34 weeks

    (C) 26 weeks

    (D) 32 weeks

88. Which of the following correctly describes omphalocele?

    (A) It is due to occlusion of the omphalomesenteric artery.

    (B) About 40 to 60% of patients have associated anomalies.

    (C) The defect is periumbilical.

    (D) Incidence is approximately 1 in 15,000 births.

89. What finding is most likely during preoperative examination of an awake and alert patient with a posterior cerebral artery aneurysm?

    (A) Brown-Séquard syndrome

    (B) Abnormal gaze or pupil response

    (C) Decorticate posturing

    (D) Hypertensive crisis

90. During a repeat cesarean section a term infant is delivered. One minute following delivery, the infant has a heart rate of 90, blue extremities, whimpering to stimulus, breathing regularly, and active with good muscle tone. What is the 1-minute Apgar score?

    (A) 5

    (B) 6

    (C) 7

    (D) 8

91. Which complication is most concerning following carotid endarterectomy?

    (A) Rapid emergence
    (B) Hypoxemia
    (C) Hypotension
    (D) Delayed emergence

92. Cleft palate, micrognathia, glossoptosis, and congenital heart disease are key characteristics of which *one* of the following syndromes?

    (A) Treacher Collins
    (B) VATER
    (C) Pierre-Robin
    (D) Prader-Willi

93. Which induction agent produces effects desirable for patients with Tetralogy of Fallot?

    (A) Etomidate
    (B) Ketamine
    (C) Midazolam
    (D) Propofol

94. Which of the following is true regarding a transplanted heart?

    (A) No response to atropine
    (B) No response to isoproterenol
    (C) No response to milrinone
    (D) No response to epinephrine

95. Which inhalational agent is most suitable for a pediatric inhalation induction?

    (A) Isoflurane
    (B) Desflurane
    (C) Sevoflurane
    (D) Halothane

96. Which of the following variables is not associated with aging?

    (A) Increased volume of distribution for lipid soluble drugs
    (B) Reduced plasma volume
    (C) Decreased volume of distribution for lipid soluble drugs
    (D) Reduced plasma protein binding

97. An elderly patient with decreased albumin and coronary artery disease is scheduled for an umbilical hernia repair. What do you expect when administering an intravenous induction dose of propofol?

    (A) Higher free drug fraction
    (B) Decreased drug effect
    (C) Lower free drug fraction
    (D) Similar drug effect

98. What is the effect of aging on the minimum alveolar concentration (MAC)?

    (A) MAC of volatile anesthetics increases 50% after age 60.
    (B) MAC of volatile anesthetics decreases 10% after age 50.
    (C) MAC of volatile anesthetics decreases 6% per decade after 40 years of age.
    (D) MAC of volatile anesthetics increases 4% per decade after 40 years of age.

99. What is the best induction dose for an 80-year-old weighing 100 kg?

    (A) Propofol 75 mg
    (B) Sodium pentothal 250 mg
    (C) Etomidate 40 mg
    (D) Ketamine 100 mg

100. What is the definition of premature birth?

    (A) Birth prior to 42 weeks gestation
    (B) Birth prior to 37 weeks gestation
    (C) Birth prior to 32 weeks gestation
    (D) Birth prior to 35 weeks gestation

101. Which body mass index (BMI) is categorized as moderate obesity?

    (A) 18.5%
    (B) 24.9%
    (C) 29.9%
    (D) 32.1%

102. Total body water will be the largest percentage of body weight in which patient?

    (A) A preterm newborn
    (B) An infant
    (C) A toddler
    (D) A school-age child

103. Which sign is associated with metabolic syndrome?

    (A) High levels of high-density lipoprotein cholesterol
    (B) Hypotension
    (C) High triglyceride levels
    (D) Small waist circumference

104. The patient is undergoing a latissimus dorsi myocutaneous flap for reconstruction of the breast. What is the desired mean arterial pressure?

    (A) MAP > 55 mmHg
    (B) MAP > 60 mmHg
    (C) MAP > 65 mmHg
    (D) MAP > 70 mmHg

105. Which patient appropriately fasted for an anesthetic to begin at 1000?

    (A) A child who had cereal at 0800
    (B) A child who had clear liquids at 0900
    (C) An infant who breast fed at 0500
    (D) An infant who had formula at 0700

106. Which dose of morphine is appropriate for intrathecal postcesarean section analgesia?

    (A) 2.5 mg
    (B) 50 µg
    (C) 0.2 mg
    (D) 100 µg

107. When is it best to avoid teratogenic drugs?

    (A) 1 to 2 weeks gestation
    (B) 3 to 10 weeks gestation
    (C) 12 to 15 weeks gestation
    (D) 20 to 25 weeks gestation

108. Which variable is not linked to postdural puncture headache following placement of a spinal anesthetic for cesarean section?

    (A) 26 g needle
    (B) Cutting needles
    (C) 20 g needle
    (D) Beveled needles

109. Which symptoms are associated with pregnant patients in the supine position?

    (A) Hypotension, nausea
    (B) Nausea, hypertension
    (C) Normotension, nausea
    (D) Hypertension, vomiting

110. Which of the following physiologic changes occur during pregnancy?

    (A) Hypocoagulation
    (B) Plasma volume decreases
    (C) Hypercoagulation
    (D) Red cell mass decreases

111. The patient requests an epidural for abdominal hysterectomy. Which sensory level is needed for epidural anesthesia?

    (A) T-12
    (B) T-10
    (C) T-8
    (D) T-6

112. The patient is scheduled for a laparoscopic cholecystectomy. Which of the following is true?

    (A) Central venous pressure decreases.
    (B) Lung compliance increases.
    (C) Intraabdominal pressure decreases.
    (D) Functional residual capacity decreases.

113. During a laparoscopic hernia repair, you notice a sudden drop in blood pressure and oxygen saturation and decreased end-tidal carbon dioxide. What is the most likely cause?

    (A) CO_2 embolus
    (B) Tension pneumothorax
    (C) Hemorrhage
    (D) Pneumomediastinum

114. Which of the following is true about the infant airway?

    (A) The tongue is small in relation to the mandible.
    (B) The larynx is located at the C2–C3 vertebrae.
    (C) The epiglottis is stiff and flat.
    (D) The larynx is located at C5–C6.

115. While reversing heparin, the anesthetist notes that the blood pressure has dropped precipitously to 42/23 mmHg. What will you do first?

    (A) Administer 100 mcg of epinephrine IV.
    (B) Administer 100 mcg of epinephrine IV.
    (C) Administer 50 mg of Benadryl and 125 mg of methylprednisolone IV.
    (D) Begin chest compressions.

116. By how much are neuraxial requirements for cesarean section decreased?

    (A) 60%
    (B) 40%
    (C) 30%
    (D) 50%

117. Which of the following is not a normal physiological change associated with pregnancy?

    (A) MAC decreases by 20%.
    (B) Functional residual capacity decreases by 20%.
    (C) Hemoglobin decreases by 20%
    (D) Plasma volume increases by 55%.

118. What is the best size endotracheal tube used for a patient undergoing general anesthesia for cesarean section?

    (A) 5.5 mm
    (B) 6.5 mm
    (C) 7.5 mm
    (D) 8.5 mm

119. How does propofol affect uterine blood flow (UBF)?

    (A) Decreases UBF
    (B) No change on UBF
    (C) Dose-related increase in UBF
    (D) Dose-related decrease in UBF

120. What statement is false regarding the use of metoclopramide in pregnant patients?

    (A) Speeds gastric emptying
    (B) Increases pH
    (C) Decreases gastric volume
    (D) Increases lower esophageal sphincter tone

121. A patient is scheduled for a radical neck dissection. History includes neck radiation. How will you manage this patient's airway?

    (A) Standard IV induction
    (B) Rapid sequence induction
    (C) Laryngeal mask airway
    (D) Awake fiberoptic intubation

122. Less than 1 minute following an epidural test dose, the patient complains of heavy legs. What is the most likely cause?

    (A) Intravascular injection
    (B) Incomplete epidural analgesia
    (C) Unintentional intrathecal block
    (D) Local anesthetic toxicity

123. The patient is receiving echothiophate eye drops for glaucoma. You plan to use succinylcholine. What should you expect?

    (A) Shortened onset of action
    (B) Shortened duration of action
    (C) Prolonged duration of action
    (D) Prolonged onset of action

124. The patient has severe preeclampsia. When will you avoid regional anesthesia?

    (A) Platelet count 100,000/uL
    (B) Platelet count 150,000/uL
    (C) Platelet count 125,000/uL
    (D) Platelet count 75,000/uL

125. What fetal monitoring pattern is associated with umbilical cord compression?

    (A) Variable decelerations
    (B) Late decelerations
    (C) Early decelerations
    (D) Increased variability

126. During labor the patient experiences an abrupt onset of constant abdominal pain accompanied by hypotension. What is the most likely cause?

    (A) Uterine rupture
    (B) Placenta previa
    (C) Placenta abruption
    (D) Hemorrhage

127. Which of the following increases intraocular pressure?

    (A) Hypotension
    (B) Hypoventilation
    (C) Decreased CVP
    (D) Hyperventilation

128. During radical neck dissection you observe new onset bradycardia, arrhythmias, and prolonged QT intervals. What is the most likely cause of these symptoms?

    (A) Denervation of carotid sinus
    (B) Manipulation of the carotid sinus
    (C) Venous air embolism
    (D) Denervation of carotid bodies

129. The patient is scheduled for laser removal of vocal cord papilloma. What will you avoid?

    (A) Eye protection with colored glasses
    (B) Nitrous oxide
    (C) Eye protection with wet gauze
    (D) Oxygen and air mixture

130. Fifteen minutes ago you transported a patient to the postanesthesia care unit following tonsillectomy. The patient is bleeding. How will you induce this patient?

    (A) Rapid sequence induction
    (B) Standard induction
    (C) Awake intubation
    (D) Standard induction with a glidescope

131. Which of the following is not associated with a peribulbar block?

    (A) Intraconal procedure
    (B) When 5 to 8 mL local anesthetic is used
    (C) Extraconal procedure
    (D) When patient gaze is straight ahead

132. Which statement is true regarding the use of inhalational agents during pregnancy?

    (A) Uterine blood flow is increased.
    (B) Uteroplacental blood flow is increased.
    (C) Uteroplacental blood flow is decreased.
    (D) Uterine blood flow is unchanged.

133. The patient is scheduled for endoscopic sinus surgery. Which of the following will not minimize blood loss?

    (A) Head-up position
    (B) Cocaine 4%
    (C) Supine position
    (D) Hypotensive technique

134. A patient is scheduled for surgery involving a LeFort II fracture. During the preoperative interview, periorbital edema and raccoon eyes hematoma are noted. What is your main anesthetic concern?

    (A) Securing the airway
    (B) Bleeding
    (C) Emergence with a wired jaw
    (D) Postoperative respiratory compromise

135. Which of the following is not a clinical sign of hyperthyroidism?

    (A) Polyuria
    (B) Weight loss
    (C) Muscle fatigue
    (D) Hypoactive reflexes

136. What is the anesthetic priority for management of an unrepaired aortic dissection?

(A) Decrease blood pressure with arterial vasodilators to decrease risk of rupture or further dissection.

(B) Increase blood pressure to ensure adequate perfusion distal to the aneurysm.

(C) Decrease shear force on the aneurysm using beta-blockers to decrease risk of rupture of further dissection.

(D) Decrease heart rate with medications to decrease myocardial oxygen demand.

137. The patient is scheduled for a laryngeal endoscopy. Jet ventilation is planned. What statement is false regarding jet ventilation?

(A) High-pressure (30-60 psi) is used.

(B) FiO_2 of 30% or less is used.

(C) End-tidal CO_2 is accurate.

(D) Expiration is passive.

138. A patient undergoing repair of a descending thoracic aortic aneurysm is found postoperatively to exhibit loss of lower extremity motor function bilaterally. What is the most likely cause?

(A) Blood flow to the motor cortex of the brain was decreased during cross-clamp.

(B) Blood flow to the anterior spinal cord was damaged during the surgery.

(C) Blood flow to the posterior spinal cord was damaged during the surgery.

(D) This is a normal occurrence when blood flow to the lower extremities has been restricted as in aortic cross-clamping.

139. The patient is undergoing a mediastinoscopy. What will you consider for this patient?

(A) Blood pressure in the left arm

(B) Small bore IV

(C) Blood pressure in the right arm

(D) Tachycardia

140. What statement is true regarding cardioversion?

(A) 50 to 100 Joules are used initially for atrial flutter.

(B) 200 to 300 Joules are used initially to convert atrial flutter.

(C) Electrical shock is asynchronous.

(D) Electrical shock is synchronized with the "Q" wave.

141. What do you anticipate with distention of the bowel during colonoscopy?

(A) Tachycardia

(B) Hypertension

(C) Bradycardia

(D) EKG changes

142. The patient is scheduled for computerized tomography (CT) scan with intravenous contrast media (ICM). What is your main concern?

(A) Patient must not move during the CT

(B) Patient anxiety

(C) Hypothermia

(D) Allergic reaction

143. A patient is scheduled for electroconvulsive therapy (ECT). What is your main anesthetic concern when calculating dosages for induction agents?

(A) Anterograde amnesia

(B) Seizure quality

(C) Parasympathetic stimulation

(D) Sympathetic stimulation

144. A patient with an intestinal obstruction is scheduled for surgery. The patient's history includes pancreatitis and gastroesophageal reflux disease (GERD). What is the best approach to airway management?

(A) Awake fiberoptic intubation

(B) Endotracheal intubation

(C) LMA

(D) Intubating LMA

145. When is cardiac output the greatest?

   (A) Immediately following delivery
   (B) Third trimester
   (C) Second trimester
   (D) First trimester

146. Which of the following would be the most appropriate induction technique for a patient undergoing drainage of a severe cardiac tamponade via subxiphoid approach or pericardiocentesis?

   (A) Propofol, high-dose fentanyl, succinylcholine, and intubate. Maintain with light sevoflurane and positive pressure ventilation.
   (B) Ketamine, high-dose fentanyl, succinylcholine, and intubate. Maintain with light sevoflurane.
   (C) Inhalational induction, LMA insertion, light maintenance with sevoflurane, ketamine supplementation.
   (D) High-dose fentanyl, midazolam, and mask ventilate patient.

147. A sedated patient experiences headache, nausea, and vomiting during stereotactic Gamma Knife surgery. What is the most likely cause?

   (A) Hemorrhage
   (B) Perforated aneurysm
   (C) Radiocontrast reaction
   (D) Embolization

148. Which of the following medications shortens the duration of a seizure during electroconvulsive therapy (ECT)?

   (A) Caffeine
   (B) Etomidate
   (C) Ketamine
   (D) Propofol

149. The patient is undergoing a mastectomy. During surgery, isosulfan blue dye is injected. What do you expect?

   (A) Tachycardia
   (B) Increased oxygen saturation
   (C) Bradycardia
   (D) Decreased oxygen saturation

150. Following cystoscopy the patient's blood pressure falls. What is the most likely cause?

   (A) Sympathectomy
   (B) Blood loss
   (C) Vasoconstriction due to spinal anesthesia
   (D) Lowering legs from lithotomy position

151. Pain relief during the second stage of labor requires neural blockade at what sensory level?

   (A) T_{10} to T_{12}
   (B) T_{12} to S_1
   (C) T_{10} to S_1
   (D) T_{10} to S_4

152. Which condition benefits most from epidural steroid injections?

   (A) Radiculopathy
   (B) Intractable cancer pain
   (C) Intraabdominal neoplasms
   (D) Phantom limb pain

153. Which drug has mainly analgesic and antipyretic properties?

   (A) Acetaminophen
   (B) Ketorolac
   (C) Fentanyl
   (D) Codeine

154. Which statement regarding the use of epidural analgesia and anesthesia for preeclamptic patients is true?

   (A) Circulating catecholamines are decreased.
   (B) Decreases intervillous blood flow.
   (C) Epidural block should be avoided.
   (D) Epidural blocks are difficult to place.

155. A patient taking duloxetine and fluoxetine for chronic neuropathic pain complains of fever, agitation, sweating, and anxiety. What is the most likely cause?

   (A) Duloxetine overdose
   (B) Fluoxetine sensitivity
   (C) Combined use of fluoxetine and duloxetine
   (D) Allergic reaction to duloxetine

156. A patient is receiving tocolytic therapy for preterm labor. Which of the following is most concerning for this patient?

    (A) Hyperkalemia

    (B) Hypoglycemia

    (C) Pulmonary Edema

    (D) Increased systemic vascular resistance

157. Which of the following is a systemic effect of hydrocortisone?

    (A) Adrenal-pituitary insufficiency

    (B) Hypoglycemia

    (C) Hypotension

    (D) Sodium depletion

158. How is the renal system affected by pregnancy?

    (A) Renal plasma flow decreases

    (B) Glomerular filtration rate increases

    (C) Tubular absorption of glucose increases

    (D) Renal blood flow decreases

159. When giving epidural steroid injections what dose will you use to avoid systemic effects?

    (A) Methylprednisolone acetate 40 mg

    (B) Triamcinolone diacetate 100 mg

    (C) Methylprednisolone acetate 20 mg

    (D) Triamcinolone diacetate 120 mg

160. The patient is scheduled for in vitro fertilization (IVF). Which medication is considered safe for this patient?

    (A) Morphine

    (B) Fentanyl

    (C) Isoflurane

    (D) NSAIDs

161. Which statement is false regarding open breast biopsy?

    (A) Postoperative nausea and vomiting increases.

    (B) Smooth emergence minimizes hematoma formation.

    (C) Monitor the EKG for ST-segment changes when local anesthetic with epinephrine is used.

    (D) The blood pressure cuff is placed on the nonoperative arm and IV placed on the operative side.

162. The patient is undergoing a modified radical mastectomy. When planning the general anesthetic, why would you check with the surgeon?

    (A) Determine the patient's risk for postoperative nausea and vomiting

    (B) To type and cross-match preoperatively

    (C) Determine what if any neuromuscular blockers will be used

    (D) Determine when to give antiemetics

163. What is your primary concern when caring for a patient undergoing hysteroscopy?

    (A) Vasovagal response to uterine traction

    (B) Postoperative pain

    (C) Lithotomy positioning

    (D) Absorption of glycine or saline solution

164. The patient is scheduled for a total abdominal hysterectomy. Why is the patient most likely to become hypotensive following induction?

    (A) Bowel prep

    (B) Chronic bleeding

    (C) Anemia

    (D) Position changes

165. During a cystoscopy, the patient becomes diaphoretic and complains of upper abdominal pain and nausea. What is the most likely cause?

    (A) Bladder perforation

    (B) Stent placement

    (C) Biopsy

    (D) Stone removal

166. What medication(s) should be immediately available for penile surgery?

    (A) Midazolam

    (B) Propofol

    (C) Fentanyl

    (D) Glycopyrrolate

167. What is a primary concern for patients undergoing rectal surgery?

(A) Postoperative pain

(B) Relaxation of the anal sphincter

(C) Fluid and electrolyte balance

(D) Postoperative nausea and vomiting

168. During total knee arthroplasty with spinal anesthesia, the patient develops hypotension, arrhythmias and loses consciousness. What is the most likely rationale?

(A) Hemorrhage

(B) Fluid imbalance

(C) Tourniquet pain

(D) Methyl methacrylate

169. Which is the preferred method of airway management in a child with acute epiglottitis?

(A) Rapid sequence induction followed by laryngoscopy

(B) Awake laryngoscopy

(C) Inhalation induction maintaining spontaneous respiration

(D) Urgent tracheostomy

170. Which factor does not contribute to decreased uterine blood flow?

(A) Systemic hypotension

(B) Uterine vasoconstriction

(C) Uterine contractions

(D) Uterine vasodilation

171. Which of the following physiologic changes occur with limb tourniquets?

(A) Cellular acidosis

(B) Metabolic alkalosis

(C) Cellular alkalosis

(D) Metabolic acidosis

172. While undergoing a shoulder arthroscopy with regional anesthesia the patient exhibits tachycardia, agitation, diaphoresis, hypotension, and jugular vein distention. What is the most likely cause?

(A) Tension pneumothorax

(B) Subcutaneous emphysema

(C) Pneumomediastinum

(D) Failed regional block

173. Which of the following risk factors is not linked to postoperative vision loss (POVL)?

(A) Thin

(B) Obese

(C) Male

(D) <18 years

174. The patient is scheduled for total hip arthroplasty. What are your anesthetic concerns?

(A) Hemorrhage

(B) Thromboembolism

(C) Tourniquet pain

(D) Bone cement implantation syndrome

175. How are hypotensive bradycardic episodes (HBEs) that occur during shoulder surgery defined?

(A) Heart rate <50 bpm and systolic blood pressure <90 mmHg

(B) Systolic blood pressure >90 mmHg

(C) Heart rate decreases 30 bpm in 3 minutes

(D) Heart rate decreases 20 bpm in 5 minutes

176. Your patient is undergoing an elective coronary artery bypass graft (CABG). The patient was managed on heparin therapy for 5 days preoperatively. The patient is now on cardiopulmonary bypass and the perfusionist is having difficulty maintaining total heparinization. What is the most likely cause?

(A) Antithrombin deficiency

(B) Factor V deficiency

(C) Factor VIII deficiency

(D) Factor IV deficiency

177. Which condition is associated with carbamazepine taken during pregnancy?

    (A) Spina bifida
    (B) Pyloric stenosis
    (C) Biliary atresia
    (D) Hypospadias

178. A patient is undergoing an elective abdominal aortic aneurysm (AAA) repair. What drug are you most likely to administer after aortic clamping?

    (A) Nitroglycerin
    (B) Phenylephrine
    (C) Milrinone
    (D) Dopamine

179. A 5-year-old requires endotracheal intubation for an exploratory laparotomy. What size ETT will you select?

    (A) 6
    (B) 5
    (C) 4
    (D) 3

180. Which of the following is linked to late decelerations?

    (A) Fetal head compression
    (B) Begins 10 to 30 seconds following the peak of a contraction
    (C) Begin with the contraction
    (D) Umbilical cord compression

181. Which neurosurgical procedure places the patient at highest risk for postoperative diabetes insipidus?

    (A) Resection of intracranial aneurysm in the anterior circle of Willis
    (B) Stereotactic biopsy of a lesion in the parietal lobe
    (C) Tumor resection within the posterior fossa
    (D) Transsphenoidal hypophysectomy

182. Which of the following agents will cause the greatest decrease in preload?

    (A) Verapamil
    (B) Nicardipine
    (C) Metoprolol
    (D) Nitroglycerine

183. What is the correct placement of a precordial Doppler to monitor for venous air embolism?

    (A) Midclavicular line at the first intercostal space
    (B) Right sternal border at the third intercostal space
    (C) Right midaxillary line at the fifth intercostal space
    (D) Left sternal border at the fifth intercostal space

184. What is average total cerebral blood flow?

    (A) 550 mL/min
    (B) 650 mL/min
    (C) 750 mL/min
    (D) 950 mL/min

185. How is minimum alveolar concentration (MAC) affected for inhaled anesthetics during pregnancy?

    (A) MAC is increased by 30%.
    (B) MAC is decreased by 15%.
    (C) MAC is increased by 25%.
    (D) MAC is decreased by 40%.

186. Calculate cerebral perfusion pressure (CPP) using the information provided and correctly interpret the result. Blood pressure is 130/90 mmHg, intracranial pressure is 12 mmHg, and central venous pressure is 6 mmHg.

    (A) CPP = 110 mmHg, high
    (B) CPP = 97 mmHg, normal
    (C) CPP = 105 mmHg, high
    (D) CPP = 91 mmHg, normal

187. Inhalational anesthetic agents have what effect on cardiac conduction?

    (A) Decrease AV node refractoriness
    (B) Suppress SA node automaticity
    (C) Increases pacing thresholds
    (D) All of the above

188. For Frank-Starling's law what do the x-axis and y-axis represent?

    (A) Heart rate; cardiac output

    (B) Ventricular end-diastolic volume; cardiac output

    (C) Cardiac output; ventricular end-diastolic volume

    (D) Afterload; systemic vascular resistance

189. The fetal scalp pH is 7.25. How would you interpret this value?

    (A) Normal infant pH

    (B) Abnormal infant pH

    (C) Needs to be repeated to ensure accuracy

    (D) Requires neonatal resuscitation

190. What does the formula,

$$\frac{\text{(end-diastolic volume)} - \text{(end-systolic volume)}}{\text{end-diastolic volume}}, \text{represent?}$$

    (A) Stroke volume

    (B) Cardiac index

    (C) Cardiac output

    (D) Ejection fraction

191. A pacemaker is placed in a patient with symptomatic sinus bradycardia with a normally functioning atrioventricular node. What settings would be most appropriate?

    (A) AAI

    (B) AOO

    (C) DDD

    (D) DDI

192. Which of the following agents possesses combined alpha- and beta-adrenergic blocking effects?

    (A) Metoprolol

    (B) Esmolol

    (C) Atenolol

    (D) Labetalol

193. Which anesthesia-induction technique would be appropriate for a severely hypertensive patient with coronary artery disease and moderate ventricular dysfunction?

    (A) Inhalational induction with sevoflurane

    (B) Inhalational induction with desflurane

    (C) Intravenous induction with ketamine

    (D) Intravenous induction with propofol

194. Which arrhythmia is best treated with magnesium sulfate?

    (A) Ventricular fibrillation

    (B) Polymorphic ventricular tachycardia in the presence of prolonged QT syndrome

    (C) Atrioventricular nodal reentrant tachycardia

    (D) Polymorphic ventricular tachycardia in the absence of prolonged QT syndrome

195. What is the goal of hemodynamic management for the patient with severe mitral valve regurgitation?

    (A) Aggressive volume resuscitation

    (B) Inotropic support

    (C) Afterload reduction

    (D) Maintenance of moderate bradycardia

196. Which patient is most at risk for catastrophic bleeding upon midline sternotomy?

    (A) Patient with ischemic cardiomyopathy on multiple vasopressor therapies undergoing aortic valve replacement

    (B) Patient with heparin-induced thrombocytopenia to be treated with argatroban for cardiopulmonary bypass undergoing coronary artery bypass grafts

    (C) Patient with previous coronary artery bypass grafting undergoing mitral valve repair

    (D) Obese patient with severe aortic stenosis undergoing aortic valve replacement

197. What is the approximate mean arterial blood pressure for the patient whose pressure reads 115/70 mmHg?

    (A) 100 mmHg

    (B) 85 mmHg

    (C) 92.5 mmHg

    (D) 80 mmHg

198. In which valvular disorder is the left ventricular volume approximately normal, but left ventricular pressures are higher than normal?

    (A) Mitral stenosis
    (B) Aortic stenosis
    (C) Mitral regurgitation
    (D) Aortic regurgitation

199. Measured systolic and pulse pressure will appear greatest when transduced and measured at which point?

    (A) Aortic root
    (B) Brachial artery
    (C) Radial artery
    (D) Dorsalis pedis

200. Which of the following is a relative contraindication to pulmonary artery catheter placement?

    (A) Atrial fibrillation
    (B) Left bundle branch block
    (C) Complete heart block
    (D) First degree block

201. Which of the following is not associated with rhabdomyolysis?

    (A) Compartment syndrome
    (B) Renal failure
    (C) Increased muscle enzymes
    (D) Decreased muscle enzymes

202. Which law explains the effect of post-intubation airway edema in children?

    (A) Poiseuille's equation
    (B) Dalton's law
    (C) The ideal gas law
    (D) Avogadro's number

203. Which medication used for preeclampsia may extend the duration of rocuronium?

    (A) Nitroglycerin
    (B) Hydralazine
    (C) Labetalol
    (D) Magnesium

204. What is the normal fetal heart rate?

    (A) 80 to 100
    (B) 100 to 110
    (C) 110 to 160
    (D) >160

205. What is the best intervention to improve hypotension resulting from aortocaval compression?

    (A) Give oxygen via facemask
    (B) Turn the patient on their side
    (C) Give ephedrine
    (D) Give neosynephrine

206. Which opioid causes the greatest respiration depression in newborns?

    (A) Demerol
    (B) Morphine
    (C) Fentanyl
    (D) Remifentanil

207. The patient is scheduled for a parathyroidectomy. How might neuromuscular blockade (NMB) affect hyperparathyroid patients?

    (A) May require decreasing the NMB dose
    (B) May require careful titration
    (C) Effect of NMB not significant
    (D) No change in the response to NMB

208. A patient undergoes bronchoscopy for removal of a foreign body. What neuromuscular blocker (NMB) is the best choice for this procedure?

    (A) Succinylcholine
    (B) Vecuronicum
    (C) Cis-atracurium
    (D) Atracrium

209. What increases stroke volume?

    (A) Increased ventricular end-diastolic volume
    (B) Increased pulmonary vascular resistance
    (C) Increased heart rate
    (D) Mitral regurgitation

210. Which inhaled agent is most associated with emergence delirium in children?

 (A) Sevoflurane

 (B) Isoflurane

 (C) Desflurane

 (D) Nitrous oxide

211. When does blood volume return to pre-pregnancy levels?

 (A) 7 to 14 days after delivery

 (B) 24 hours after delivery

 (C) 36 hours after delivery

 (D) 21 days after delivery

212. An octogenarian is scheduled for a laparoscopic cholecystectomy. You plan to adjust the dosage of neuromuscular blockers. What is your rationale for this decision?

 (A) Renal function declines with aging

 (B) Renal clearance increases with aging

 (C) Hepatic blood flow increases with aging

 (D) Total body water increases by 10% to 15% with aging

213. Which of the following is not associated with retinopathy of prematurity?

 (A) High oxygen tension in vessels of the retina

 (B) Low oxygen tension in vessels of the retina

 (C) Wide swings in oxygen tension

 (D) Ventilated premature infants with sepsis

214. Which of the following is not a concern for the anesthetists when caring for patients with omphalocele and gastroschisis?

 (A) Severe dehydration

 (B) Fluid loss

 (C) Heat loss

 (D) Low abdominal pressure with closure

215. Which of the following is not an anesthetic goal when caring for patients with Tetralogy of Fallot?

 (A) Increase systemic vascular resistance (SVR)

 (B) Avoid acidosis

 (C) Maintain intravascular volume

 (D) Maintain SVR

216. Which feature is not associated with dementia?

 (A) Acute onset

 (B) Memory impairment

 (C) Disorientation

 (D) Slow onset

217. Why is there an initial increase in plasma concentration following intravenous induction in geriatric patients?

 (A) Total body water increases

 (B) Central compartment volume increases

 (C) Total body water decreases

 (D) Body fat decreases

218. Which of the following anesthetic implications should be considered when caring for obese patients?

 (A) Caution when administering respiratory depressants

 (B) Low gastric volume

 (C) High gastric volume

 (D) Low pH

219. Which of the following guidelines for management of patients with obstructive sleep apnea is false?

 (A) Consider regional techniques.

 (B) Consider nonsteroidal anti-inflammatory agents to reduce opioid requirements.

 (C) Standard use of opioids should be considered when using regional techniques.

 (D) Consider the risks and benefits of using opioids in combination with regional techniques.

220. Which of the following is an advantage of the sitting position for orthopedic surgery?

 (A) Risk of injury to the brachial plexus and forearm neuropathies decreases.

 (B) Risk of injury to the brachial plexus and forearm neuropathies increases.

 (C) Arm weight distorts the shoulder joint anatomy.

 (D) Arm weight distorts the intra-articular anatomy.

Answers and Explanations: Advanced Principles

1. During induction of general anesthesia the pregnant patient quickly desaturates. Which factors most likely caused the desaturation?

   (A) Increased functional residual capacity and increased oxygen consumption
   (B) Decreased residual volume and increased expiratory reserve volume
   (C) Decreased functional residual capacity and increased oxygen consumption

TABLE 4-1. Average maximum physiological changes associated with pregnancy.

Parameter	Change
Neurological	
MAC	−40%
Respiratory	
Oxygen consumption	+20 to 50%
Airway resistance	−35%
FRC	−20%
Minute ventilation	+50%
Tidal volume	+40%
Respiratory rate	+15%
PaO_2	+10%
$PaCO_2$	−15%
HCO_3	−15%
Cardiovascular	
Blood volume	+35%
Plasma volume	+55%
Cardiac output	+40%
Stroke volume	+30%
Heart rate	+20%
Systolic blood pressure	−5%
Diastolic blood pressure	−15%
Peripheral resistance	−15%
Pulmonary resistance	−30%
Hematological	
Hemoglobin	−20%
Platelets	−10%
Clotting factors[1]	+30 to 250%
Renal	
GFR	+50%

[1]Varies with each factor.
FRC, functional residual capacity; GFR, glomerular filtration rate; MAC, minimum alveolar concentration.
(Reproduced with permission from Butterworth JF IV, Mackey DC, Wasnick JD, eds. *Morgan & Mikhail's Clinical Anesthesiology*. 7th ed. New York: McGraw Hill; 2022.)

   (D) Increased residual volume and decreased expiratory reserve volume

Rationale: Respiratory changes of pregnancy include decreased functional residual capacity (FRC), increased oxygen consumption, and decreased residual and expiratory reserve volumes. Decreased FRC and increased oxygen consumption leads to a rapid decrease in oxygen saturation.

References: Butterworth JF IV, Mackey DC, Wasnick JD, eds. *Morgan & Mikhail's Clinical Anesthesiology*. 7th ed. New York, NY: McGraw Hill; 2022: Chapter 40.
Longnecker DE, Mackey SC, Newman MF, Sandberg WS, Zapol WM, eds. *Anesthesiology*. 3rd ed. McGraw Hill; 2018: Chapter 18.

2. Which cardiac variable leads to heart failure due to obesity?

   (A) Decreased preload
   (B) Left ventricular systolic dysfunction
   (C) Decreased afterload
   (D) Hypotension

Rationale: Volume overload and vascular stiffness result from obesity. Increased preload, increased afterload, and hypertension lead to left ventricular systolic dysfunction.

Reference: Hines RL, Marschall KE. *Stoelting's Anesthesia and Co-existing Disease*. 7th ed. Philadelphia, PA: Elsevier Saunders; 2018: Chapter 19.

3. What is the average weight of a 6-year-old?

   (A) 15 kg
   (B) 18 kg
   (C) 21 kg
   (D) 24 kg

Rationale: A simple estimation of body weight by age is the addition of 9 to twice the age.

Reference: Butterworth JF IV, Mackey DC, Wasnick JD, eds. *Morgan & Mikhail's Clinical Anesthesiology*. 7th ed. New York, NY: McGraw Hill; 2022: Chapter 42.

4. Which of the following is not a symptom of fat embolism associated with a long bone fracture?

   (A) Dyspnea

   (B) Confusion

   (C) Petechiae

   (D) Decreased free fatty acids

Rationale: Signs of fat embolism following a long bone fracture generally occur within 72 hours of the event. Increased free fatty acids lead to capillary-alveolar membrane disturbance. Neurological symptoms result due to cerebral circulation damage and edema.

Reference: Butterworth JF IV, Mackey DC, Wasnick JD, eds. *Morgan & Mikhail's Clinical Anesthesiology.* 7th ed. New York, NY: McGraw Hill; 2022: Chapter 38.

5. An 80-year-old female with moderate aortic stenosis is undergoing an emergent open reduction and internal fixation of her left hip. Preoperative vital signs include a blood pressure of 175/95 mmHg and a heart rate in sinus rhythm of 65 beats/min. Shortly after induction with propofol and general anesthesia maintained with sevoflurane, the patient's heart rate increases to an irregular 133 beats/min. The blood pressure decreases to 69/55 mmHg. What would be the most effective action to restore a stable hemodynamic profile?

   (A) Administer 100 mcg of phenylephrine intravenously.

   (B) Request that the surgery begin immediately in order that a painful stimulus may increase blood pressure.

   (C) Cardiovert the patient with a synchronized transthoracic shock of 170 joules.

   (D) Administer a 500 mL bolus of lactated ringers.

Rationale: The irregular accelerated heart rate is likely atrial fibrillation. Loss of atrial synchronized contraction can reduce ventricular filling by 20% to 30%. An elderly patient with atrial stenosis has a fixed outflow obstruction and can be expected to have hypertrophy, resulting in decreased ventricular compliance. The increased heart rate and decreased atrial "kick" all combine to significantly decrease this patient's left ventricular end-diastolic volume. Hemodynamic consequences to a reduced ventricular end-diastolic volume will be most profoundly seen in a patient with concomitant reduced ventricular compliance. While all the interventions mentioned may increase blood pressure, only synchronized cardioversion solves the underlying problem.

Reference: Butterworth JF IV, Mackey DC, Wasnick JD, eds. *Morgan & Mikhail's Clinical Anesthesiology.* 7th ed. New York, NY: McGraw Hill; 2022: Chapter 20.

6. What finding may be identified during preoperative examination of an awake and alert patient with a posterior cerebral artery aneurysm?

   (A) Brown-Séquard syndrome

   (B) Abnormal gaze or pupil response

   (C) Decorticate posturing

   (D) Hypertensive crisis

Rationale: Oculomotor palsy may result from an aneurysm in this area due to proximity of these structures.

References: Butterworth JF IV, Mackey DC, Wasnick JD, eds. *Morgan & Mikhail's Clinical Anesthesiology.* 7th ed. New York, NY: McGraw Hill; 2022: Chapter 27.

Moore KL, Agur AMR, Dalley AF. *Moore's Essential Clinical Anatomy.* 6th ed. Philadelphia, PA: Wolters Kluwer; 2019: Chapter 8.

7. What is the uterine blood flow at term?

   (A) 200 to 300 mL/min

   (B) 300 to 400 mL/min

   (C) 400 to 500 mL/min

   (D) 600 to 700 mL/min

Rationale: The normal uterine blood flow in the nonpregnant female is 50 mL/min. At term, the blood flow increases to approximately 10% of the cardiac output.

References: Butterworth JF IV, Mackey DC, Wasnick JD, eds. *Morgan & Mikhail's Clinical Anesthesiology.* 7th ed. New York, NY: McGraw Hill; 2022: Chapter 41.

Longnecker DE, Mackey SC, Newman MF, Sandberg WS, Zapol WM, eds. *Anesthesiology.* 3rd ed. McGraw Hill; 2018: Chapter 18.

8. What is resting cerebral oxygen consumption?

   (A) 3.5 mL/100 g/min

   (B) 5 mL/100 g/min

   (C) 100 mL/min

   (D) 250 mL/min

Rationale: Resting cerebral oxygen demand averages 3.5 mL/100 g/min.

References: Butterworth JF IV, Mackey DC, Wasnick JD, eds. *Morgan & Mikhail's Clinical Anesthesiology.* 7th ed. New York, NY: McGraw Hill; 2022: Chapter 27.

Hall JE. *Guyton and Hall Textbook of Medical Physiology.* 14th ed. Philadelphia, PA: Saunders Elsevier; 2021: Chapter 62.

9. What dose of protamine sulfate would be appropriate to reverse 5,000 units of heparin?

   (A) 500 mcg
   (B) 5 mg
   (C) 50 mg
   (D) 5 mcg

   Rationale: Protamine is a positively charged protein that binds to and inactivates heparin. The dose of protamine is calculated according to the dose of heparin given and not the degree of anticoagulation obtained. Generally, 1 mg of protamine is administered for every 100 units of heparin in circulation. Therefore, this patient needs 5,000/100 = 50 mg of protamine IV.

   Reference: Butterworth JF IV, Mackey DC, Wasnick JD, eds. *Morgan & Mikhail's Clinical Anesthesiology.* 7th ed. New York, NY: McGraw Hill; 2022: Chapter 22.

10. Which of the following is not harmful when in proximity to the magnetic resonance imaging (MRI) machine?

    (A) Implanted medication pumps
    (B) Pacing wires
    (C) Cardiac pacemakers
    (D) Pulse oximeter

    Rationale: Items containing iron (ferromagnetic) are strongly attracted to the MRI magnet. MRI-compatible equipment lists items that are acceptable for use for patients undergoing MRI.

    Reference: Elisha S, Heiner JS, Nagelhout JJ. *Nurse Anesthesia.* 7th ed. St. Louis, MO: Elsevier Saunders; 2023: Chapter 58.

11. A patient is scheduled for bariatric surgery. What is the recommended induction dose for propofol?

    (A) Dose based on ideal body weight
    (B) Dose based on total body weight
    (C) Dose based on obesity scale
    (D) Dose based on morbid obesity

    Rationale: The induction dose of propofol for an obese patient is based on the lean body weight (LBW). A maintenance dose of propofol is based on the total body weight.

    Reference: Elisha S, Heiner JS, Nagelhout JJ. *Nurse Anesthesia.* 7th ed. St. Louis, MO: Elsevier Saunders; 2023: Chapter 48.

12. What is an indication of significant venous air embolism during a seated craniotomy?

    (A) Increased end-tidal carbon dioxide
    (B) Unchanged end-tidal carbon dioxide
    (C) Decreased end-tidal carbon dioxide
    (D) Hypertension

    Rationale: Entraining large amounts of air into the venous system results in a sudden decreased end-tidal carbon dioxide. Hypotension is associated with a venous air embolism.

    References: Butterworth JF IV, Mackey DC, Wasnick JD, eds. *Morgan & Mikhail's Clinical Anesthesiology.* 7th ed. New York, NY: McGraw Hill; 2022: Chapter 27.

    Pardo MC Jr, ed. *Basics of Anesthesia.* 8th ed. Philadelphia, PA: Elsevier Saunders; 2023: Chapter 30.

13. Which of the following is not associated with pulseless electrical activity?

    (A) Hypovolemia
    (B) Hypoxia
    (C) Hyperkalemia
    (D) Hyperthermia

    Rationale: A review for differential diagnosis for pulseless electrical activity includes hypovolemia, hypoxia, hydrogen ion-acidosis, hyper-/hypokalemia, hypothermia, toxins, tamponade, tension pneumothorax, thrombosis (coronary and pulmonary).

    Reference: Butterworth JF IV, Mackey DC, Wasnick JD, eds. *Morgan & Mikhail's Clinical Anesthesiology.* 7th ed. New York, NY: McGraw Hill; 2022: Chapter 55.

14. A patient with dysmenorrhea is scheduled for dilation and curettage (D&C). What preoperative testing is required?

    (A) CBC
    (B) Electrolyte panel
    (C) Chest x-ray
    (D) HCG

    Rationale: A pregnancy test is needed prior to D&C.

    Reference: Macksey LF. *Surgical Procedures and Anesthetic Implications.* 2nd ed. Sudbury, MA: Jones & Bartlett Learning; 2018: Chapter 20.

15. The addition of an intravenous inotrope will move the Frank-Starling curve in which direction?

    (A) Up
    (B) Down
    (C) Left
    (D) Right

    Rationale: Frank-Starling's law relates preload (ventricular end-diastolic volume) with stroke volume (or cardiac output) when heart rate and contractility remain constant. If an inotrope exerts its influence on the ventricular myocardium, contractility will increase independently from preload effects. The stroke volume and cardiac output will be higher for a given ventricular end-diastolic pressure.

Reference: Butterworth JF IV, Mackey DC, Wasnick JD, eds. *Morgan & Mikhail's Clinical Anesthesiology.* 7th ed. New York, NY: McGraw Hill; 2022: Chapter 20.

16. During an uncomplicated vaginal delivery, what is the expected blood loss?

    (A) 250 mL
    (B) 400 mL
    (C) 750 mL
    (D) 800 mL

    Rationale: The normal blood loss of vaginal delivery is 400 to 500 mL whereas the normal blood loss during cesarean section is 700 to 750 mL.

    Reference: Longnecker DE, Mackey SC, Newman MF, Sandberg WS, Zapol WM, eds. *Anesthesiology.* 3rd ed. McGraw Hill; 2018: Chapter 18.

17. What should the activated clotting time be prior to initiation of cardiopulmonary bypass (CPB)?

    (A) <150 seconds
    (B) >200 seconds but <350 seconds
    (C) >350 seconds but <450 seconds
    (D) >400 seconds

    Rationale: Initiation of cardiopulmonary bypass can begin after the ACT is greater than 400 to 480 seconds. Failure to establish adequate anticoagulation will result in disseminated intravascular coagulation and formation of clots in the CPB pump.

    Reference: Butterworth JF IV, Mackey DC, Wasnick JD, eds. *Morgan & Mikhail's Clinical Anesthesiology.* 7th ed. New York, NY: McGraw Hill; 2022: Chapter 22.
    Elisha S, Heiner JS, Nagelhout JJ. *Nurse Anesthesia.* 7th ed. St. Louis, MO: Elsevier Saunders; 2023: Chapter 26.

18. What level of neural blockade is needed for analgesia during the first stage of labor?

    (A) T_{10}-L_1 motor level
    (B) T_{10}-S_4 sensory level
    (C) T_{10}-L_1 sensory level
    (D) T_{10}-S_4 motor level

    Rationale: A sensory level T_{10}-L_1 is needed for adequate analgesia during the first stage of labor. During the second stage of labor additional sensory levels T_{10}-S_4 require neural blockade.

    Reference: Butterworth JF IV, Mackey DC, Wasnick JD, eds. *Morgan & Mikhail's Clinical Anesthesiology.* 7th ed. New York, NY: McGraw Hill; 2022: Chapter 41.

19. How is cardiac index calculated?

    (A) $\dfrac{Cardiac\ Output}{Stroke\ Volume}$

    (B) $\dfrac{Cardiac\ Output}{Systemic\ Vascular\ Resistance}$

    (C) $\dfrac{Cardiac\ Output}{Body\ Surface\ Area}$

    (D) $\dfrac{Cardiac\ Output}{Heart\ Rate}$

    Rationale: Cardiac index is a measure of cardiac output comparable among individuals of differing body habitus. Cardiac index is calculated by dividing the cardiac output by the body surface area.

    Reference: Butterworth JF IV, Mackey DC, Wasnick JD, eds. *Morgan & Mikhail's Clinical Anesthesiology.* 7th ed. New York, NY: McGraw Hill; 2022: Chapter 20.

20. What is the goal of hemodynamic management for patients with mitral stenosis?

    (A) Avoiding bradycardia
    (B) Maintenance of sinus rhythm
    (C) Aggressive volume resuscitation
    (D) Inotropic support with phosphodiesterase inhibitors

    Rationale: The patient with mitral stenosis has impaired left ventricular filling. Sinus rhythm's atrial contractions help optimize left ventricular filling. Maintenance of sinus rhythm at a normal rate should be a perioperative goal. Tachycardia should be avoided as it will decrease diastolic left ventricular filling time and left ventricular end diastolic pressure. Mitral stenosis is associated with left atrial and pulmonary hypertension due to the stenotic transvalvular pressure gradient. Phosphodiesterase inhibitors cause vasodilation and increase left ventricular emptying which will result in severe hypotension. Noninotropic vasopressors such as vasopressin or phenylephrine should be used in the presence of hypotension.

    Reference: Butterworth JF IV, Mackey DC, Wasnick JD, eds. *Morgan & Mikhail's Clinical Anesthesiology.* 7th ed. New York, NY: McGraw Hill; 2022: Chapter 20.

21. A peribulbar block was performed. There was notable resistance during the injection. The patient becomes agitated and complains of pain. What do you suspect?

(A) Retrobulbar hemorrhage

(B) Globe puncture

(C) Extraocular muscle palsy

(D) Intravascular injection

Rationale: Globe puncture is associated with increased IOP, resistance during injection, patient agitation and pain, and hemorrhage. In a retrobulbar hemorrhage, the eye moves forward. There may be subconjunctival bleeding. Extraocular muscle palsy results in diplopia. Intravascular injection of local anesthetic during eye blocks result in seizures.

References: Butterworth JF IV, Mackey DC, Wasnick JD, eds. *Morgan & Mikhail's Clinical Anesthesiology.* 7th ed. New York, NY: McGraw Hill; 2022: Chapter 36.

Elisha S, Heiner JS, Nagelhout JJ. *Nurse Anesthesia.* 7th ed. St. Louis, MO: Elsevier Saunders; 2023: Chapter 44.

22. Which sign is associated with placenta previa?

(A) Painless vaginal bleeding

(B) Uterine irritability

(C) Painful vaginal bleeding

(D) Coagulopathy

Rationale: Placenta previa is associated with painless vaginal bleeding and in part by malpresentation of the fetus. In contrast, placenta abruption results in painful vaginal bleeding, uterine irritability and is associated with coagulopathy.

Reference: Butterworth JF IV, Mackey DC, Wasnick JD, eds. *Morgan & Mikhail's Clinical Anesthesiology.* 7th ed. New York, NY: McGraw Hill; 2022: Chapter 41.

23. What sign is not an effect of hyperparathyroidism?

(A) Hypertension

(B) Ventricular arrhythmias

(C) Muscle weakness

(D) Hypochloremic metabolic acidosis

Rationale: Hyperchloremic metabolic acidosis is a renal effect of hyperparathyroidism.

References: Butterworth JF IV, Mackey DC, Wasnick JD, eds. *Morgan & Mikhail's Clinical Anesthesiology.* 7th ed. New York, NY: McGraw Hill; 2022: Chapter 35.

Elisha S, Heiner JS, Nagelhout JJ. *Nurse Anesthesia.* 7th ed. St. Louis, MO: Elsevier Saunders; 2023: Chapter 37.

TABLE 4-2. Effects of hyperparathyroidism.

Cardiovascular
Hypertension
Ventricular arrhythmias
ECG changes (shortened QT interval,[1] widened T wave)

Renal
Polyuria
Impaired renal concentrating ability
Kidney stones
Hyperchloremic metabolic acidosis
Dehydration
Polydipsia
Kidney failure

Gastrointestinal
Constipation
Nausea and vomiting
Anorexia
Pancreatitis
Peptic ulcer disease

Musculoskeletal
Muscle weakness
Osteoporosis

Neurological
Mental status change (e.g., delirium, psychosis, coma)

[1]The QT interval may be prolonged at serum calcium concentrations >16 mg/dL. ECG, electrocardiogram.
(Reproduced with permission from Butterworth JF IV, Mackey DC, Wasnick JD, eds. *Morgan & Mikhail's Clinical Anesthesiology.* 7th ed. New York: McGraw Hill; 2022.)

24. Which factor does not contribute to respiratory fatigue in neonates and infants?

(A) Weaker intercostal muscles

(B) More horizontal ribs

(C) Sunken abdomen

(D) Decreased chest wall compliance

Rationale: Factors contributing to respiratory fatigue in neonates and infants include a weaker diaphragm and intercostal muscles due to fewer Type I muscle fibers. Neonates and infants also have more horizontal and pliable ribs as well as a protuberant abdomen that affect efficient ventilation.

References: Butterworth JF IV, Mackey DC, Wasnick JD, eds. *Morgan & Mikhail's Clinical Anesthesiology.* 7th ed. New York, NY: McGraw Hill; 2022: Chapter 42.

Hall JE. *Guyton and Hall Textbook of Medical Physiology.* 14th ed. Philadelphia, PA: Saunders Elsevier; 2021: Chapter 84.

25. Which valvular disorder leads to left ventricular volume?

(A) Mitral stenosis

(B) Aortic stenosis

(C) Mitral regurgitation

(D) Aortic regurgitation

Rationale: This question is an application of the left-ventricular pressure-volume loops for patients with valvular heart disease. Aortic regurgitation causes volume overload of the left ventricle.

Reference: Butterworth JF IV, Mackey DC, Wasnick JD, eds. *Morgan & Mikhail's Clinical Anesthesiology.* 7th ed. New York, NY: McGraw Hill; 2022: Chapter 21.

26. Which narcotic analgesic is not used for patient-controlled analgesia (PCA)?

(A) Meperidine

(B) Morphine

(C) Fentanyl

(D) Hydromorphone

Rationale: The demerol metabolite normeperidine is neurotoxic. Therefore, it is not recommended for PCA.

Reference: Elisha S, Heiner JS, Nagelhout JJ. *Nurse Anesthesia.* 7th ed. St. Louis, MO: Elsevier Saunders; 2023: Chapter 51.

27. With which patient would the anesthetist most want to maintain spontaneous ventilation while under general anesthesia?

(A) Severe aortic stenosis

(B) Severe mitral regurgitation

(C) Acute pulmonary edema

(D) Mitral valve prolapse

Rationale: Positive pressure ventilation decreases the heart's preload. Severe aortic stenosis leads to left ventricular diastolic dysfunction secondary to left ventricular hypertrophy. This diastolic dysfunction combined with outflow obstruction makes patients with aortic stenosis extremely sensitive to decreases in preload (left ventricular end diastolic volume). Mitral regurgitation and pulmonary edema may benefit from positive pressure ventilation.

Reference: Butterworth JF IV, Mackey DC, Wasnick JD, eds. *Morgan & Mikhail's Clinical Anesthesiology.* 7th ed. New York, NY: McGraw Hill; 2022: Chapter 21.

28. The a-wave on the central venous pressure tracing corresponds to which on the EKG tracing?

(A) P wave

(B) QRS wave

(C) QT interval

(D) T wave

Rationale: The a-wave on the venous tracing corresponds to atrial contraction. The P wave corresponds to atrial depolarization couple to atrial contraction.

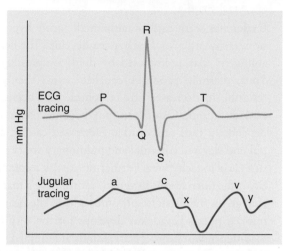

FIG. 4-1. The upward waves (*a, c, v*) and the downward descents (*x, y*) of a central venous tracing in relation to the electrocardiogram (ECG). (Reproduced with permission from Butterworth JF IV, Mackey DC, Wasnick JD, eds. *Morgan & Mikhail's Clinical Anesthesiology.* 7th ed. New York: McGraw Hill; 2022.)

Reference: Butterworth JF IV, Mackey DC, Wasnick JD, eds. *Morgan & Mikhail's Clinical Anesthesiology.* 7th ed. New York, NY: McGraw Hill; 2022: Chapter 5.

29. What do you anticipate during laparoscopic cholecystectomy for an obese patient?

(A) Increased functional residual capacity

(B) Increased closing capacity

(C) Decreased functional residual capacity

(D) Decreased peak inspiratory pressure

Rationale: Obesity results in decreased vital capacity, inspiratory capacity, and expiratory reserve volume. Due to insufflation with carbon dioxide, the functional residual capacity and closing capacity are decreased. The peak inspiratory pressure is increased. Respiratory compliance and lung volumes are low.

References: Gropper MA, Cohen NH, Eriksson LI, et al, eds. *Miller's Anesthesia.* 9th ed. Philadelphia, PA: Churchill Livingstone Elsevier; 2020: Chapter 58.

Elisha S, Heiner JS, Nagelhout JJ. *Nurse Anesthesia.* 7th ed. St. Louis, MO: Elsevier Saunders; 2023: Chapter 48.

30. Which of the following symptoms is consistent with Cardiac tamponade?

(A) Hypotension, tachycardia, tachypnea, muffled heart sounds, and pulsus paradoxus

(B) Hypertension, tachycardia, tachypnea, and widened pulse pressure

(C) Jugular venous distension, muffled heart sounds, and bradycardia

(D) Hypotension, widened pulse pressure, and tachycardia

Rationale: With cardiac tamponade, acute hypotension, tachycardia, and tachypnea develop. The heart's ability to relax is impaired by fluid compressing it. Thus, diastolic pressures equalize across the heart resulting in decreased stroke volume and decreased cardiac output. Cardiac output becomes heart rate dependent, thus tachycardia. Decreased cardiac output and elevated left atrial and pulmonary artery pressures lead to tachypnea. Furthermore, with respiratory effort the fluctuations in venous return have a marked change on the diastolic pressures within the heart. A marked pulsus paradoxus develops for the very preload-dependent heart. Heart sounds are muffled.

Reference: Butterworth JF IV, Mackey DC, Wasnick JD, eds. *Morgan & Mikhail's Clinical Anesthesiology.* 7th ed. New York, NY: McGraw Hill; 2022: Chapter 21.

31. Which of the following is an absolute contraindication for electroconvulsive therapy (ECT)?

(A) Myocardial infarction <6 weeks

(B) Intercranial mass

(C) Glaucoma

(D) Pregnancy

Rationale: A recent myocardial infarction <3 months and stroke <1 month are contraindications for ECT. Absolute contraindications also include intracranial mass and/or surgery, and cervical spine instability. Glaucoma and pregnancy are relative contraindications to ECT. Other relative contraindications include cardiac dysfunction (angina, CHF), bone fractures, thrombophlebitis, retinal detachment, and pulmonary disease.

Reference: Butterworth JF IV, Mackey DC, Wasnick JD, eds. *Morgan & Mikhail's Clinical Anesthesiology.* 7th ed. New York, NY: McGraw Hill; 2022: Chapter 28.

32. What is the most common cause of acute epiglottitis?

(A) *Streptococcus pneumoniae*

(B) Allergic reaction

(C) *Haemophilus influenza B*

(D) COVID-19 infection

Rationale: *Haemophilus influenza B* bacteria most commonly cause acute epiglottitis.

References: Butterworth JF IV, Mackey DC, Wasnick JD, eds. *Morgan & Mikhail's Clinical Anesthesiology.* 7th ed. New York, NY: McGraw Hill; 2022: Chapter 42.

Pardo MC Jr, ed. *Basics of Anesthesia.* 8th ed. Philadelphia, PA: Elsevier Saunders; 2023: Chapter 31.

33. The patient is scheduled for a thyroidectomy. Which of the following is not a primary anesthetic concern?

(A) Arrhythmias

(B) Tachycardia

(C) Body temperature

(D) Hypotension

Rationale: Each of the options should concern the anesthetist when caring for a hyperthyroid patient. However, the primary concerns focus on decreasing sympathetic stimulation that leads to cardiac arrhythmias, hypertension, tachycardia, and increased body temperature. Corneal abrasion is possible in patients with exophthalmos. Hypotension may result from chronic hypovolemia.

References: Butterworth JF IV, Mackey DC, Wasnick JD, eds. *Morgan & Mikhail's Clinical Anesthesiology.* 7th ed. New York, NY: McGraw Hill; 2022: Chapter 35.

Elisha S, Heiner JS, Nagelhout JJ. *Nurse Anesthesia.* 7th ed. St. Louis, MO: Elsevier Saunders; 2023: Chapter 37.

34. What is the lowest recommended $PaCO_2$ if hyperventilation is used during intracranial tumor resection?

(A) 35 mmHg

(B) 30 mmHg

(C) 25 mmHg

(D) 20 mmHg

Rationale: The recommended $PaCO_2$ range during induced hypocapnia is 30 to 35 mmHg.

References: Butterworth JF IV, Mackey DC, Wasnick JD, eds. *Morgan & Mikhail's Clinical Anesthesiology.* 7th ed. New York, NY: McGraw Hill; 2022: Chapter 27.

Elisha S, Heiner JS, Nagelhout JJ. *Nurse Anesthesia.* 7th ed. St. Louis, MO: Elsevier Saunders; 2023: Chapter 31.

35. How is coronary perfusion pressure defined?

(A) Difference between mean arterial pressure and central venous pressure

(B) Difference between aortic diastolic pressure and left-ventricular end-diastolic pressure

(C) Difference between aortic systolic pressure and left-ventricular end-diastolic pressure

(D) Difference between systolic pressure and central venous pressure

Rationale: Left-ventricular perfusion mostly occurs during diastole, when the force of the aortic diastolic pressure drives blood through the coronary arteries, overcoming the intramural left-ventricular end-diastolic pressure. During systole, aortic pressure is unable to overcome the higher left-ventricular systolic pressures to generate flow.

Reference: Butterworth JF IV, Mackey DC, Wasnick JD, eds. *Morgan & Mikhail's Clinical Anesthesiology.* 7th ed. New York, NY: McGraw Hill; 2022: Chapter 21.

36. What results when a limb tourniquet is released?

    (A) Hypokalemia
    (B) Metabolic acidosis
    (C) Metabolic alkalosis
    (D) Bradycardia

    Rationale: When a tourniquet is released products of cellular metabolic waste enter the circulation. Hypotension, tachycardia, and increased minute ventilation occur. The end-tidal CO_2 serum potassium and lactate increase. Hyperkalemia, myoglobinuria, and renal failure may occur.

    References: Butterworth JF IV, Mackey DC, Wasnick JD, eds. *Morgan & Mikhail's Clinical Anesthesiology.* 7th ed. New York, NY: McGraw Hill; 2022: Chapter 38.
    Elisha S, Heiner JS, Nagelhout JJ. *Nurse Anesthesia.* 7th ed. St. Louis, MO: Elsevier Saunders; 2023: Chapter 45.

37. Which patient faces the greatest risk of complete cardiovascular collapse?

    (A) 75-year-old female with bilateral carotid artery disease with an aortic valve area of 1.1 cm^2 undergoing left carotid endarterectomy
    (B) 82-year-old male with severe mitral regurgitation and severe tricuspid regurgitation with atrial fibrillation undergoing bowel resection for colon cancer
    (C) 67-year-old male with aortic valve area of 0.7 cm^2 undergoing left carotid endarterectomy
    (D) 59-year-old male with aortic valve area of 0.7 cm^2 undergoing colon resection for ischemic colon

    Rationale: Aortic valve area of 0.7 cm^2 is indicative of severe aortic stenosis. In severe aortic stenosis, changes in intravascular volume and decreases in afterload can lead to critical coronary ischemia. Patients with advanced aortic stenosis are particularly sensitive to hypotension. Aortic stenosis leads to left ventricular hypertrophy due to elevated left ventricular pressures. This, in turn, leads to both an increase in oxygen

demand (due to hypertrophy and increased left ventricular systolic pressures) and a decrease in myocardial perfusion (due to left ventricular end-diastolic pressure). Abdominal surgeries in general, and colon resections (especially with ischemia which can lead to septic shock like states) in particular, are known for fluid shifts and decreases in afterload secondary to release of vasodilatory substances. Hypotension can quickly deteriorate to ventricular dysrhythmias and complete cardiovascular collapse necessitating cardiopulmonary resuscitation, even resulting in death.

Reference: Butterworth JF IV, Mackey DC, Wasnick JD, eds. *Morgan & Mikhail's Clinical Anesthesiology.* 7th ed. New York, NY: McGraw Hill; 2022: Chapter 21.

38. What risk factor places patients at greater risk of perioperative vision loss (POVL)?

    (A) Low estimated blood loss
    (B) Prolonged surgery in the head down position
    (C) Controlled hypertension
    (D) Thin stature

    Rationale: POVL may occur in prolonged spine surgery in the head down position. Large blood loss, hypotension, smoking, obesity, and diabetes are contributing factors. Ischemic optic neuropathy, perioperative glaucoma, cortical hypotension, and embolism are precursors to POVL.

    Reference: Butterworth JF IV, Mackey DC, Wasnick JD, eds. *Morgan & Mikhail's Clinical Anesthesiology.* 7th ed. New York, NY: McGraw Hill; 2022: Chapter 27.

39. While observing the fetal heart monitor during labor you note a decreased fetal heart rate. What is the probable cause?

    (A) Epidural opioids
    (B) Terbutaline
    (C) Ritodrine
    (D) Atropine

    Rationale: Fetal tachycardia is linked to beta-adrenergic agonists (ritodrine, terbutaline), atropine, and epinephrine. Epidural or intrathecal analgesia contributes to lowering the fetal heart rate particularly with repeated dosing. This occurs indirectly most often due to maternal hypotension.

    Reference: Chestnut DH, Wong CA, Tsen LC, et al, eds. *Chestnut's Obstetric Anesthesia Principles and Practice.* 6th ed. Philadelphia, PA: Mosby Elsevier; 2020: Chapter 13.

40. Estimate the total difference in cerebral blood flow if $PaCO_2$ is decreased from 40 mmHg to 34 mmHg. Assume total brain weight is 1,400 g.

(A) 0 to 50 mL/min

(B) 30 to 60 mL/min

(C) 60 to 120 mL/min

(D) 90 to 180 mL/min

Rationale: The change in cerebral blood flow is 1 or 2 mL/100 g/min for every 1 mmHg change in $PaCO_2$.

References: Butterworth JF IV, Mackey DC, Wasnick JD, eds. *Morgan & Mikhail's Clinical Anesthesiology.* 7th ed. New York, NY: McGraw Hill; 2022: Chapter 26.

Gropper MA, Cohen NH, Eriksson LI, et al, eds. *Miller's Anesthesia.* 9th ed. Philadelphia, PA: Churchill Livingstone Elsevier; 2020: Chapter 11.

41. Which of the following rate control agents should be avoided in a patient undergoing general anesthesia with acute onset wide-complex supraventricular tachycardia (SVT)?

(A) Digitalis

(B) Adenosine

(C) Esmolol

(D) Amiodarone

Rationale: The type of SVT is unknown. If a reentrant pathway is present, blocking the AV node digoxin may exacerbate tachycardia while limiting other treatment options.

Reference: Butterworth JF IV, Mackey DC, Wasnick JD, eds. *Morgan & Mikhail's Clinical Anesthesiology.* 7th ed. New York, NY: McGraw Hill; 2022: Chapter 21.

42. Which factor contributes to the rapid development of hypoxia seen during apnea in neonates?

(A) High functional residual capacity

(B) Low basal metabolic rate

(C) High oxygen reserve

(D) High oxygen demand

Rationale: Neonates and infants have relatively low functional residual capacity coupled with increased oxygen demand.

References: Butterworth JF IV, Mackey DC, Wasnick JD, eds. *Morgan & Mikhail's Clinical Anesthesiology.* 7th ed. New York, NY: McGraw Hill; 2022: Chapter 42.

Elisha S, Heiner JS, Nagelhout JJ. *Nurse Anesthesia.* 7th ed. St. Louis, MO: Elsevier Saunders; 2023: Chapter 52.

43. What is cerebral metabolic rate?

(A) 3.5 mL/100 g/min

(B) 5 mL/100 g/min

(C) 100 mL/min

(D) 250 mL/min

Rationale: The cerebral metabolic rate averages from 3 to 3.8 mL/100 g/min.

References: Butterworth JF IV, Mackey DC, Wasnick JD, eds. *Morgan & Mikhail's Clinical Anesthesiology.* 7th ed. New York, NY: McGraw Hill; 2022: Chapter 26.

Hall JE. *Guyton and Hall Textbook of Medical Physiology.* 14th ed. Philadelphia, PA: Saunders Elsevier; 2021: Chapter 62.

44. A 100-kg patient is administered 40,000 units of heparin. Five minutes later the ACT was measured to be 182 seconds. What is the next step?

(A) Proceed with cardiopulmonary bypass.

(B) Wait 5 more minutes and recheck ACT.

(C) Administer an additional 40,000 units of heparin.

(D) Administer two units of fresh frozen plasma.

Rationale: The dose administered is appropriate (300-400 units/kg) to obtain an ACT necessary for initiating cardiopulmonary bypass, 400 to 800 seconds. Typically, this therapeutic anticoagulation is obtained and verified within 3 to 5 minutes of administration. A patient may have an antithrombin III deficiency that renders them resistant to the effects of heparin. Recombinant antithrombin III can be administered, but more commonly two units of fresh frozen plasma are administered to provide the antithrombin III necessary to achieve adequate anticoagulation.

Reference: Butterworth JF IV, Mackey DC, Wasnick JD, eds. *Morgan & Mikhail's Clinical Anesthesiology.* 7th ed. New York, NY: McGraw Hill; 2022: Chapter 22.

45. Because you are concerned with factors contributing to cerebral ischemia during mediastinoscopy, where will you place the blood pressure cuff and arterial line?

(A) Blood pressure cuff on right arm, arterial line in left hand

(B) Blood pressure cuff on right arm, pulse oximeter on right hand

(C) Blood pressure cuff on left arm, arterial line in right hand

(D) Blood pressure cuff on left arm, pulse oximeter on left hand

Rationale: Because there may be compression of the innominate artery as it passes through the upper thorax, there is concern about decreased blood flow to the right common carotid artery, to the right vertebral artery and a decrease in subclavian flow to the right hand. Therefore, monitoring perfusion to the right hand with either a pulse oximeter waveform or radial arterial waveform can detect decreased flow to the right arm.

References: Butterworth JF IV, Mackey DC, Wasnick JD, eds. *Morgan & Mikhail's Clinical Anesthesiology.* 7th ed. New York, NY: McGraw Hill; 2022: Chapter 25.

Elisha S, Heiner JS, Nagelhout JJ. *Nurse Anesthesia.* 7th ed. St. Louis, MO: Elsevier Saunders; 2023: Chapter 30.

46. Which symptom is not present in advanced aortic stenosis?

   (A) Angina

   (B) Dyspnea on exertion

   (C) Orthostatic syncope

   (D) Dyspnea at rest

Rationale: Angina, dyspnea on exertion, orthostatic, and/or exertional syncope are the classic triad of aortic stenosis symptoms.

Reference: Butterworth JF IV, Mackey DC, Wasnick JD, eds. *Morgan & Mikhail's Clinical Anesthesiology.* 7th ed. New York, NY: McGraw Hill; 2022: Chapter 21.

47. Which nerve is at greatest risk for injury during thyroid surgery?

   (A) Recurrent laryngeal nerve

   (B) Superior laryngeal nerve

   (C) Facial nerve

   (D) Glossopharyngeal nerve

Rationale: Injury is greatest for surgery involving the superior laryngeal nerve.

References: Butterworth JF IV, Mackey DC, Wasnick JD, eds. *Morgan & Mikhail's Clinical Anesthesiology.* 7th ed. New York, NY: McGraw Hill; 2022: Chapter 37.

Elisha S, Heiner JS, Nagelhout JJ. *Nurse Anesthesia.* 7th ed. St. Louis, MO: Elsevier Saunders; 2023: Chapter 37.

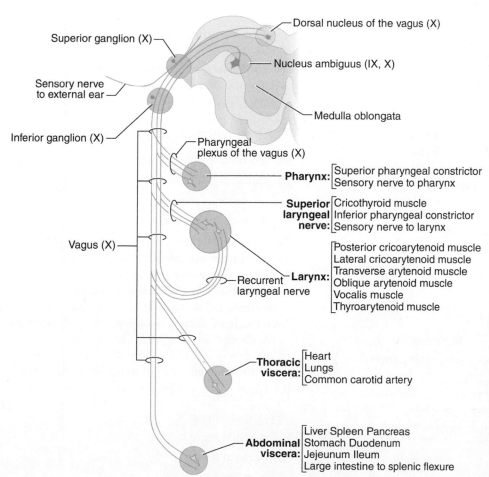

FIG. 4-2. The **vagus nerve** (cranial nerve X) originates in the medulla oblongata and then ramifies in the superior and inferior vagal ganglia in the neck. Its first major branch is the pharyngeal plexus of the vagus. The **superior laryngeal nerve** divides into the external and internal laryngeal nerves. The *internal branch* supplies sensory innervation of the laryngeal mucosa above the vocal cords, and the *external branch* innervates the inferior pharyngeal constrictor muscles and the cricothyroid muscle of the larynx. Cricothyroid muscle contraction increases the voice pitch by lengthening, tensing, and adducting the vocal folds. The superior laryngeal nerve is at risk of damage during operations of the anterior neck, especially thyroid surgery, and injury to this nerve may result in hoarseness and loss of vocal volume. The next branch of the vagus is the **recurrent laryngeal nerve**, which innervates all of the muscles of the larynx except the cricothyroid, and is responsible for phonation and glottic opening. The recurrent laryngeal nerve runs immediately behind the thyroid gland and thus is the nerve at greatest risk for injury during thyroid surgery. Unilateral recurrent laryngeal nerve damage may result in vocal changes or hoarseness, and bilateral nerve damage may result in aphonia and respiratory distress. Inferior to this nerve, the vagus nerve provides autonomic motor and sensory nerve fibers to the thoracic and abdominal viscera. (Reproduced with permission from Dillon FX. Electromyographic (EMG) neuromonitoring in otolaryngology-head and neck surgery. *Anesthesiol Clin.* 2010;28(3):423-442.)

48. Which statement is true regarding gastrointestinal changes during pregnancy?

(A) Pregnant patients are not considered a "full stomach."

(B) Gastric acid increases.

(C) Gastric volume increases.

(D) Lower esophageal sphincter relaxation occurs due to progesterone and estrogen.

Rationale: Gastric acid and gastric volume are unaffected by pregnancy. Mechanical changes that affect the stomach and lower esophageal sphincter place the parturient at high risk for aspiration.

References: Butterworth JF IV, Mackey DC, Wasnick JD, eds. *Morgan & Mikhail's Clinical Anesthesiology*. 7th ed. New York, NY: McGraw Hill; 2022: Chapter 40.

Suresh MS, Segal BS, Preston RL, Fernando R, Mason CL, eds. *Shnider and Levinson's Anesthesia for Obstetrics*. 5th ed. Philadelphia, PA: Lippincott Williams & Wilkins; 2013: Chapter 1.

49. What is the cervical level of the larynx in a child?

(A) C_1–C_3

(B) C_2–C_4

(C) C_3–C_5

(D) C_4–C_7

Rationale: The larynx in a small child is adjacent to cervical vertebrae 2-4 with the glottis adjacent to C_4.

References: Butterworth JF IV, Mackey DC, Wasnick JD, eds. *Morgan & Mikhail's Clinical Anesthesiology*. 7th ed. New York, NY: McGraw Hill; 2022: Chapter 42.

Pardo MC Jr, ed. *Basics of Anesthesia*. 8th ed. Philadelphia, PA: Elsevier Saunders; 2023: Chapter 34.

50. How does general anesthesia affect the functional residual capacity (FRC)?

(A) Increases FRC by 50%

(B) Decreases FRC by 20%

(C) Increases FRC by 20%

(D) Decreases FRC by 50%

Rationale: A 20% decrease in FRC exists for non-obese patients. For obese patients undergoing general anesthesia, FRC decreases by 50%.

Reference: Butterworth JF IV, Mackey DC, Wasnick JD, eds. *Morgan & Mikhail's Clinical Anesthesiology*. 7th ed. New York, NY: McGraw Hill; 2022: Chapter 23.

51. Which is least adaptive in an infant as compared to an adult?

(A) Heart rate

(B) Cardiac output

(C) Stroke volume

(D) Chest wall

Rationale: Stroke volume in neonates and infants is less adaptive than in an adult. Increasing heart rate is the means of increasing cardiac output.

References: Butterworth JF IV, Mackey DC, Wasnick JD, eds. *Morgan & Mikhail's Clinical Anesthesiology*. 7th ed. New York, NY: McGraw Hill; 2022: Chapter 42.

Pardo MC Jr, ed. *Basics of Anesthesia*. 8th ed. Philadelphia, PA: Elsevier Saunders; 2023: Chapter 34.

52. A spinal anesthetic is planned for an obese patient. How will you adjust the dose of local anesthetic?

(A) Decrease by 20%

(B) Increase by 20%

(C) Decrease by 10%

(D) Increase by 10%

Rationale: The dose of local anesthetic used for spinal or epidural anesthesia in obese patients is decreased by 20% to 25%.

Reference: Elisha S, Heiner JS, Nagelhout JJ. *Nurse Anesthesia*. 7th ed. St. Louis, MO: Elsevier Saunders; 2023: Chapter 48.

53. What is the primary determinant of cerebral perfusion?

(A) Position

(B) Mean arterial pressure

(C) Intracranial pressure

(D) Central venous pressure

Rationale: All of these can impact cerebral perfusion, but the primary variable is the mean arterial pressure.

References: Butterworth JF IV, Mackey DC, Wasnick JD, eds. *Morgan & Mikhail's Clinical Anesthesiology*. 7th ed. New York, NY: McGraw Hill; 2022: Chapter 26.

Pardo MC Jr, ed. *Basics of Anesthesia*. 8th ed. Philadelphia, PA: Elsevier Saunders; 2023: Chapter 30.

54. What is the efferent limb of the oculocardiac reflex?

(A) Cranial nerve V

(B) Cranial nerve X

(C) Cranial nerve I

(D) Cranial nerve III

Rationale: Trigeminal (CN V) afferent and vagal (CN X) efferent pathways comprise the oculocardiac reflex.

References: Butterworth JF IV, Mackey DC, Wasnick JD, eds. *Morgan & Mikhail's Clinical Anesthesiology.* 7th ed. New York, NY: McGraw Hill; 2022: Chapter 36.

Elisha S, Heiner JS, Nagelhout JJ. *Nurse Anesthesia.* 7th ed. St. Louis, MO: Elsevier Saunders; 2023: Chapter 44.

55. What factor is increased in a neonate as compared to an adult?

   (A) Surface area to weight ratio
   (B) Systolic blood pressure
   (C) Plasma protein concentration
   (D) Lung compliance

Rationale: Neonates have a relatively larger body surface area to mass ratio which contributes to the risk of hypothermia. (B), (C), and (D) are all decreased in the neonate compared to the adult.

References: Butterworth JF IV, Mackey DC, Wasnick JD, eds. *Morgan & Mikhail's Clinical Anesthesiology.* 7th ed. New York, NY: McGraw Hill; 2022: Chapter 42.

Elisha S, Heiner JS, Nagelhout JJ. *Nurse Anesthesia.* 7th ed. St. Louis, MO: Elsevier Saunders; 2023: Chapter 52.

56. When calculating medication doses for obese patients, what is the best weight parameter to use?

   (A) Total body weight
   (B) Ideal body weight
   (C) Lean body weight
   (D) Total body mass index

Rationale: High plasma concentrations result when administering IV medications to obese patients based on total body weight. This is due to poor blood flow to fat. Lean body weight is the parameter used for calculating medications for obese patients. Lean body weight does not include fat weight. Neither ideal body weight nor body mass index is used to calculate IV medications for obese patients.

Reference: Hines RL, Marschall KE. *Stoelting's Anesthesia and Co-existing Disease.* 7th ed. Philadelphia, PA: Elsevier Saunders; 2018: Chapter 19.

57. Which is true regarding morbidity and mortality in pediatric anesthesia?

   (A) Anesthetic risk is directly related to patient age.
   (B) Anesthetic risk is greatest in patients younger than 1 year.
   (C) Anesthetic risk is greater now than in the past.
   (D) Anesthetic risk is similar throughout childhood.

Rationale: Pediatric anesthetic morbidity and mortality are inversely related to age with greatest risk in patients younger than 1 year.

References: Butterworth JF IV, Mackey DC, Wasnick JD, eds. *Morgan & Mikhail's Clinical Anesthesiology.* 7th ed. New York, NY: McGraw Hill; 2022: Chapter 42.

Longnecker DE, Mackey SC, Newman MF, Sandberg WS, Zapol WM, eds. *Anesthesiology.* 3rd ed. McGraw Hill; 2018: Chapter 59.

58. With which of the following preoperative EKG findings will the anesthetist be particularly careful to avoid bradycardia?

   (A) Sinus rhythm with prolonged QT interval
   (B) Sinus rhythm with left bundle branch block
   (C) Sinus rhythm with premature ventricular complexes
   (D) Atrial fibrillation

Rationale: Long QT may precipitate torsade de pointes. QT interval is rate dependent; slow heart rate is consistent with longer QT interval. Additionally, premature ventricular complexes are more common with bradycardia.

Reference: Butterworth JF IV, Mackey DC, Wasnick JD, eds. *Morgan & Mikhail's Clinical Anesthesiology.* 7th ed. New York, NY: McGraw Hill; 2022: Chapter 21.

59. A patient is scheduled for a total knee arthroscopy under general anesthesia. The patient's history includes retina surgery using sulfur hexafluoride 2 weeks ago. What will you avoid?

   (A) Nitrous oxide
   (B) Rocuronium
   (C) Sevoflurane
   (D) Fentanyl

Rationale: Nitrous oxide expands the gas bubble and may cause intraocular hypertension. There are no other medication contraindications.

References: Butterworth JF IV, Mackey DC, Wasnick JD, eds. *Morgan & Mikhail's Clinical Anesthesiology.* 7th ed. New York, NY: McGraw Hill; 2022: Chapter 36.

Longnecker DE, Mackey SC, Newman MF, Sandberg WS, Zapol WM, eds. *Anesthesiology.* 3rd ed. McGraw Hill; 2018: Chapter 61.

60. What is the maintenance intravenous fluid replacement rate for a toddler weighing 12 kg?

(A) 48 mL/h
(B) 44 mL/h
(C) 40 mL/h
(D) 36 mL/h

Rationale: Hourly maintenance fluid rate is calculated as 4 mL/kg/h up to 10 kg of body weight, 2 mL/kg/h for the second 10 kg of body weight, and 1 mL/kg/h for every kilogram beyond 20.

References: Butterworth JF IV, Mackey DC, Wasnick JD, eds. *Morgan & Mikhail's Clinical Anesthesiology*. 7th ed. New York, NY: McGraw Hill; 2022: Chapter 42.
Elisha S, Heiner JS, Nagelhout JJ. *Nurse Anesthesia*. 7th ed. St. Louis, MO: Elsevier Saunders; 2023: Chapter 53.

61. How much intravenous replacement should be given in the first hour of the anesthetic for a child weighing 16 kg who last had anything by mouth at 0400 if the current time is 0700?

(A) 52 mL
(B) 104 mL
(C) 208 mL
(D) 130 mL

Rationale: The maintenance replacement rate is 52 mL/h. The calculated fluid deficit is 52 mL/h over 3 hours fasted (156 mL). Half of the deficit (78 mL) is given during the first hour in addition to the maintenance rate (52 mL) for a total replacement of 130 mL during the first hour.

References: Butterworth JF IV, Mackey DC, Wasnick JD, eds. *Morgan & Mikhail's Clinical Anesthesiology*. 7th ed. New York, NY: McGraw Hill; 2022: Chapter 42.
Elisha S, Heiner JS, Nagelhout JJ. *Nurse Anesthesia*. 7th ed. St. Louis, MO: Elsevier Saunders; 2023: Chapter 53.

62. Which feature of a pediatric endotracheal tube will have greatest influence on the work of breathing?

(A) External diameter
(B) Length
(C) Internal diameter
(D) Curvature

Rationale: The internal diameter of the tube has the greatest influence on resistance.

References: Butterworth JF IV, Mackey DC, Wasnick JD, eds. *Morgan & Mikhail's Clinical Anesthesiology*. 7th ed. New York, NY: McGraw Hill; 2022: Chapter 19.

Dorsch J, Dorsch S, eds. *Understanding Anesthesia Equipment*. 5th ed. Philadelphia, PA: Wolters Kluwer Lippincott Williams & Wilkins; 2008: Chapter 19.

63. During laparoscopic bariatric surgery, you add positive end expiratory pressure (PEEP). What is the recommended upper limit?

(A) 5 cm H_2O
(B) 10 cm H_2O
(C) 15 cm H_2O
(D) 20 cm H_2O

Rationale: When using large tidal volumes, oxygenation may be impaired. Limit PEEP to 15 cm H_2O.

References: Butterworth JF IV, Mackey DC, Wasnick JD, eds. *Morgan & Mikhail's Clinical Anesthesiology*. 7th ed. New York, NY: McGraw Hill; 2022: Chapter 58.
Gropper MA, Cohen NH, Eriksson LI, et al, eds. *Miller's Anesthesia*. 9th ed. Philadelphia, PA: Churchill Livingstone Elsevier; 2020: Chapter 77.

64. Which of the following agents will cause the greatest decrease on afterload?

(A) Verapamil
(B) Nicardipine
(C) Metoprolol
(D) Nitroglycerine

Rationale: All the agents mentioned decrease afterload. Nicardipine, however, is a calcium-channel blocking agent, which is very selective for vascular smooth muscle. Verapamil is a calcium-channel blocker more selective for cardiac than vascular smooth muscle. Nitroglycerine is a nitrate that causes arterial and venodilation. The dilation from nitroglycerine is more pronounced on venous vessels. Metoprolol, a beta blocker, will have minimal to no effect on afterload. From the list, nicardipine causes the most arterial vasodilation.

Reference: Butterworth JF IV, Mackey DC, Wasnick JD, eds. *Morgan & Mikhail's Clinical Anesthesiology*. 7th ed. New York, NY: McGraw Hill; 2022: Chapter 21.

65. What is the correct depth for an endotracheal tube placed in a 4-year-old?

(A) Internal diameter 3.5 mm
(B) Internal diameter 5.0 cm
(C) Internal diameter of 4.5 mm
(D) Internal diameter of 5.0 mm

Rationale: The correct internal diameter for this age is 5 mm. The internal diameter is calculated for children: 4 + Age/4. Depth is estimated to be triple the internal diameter.

Reference: Butterworth JF IV, Mackey DC, Wasnick JD, eds. *Morgan & Mikhail's Clinical Anesthesiology.* 7th ed. New York, NY: McGraw Hill; 2022: Chapter 19.

TABLE 4-3. Oral endotracheal tube size guidelines.

Age	Internal Diameter (mm)	Cut Length (cm)
Full-term infant	3.5	12
Child	$4 + \dfrac{Age}{4}$	12 + Age/2
Adult		
Female	7.0-7.5	24
Male	7.5-9.0	24

(Reproduced with permission from Butterworth JF IV, Mackey DC, Wasnick JD, eds. *Morgan & Mikhail's Clinical Anesthesiology.* 7th ed. New York: McGraw Hill; 2022.)

66. You are planning to add fentanyl to the epidural for labor. How much will you add to the local anesthetic solution?

(A) 5 mg

(B) 10 µg

(C) 50 to 150 mcg

(D) 0.5 mg

Rationale: Fentanyl 50 to 150 mcg is the appropriate dose as an addition to labor epidural analgesia. Morphine 5 mg is also useful as well as meperidine (50-100 mcg) or sufentanil (5-20 µg). However, morphine and meperidine carry a high risk of nausea and vomiting.

TABLE 4-4. Spinal opioid dosages for labor and delivery.

Agent	Intrathecal	Epidural
Morphine	0.1-0.5 mg	5 mg
Meperidine	10-15 mg	50-100 mg
Fentanyl	10-25 mcg	50-150 mcg
Sufentanil	3-10 mcg	10-20 mcg

(Reproduced with permission from Butterworth JF IV, Mackey DC, Wasnick JD, eds. *Morgan & Mikhail's Clinical Anesthesiology.* 7th ed. New York: McGraw Hill; 2022.)

References: Butterworth JF IV, Mackey DC, Wasnick JD, eds. *Morgan & Mikhail's Clinical Anesthesiology.* 7th ed. New York, NY: McGraw Hill; 2022: Chapter 41.

Chestnut DH, Wong CA, Tsen LC, et al, eds. *Chestnut's Obstetric Anesthesia Principles and Practice.* 6th ed. Philadelphia, PA: Mosby Elsevier; 2020: Chapter 23.

67. A patient with ischemic cardiomyopathy, with a preoperative ejection fraction of 15%, presents for a general anesthetic. After induction of general anesthesia, the vital signs include a blood pressure of 79/61 mmHg and a heart rate of 54 beats/min. What intravenous drip is best?

(A) Epinephrine

(B) Vasopressin

(C) Phenylephrine

(D) Milrinone

Rationale: The most effective treatment would be to restore the circulating catecholamine levels through an epinephrine or norepinephrine drip, restoring an adequate blood pressure and cardiac output. Increasing afterload without simultaneously increasing contractility (with phenylephrine or vasopressin) may raise blood pressure for a time but decrease cardiac output and increase left-ventricular end-diastolic, thereby dangerously decreasing coronary perfusion in a patient already suffering from coronary ischemia. Milrinone will increase cardiac output but will only further decrease blood pressure by exacerbating vasodilation, thereby decreasing perfusion pressure to vital organs including the heart.

Reference: Butterworth JF IV, Mackey DC, Wasnick JD, eds. *Morgan & Mikhail's Clinical Anesthesiology.* 7th ed. New York, NY: McGraw Hill; 2022: Chapter 20.

68. Which solution is appropriate for replacement of calculated fluid deficits, blood loss, or third-space loss in the pediatric patient?

(A) Lactated Ringer's

(B) 5% dextrose in water

(C) 5% dextrose in 0.45% normal saline

(D) 25% albumin

Rationale: Lactated Ringer's is a common and appropriate choice for volume replacement. To prevent hyperglycemia in children, avoid dextrose containing solutions.

References: Butterworth JF IV, Mackey DC, Wasnick JD, eds. *Morgan & Mikhail's Clinical Anesthesiology.* 7th ed. New York, NY: McGraw Hill; 2022: Chapter 42.

Gropper MA, Cohen NH, Eriksson LI, et al, eds. *Miller's Anesthesia.* 9th ed. Philadelphia, PA: Churchill Livingstone Elsevier; 2020: Chapter 77.

69. Which estimation of blood volume per kilogram is correct for a 2-week-old?

(A) 65 mL

(B) 75 mL

(C) 85 mL

(D) 95 mL

Rationale: Blood volume in the neonatal period is estimated to be between 80 and 90 mL/kg.

References: Butterworth JF IV, Mackey DC, Wasnick JD, eds. *Morgan & Mikhail's Clinical Anesthesiology.* 7th ed. New York, NY: McGraw Hill; 2022: Chapter 42.

Gropper MA, Cohen NH, Eriksson LI, et al, eds. *Miller's Anesthesia.* 9th ed. Philadelphia, PA: Churchill Livingstone Elsevier; 2020: Chapter 77.

Elisha S, Heiner JS, Nagelhout JJ. *Nurse Anesthesia.* 7th ed. St. Louis, MO: Elsevier Saunders; 2023: Chapter 53.

70. Which patient requires the highest minimum alveolar concentration (MAC)?

(A) Newborn of 35 weeks gestation

(B) A 4-month-old

(C) An 18-month-old

(D) A 3-year-old

Rationale: Infants greater than 3 to 6 months of age have the highest MAC.

References: Butterworth JF IV, Mackey DC, Wasnick JD, eds. *Morgan & Mikhail's Clinical Anesthesiology.* 7th ed. New York, NY: McGraw Hill; 2022: Chapter 42.

Gropper MA, Cohen NH, Eriksson LI, et al, eds. *Miller's Anesthesia.* 9th ed. Philadelphia, PA: Churchill Livingstone Elsevier; 2020: Chapter 77.

71. If intramuscular succinylcholine were indicated, what would be the correct dose for a 1-year-old child?

(A) 0.5 mg/kg

(B) 4.5 mg/kg

(C) 6 mg/kg

(D) 4 mg/kg

Rationale: Intramuscular succinylcholine can be administered for emergency airway management in children. The dose is 4 to 5 mg/kg for children older than 6 months.

References: Butterworth JF IV, Mackey DC, Wasnick JD, eds. *Morgan & Mikhail's Clinical Anesthesiology.* 7th ed. New York, NY: McGraw Hill; 2022: Chapter 42.

Gropper MA, Cohen NH, Eriksson LI, et al, eds. *Miller's Anesthesia.* 9th ed. Philadelphia, PA: Churchill Livingstone Elsevier; 2020: Chapter 77.

72. Why does an infant require an increased induction dose (mg/kg) of propofol than an adult?

(A) Enzyme induction

(B) Increased central volume of distribution

(C) Immature renal function

(D) Decreased adipose for redistribution

Rationale: Infants require larger per-kilogram induction doses of propofol because of a relatively larger central volume of distribution.

References: Butterworth JF IV, Mackey DC, Wasnick JD, eds. *Morgan & Mikhail's Clinical Anesthesiology.* 7th ed. New York, NY: McGraw Hill; 2022: Chapter 42.

Gropper MA, Cohen NH, Eriksson LI, et al, eds. *Miller's Anesthesia.* 9th ed. Philadelphia, PA: Churchill Livingstone Elsevier; 2020: Chapter 77.

73. What is the best means to avoid lung overdistension for obese ventilated patients?

(A) Tidal volume 10 to 15 mL/kg

(B) Tidal volume 12 to 15 mL/kg

(C) Tidal volume 6 to 10 mL/kg

(D) Tidal volume 4 to 8 mL/kg

Rationale: Methods to minimize overdistension of the lung in obese patients include increasing the ventilation rate, keeping the end-inspiratory pressure <30 cm H_2O and using a tidal volume of 6 to 10 mL/kg.

References: Butterworth JF IV, Mackey DC, Wasnick JD, eds. *Morgan & Mikhail's Clinical Anesthesiology.* 7th ed. New York, NY: McGraw Hill; 2022: Chapter 34

Elisha S, Heiner JS, Nagelhout JJ. *Nurse Anesthesia.* 7th ed. St. Louis, MO: Elsevier Saunders; 2023: Chapter 48.

74. Which patient is at greatest risk of central apnea following anesthesia?

(A) A 3-month-old born at 40 weeks gestation

(B) A 9-week-old born at 39 weeks gestation

(C) A 4-month-old born at 30 weeks gestation

(D) An 8-month-old born at 28 weeks gestation

Rationale: Calendar age plus gestational age yields post conceptual age. History of premature birth and postconceptual age less than 50 to 60 weeks pose an increase in the risk of postoperative central apnea.

References: Butterworth JF IV, Mackey DC, Wasnick JD, eds. *Morgan & Mikhail's Clinical Anesthesiology.* 7th ed. New York, NY: McGraw Hill; 2022: Chapter 42.

Pardo MC Jr, ed. *Basics of Anesthesia.* 8th ed. Philadelphia, PA: Elsevier Saunders; 2023: Chapter 34.

75. Following administration of intrathecal anesthesia for cesarean section the patient is unable to speak, loses consciousness, and is hypotensive. What is the most likely cause?

(A) High spinal

(B) Use of ropivacaine

(C) Spinal hematoma

(D) Use of bupivacaine

Rationale: Hypotension is a common side effect of intrathecal anesthesia. Causative factors for high spinals include lack of adjustment in dosages for pregnant patients as well as excessive spread of the local anesthetic. For cesarean section, a T_4 level is desired. All local anesthetics may produce a high spinal. Spinal hematoma produces symptoms including severe back and leg pain and motor weakness.

References: Butterworth JF IV, Mackey DC, Wasnick JD, eds. *Morgan & Mikhail's Clinical Anesthesiology.* 7th ed. New York, NY: McGraw Hill; 2022: Chapter 4.

Longnecker DE, Mackey SC, Newman MF, Sandberg WS, Zapol WM, eds. *Anesthesiology.* 3rd ed. McGraw Hill; 2018: Chapter 42.

76. What is the best position for optimizing airway patency during pediatric airway management?

(A) Small pad placed under the shoulders

(B) Small pad placed behind the head

(C) The "sniffing position"

(D) "Ramp" of towels behind the back

Rationale: A small pad under the shoulders compensates for the disproportionately large occiput.

References: Butterworth JF IV, Mackey DC, Wasnick JD, eds. *Morgan & Mikhail's Clinical Anesthesiology.* 7th ed. New York, NY: McGraw Hill; 2022: Chapter 42.

Longnecker DE, Mackey SC, Newman MF, Sandberg WS, Zapol WM, eds. *Anesthesiology.* 3rd ed. McGraw Hill; 2018: Chapter 59.

77. What is the best indication for a caudal block in a pediatric patient?

(A) Anesthesia or analgesia for procedures below the xyphoid process

(B) Analgesia for the first stage of labor

(C) Anesthesia or analgesia for procedures below the umbilicus

(D) Significant deformity of the sacral region

Rationale: Caudal anesthesia is indicated to supplement general anesthesia or provide analgesia for procedures below the level of the umbilicus.

References: Butterworth JF IV, Mackey DC, Wasnick JD, eds. *Morgan & Mikhail's Clinical Anesthesiology.* 7th ed. New York, NY: McGraw Hill; 2022: Chapter 42.

Gropper MA, Cohen NH, Eriksson LI, et al, eds. *Miller's Anesthesia.* 9th ed. Philadelphia, PA: Churchill Livingstone Elsevier; 2020: Chapter 77.

Chestnut DH, Wong CA, Tsen LC, et al, eds. *Chestnut's Obstetric Anesthesia Principles and Practice.* 6th ed. Philadelphia, PA: Mosby Elsevier; 2020: Chapter 12.

78. Which valve disorder most likely predisposes a patient to coronary ischemia with hypotension?

(A) Mitral stenosis

(B) Mitral regurgitation

(C) Aortic stenosis

(D) Aortic regurgitation

Rationale: Patients with advanced aortic stenosis are extremely sensitive to hypotension. Aortic stenosis leads to left ventricular hypertrophy due to elevated left ventricular pressures. This leads to both an increase in oxygen demand (hypertrophy and increased left ventricular systolic pressures) and a decrease in myocardial perfusion due to left ventricular end-diastolic pressure, which is elevated even early in disease progression.

Reference: Butterworth JF IV, Mackey DC, Wasnick JD, eds. *Morgan & Mikhail's Clinical Anesthesiology.* 7th ed. New York, NY: McGraw Hill; 2022: Chapter 21.

79. What is the hallmark laboratory finding associated with pyloric stenosis?

(A) Hypokalemic hypochloremic metabolic acidosis

(B) Hypokalemic hyperchloremic metabolic alkalosis

(C) Hyperkalemic hypochloremic metabolic acidosis

(D) Hypochloremic metabolic alkalosis

Rationale: Vomiting causes loss of stomach acid and electrolytes. Loss of potassium, chloride, hydrogen, and sodium ions results in hypochloremic metabolic alkalosis.

References: Butterworth JF IV, Mackey DC, Wasnick JD, eds. *Morgan & Mikhail's Clinical Anesthesiology.* 7th ed. New York, NY: McGraw Hill; 2022: Chapter 42.

Jaffe RA, ed. *Anesthesiologist's Manual of Surgical Procedures.* 6th ed. Lippincott Williams & Wilkins; 2020: Chapter 12.5.

80. Which of the following is true regarding a patient with septal defects?

(A) An increase in SVR relative to PVR will increase cyanosis.

(B) An increase in PVR relative to SVR favors right to left shunting.

(C) An increase in PVR relative to SVR will decrease risk of paradoxical air embolism.

(D) Eisenmenger syndrome is most often due to left ventricular hypertrophy.

Rationale: When right-sided pressures exceed left-sided pressures with septal defects, a mixing of unoxygenated venous blood with the oxygenated blood can lead to cyanotic states, a right to left shunting. This also can lead to right-sided air bubbles moving across the septum to the left, causing paradoxical air embolism to the cerebral or coronary arterial circulation. The reverse is true. An increase in SVR (with increased left-sided pressures) will reverse the right-to-left shunt and decrease cyanosis. Eisenmenger syndrome is the result of chronic left-to-right shunts which increase right-sided pressures, resulting in right-ventricular hypertrophy with elevated right-sided pressures. This will result in a reversal of the pressure gradient, reversing the shunt to become a right-to-left shunt.

Reference: Butterworth JF IV, Mackey DC, Wasnick JD, eds. *Morgan & Mikhail's Clinical Anesthesiology.* 7th ed. New York, NY: McGraw Hill; 2022: Chapters 20-21.

81. What is the most common site of herniation in congenital diaphragmatic hernia?

(A) Right foramen of Bochdalek

(B) Foramen of Morgagni

(C) Left foramen of Bochdalek

(D) Foramen of Luschka

Rationale: Herniation through the foramen of Bochdalek, specifically the left side, accounts for most cases.

References: Butterworth JF IV, Mackey DC, Wasnick JD, eds. *Morgan & Mikhail's Clinical Anesthesiology.* 7th ed. New York, NY: McGraw Hill; 2022: Chapters 20-21.

Jaffe RA, ed. *Anesthesiologist's Manual of Surgical Procedures.* 6th ed. Lippincott Williams & Wilkins; 2020: Chapter 12.5.

82. Which is the most common type of tracheoesophageal fistula?

(A) Type IIIB, esophageal atresia with a fistula between the distal esophagus and trachea

(B) Type I, proximal tracheoesophageal fistula without distal fistula between stomach and trachea

(C) Type IIIC, fistula between the trachea and both the upper and lower esophageal sections

(D) Type II, esophageal atresia without communication with the trachea

Rationale: Type IIIB is most common. The other options are incorrectly described and/or less frequent.

References: Butterworth JF IV, Mackey DC, Wasnick JD, eds. *Morgan & Mikhail's Clinical Anesthesiology.* 7th ed. New York, NY: McGraw Hill; 2022: Chapter 42.

Elisha S, Heiner JS, Nagelhout JJ. *Nurse Anesthesia.* 7th ed. St. Louis, MO: Elsevier Saunders; 2023: Chapter 53.

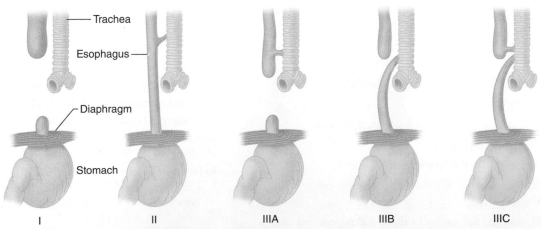

FIG. 4-3. Of the five types of tracheoesophageal fistula, type IIIB represents 90% of cases. (Reproduced with permission from Butterworth JF IV, Mackey DC, Wasnick JD, eds. *Morgan & Mikhail's Clinical Anesthesiology.* 7th ed. New York: McGraw Hill; 2022.)

83. Which statement is true regarding omphalocele and gastroschisis?

(A) Gastroschisis is less common and presents with a peritoneal covering.

(B) Omphalocele is less common and presents without peritoneal covering.

(C) Gastroschisis is more common and presents without peritoneal covering.

(D) Omphalocele is more common and presents with a peritoneal covering.

Rationale: Omphalocele occurs more frequently and is contained within a peritoneal covering.

References: Butterworth JF IV, Mackey DC, Wasnick JD, eds. *Morgan & Mikhail's Clinical Anesthesiology.* 7th ed. New York, NY: McGraw Hill; 2022: Chapter 42.

Elisha S, Heiner JS, Nagelhout JJ. *Nurse Anesthesia.* 7th ed. St. Louis, MO: Elsevier Saunders; 2023: Chapter 53.

Gropper MA, Cohen NH, Eriksson LI, et al, eds. *Miller's Anesthesia.* 9th ed. Philadelphia, PA: Churchill Livingstone Elsevier; 2020: Chapter 77.

84. Which congenital cardiac malformation is most associated with Trisomy 21 (Down syndrome)?

(A) Transposition of the great vessels

(B) Coarctation of the aorta

(C) Endocardial cushion defect

(D) Aortic stenosis

Rationale: Cardiac defects are plentiful for patients with Trisomy 21. Endocardial cushion defects are the most common congenital cardiac malformations associated with Down syndrome.

References: Butterworth JF IV, Mackey DC, Wasnick JD, eds. *Morgan & Mikhail's Clinical Anesthesiology.* 7th ed. New York, NY: McGraw Hill; 2022: Chapter 42.

Ellinas H, Matthes K, Alrayashi W, Bilge A, eds. *Clinical Pediatric Anesthesiology.* New York, NY: McGraw Hill; 2021: Chapter 40.

85. Which of the following is an anatomic characteristic of the pediatric airway that distinguishes it from the adult patient?

(A) The rima glottis is the narrowest point of the airway until the age of 5.

(B) The tongue is proportionately smaller.

(C) The larynx is located at the level of C_4.

(D) The epiglottis is flat and flexible.

Rationale: The larynx is in a more cephalad position (C_3–C_4) than the adult larynx (C_4–C_5). Because the

larynx is higher, the distance between the tongue, palate, and epiglottis are smaller and more prone to obstruction.

References: Butterworth JF IV, Mackey DC, Wasnick JD, eds. *Morgan & Mikhail's Clinical Anesthesiology.* 7th ed. New York, NY: McGraw Hill; 2022: Chapter 42.

Cote CJ, Lerman J, Anderson BJ, eds. *A Practice of Anesthesia for Infants and Children.* 6th ed. Philadelphia, PA: Elsevier Saunders; 2019: Chapter 14.

86. Which type of surgical procedure will result in the greatest increase in afterload accompanied by acute hypertension during aortic cross-clamping?

(A) Stanford Type A dissection of the ascending aorta

(B) Suprarenal descending aortic aneurysm

(C) Infrarenal descending aortic aneurysm

(D) Stanford Type B dissection

Rationale: When an aortic cross-clamp is applied, an immediate intense increase in left-ventricular afterload is experienced with a concomitant increase in blood pressure proximal to the clamp. The more proximal the clamp is applied, the more marked the effects. Since the ascending aorta is most proximal, it will experience the greatest increase in afterload if it is cross-clamped with the heart beating.

Reference: Butterworth JF IV, Mackey DC, Wasnick JD, eds. *Morgan & Mikhail's Clinical Anesthesiology.* 7th ed. New York, NY: McGraw Hill; 2022: Chapter 22.

87. At what gestational age does surfactant production begin?

(A) 30 weeks

(B) 34 weeks

(C) 26 weeks

(D) 32 weeks

Rationale: At 30 weeks pulmonary surfactant production begins. Enough surfactant for extrauterine life is usually present at 34 weeks.

References: Butterworth JF IV, Mackey DC, Wasnick JD, eds. *Morgan & Mikhail's Clinical Anesthesiology.* 7th ed. New York, NY: McGraw Hill; 2022: Chapters 41-42.

Chestnut DH, Wong CA, Tsen LC, et al, eds. *Chestnut's Obstetric Anesthesia Principles and Practice.* 6th ed. Philadelphia, PA: Mosby Elsevier; 2020: Chapter 5.

Cote CJ, Lerman J, Anderson BJ, eds. *A Practice of Anesthesia for Infants and Children.* 6th ed. Philadelphia, PA: Elsevier Saunders; 2019: Chapter 13.

88. Which of the following correctly describes omphalocele?

(A) It is due to occlusion of the omphalomesenteric artery.

(B) About 40 to 60% of patients have associated anomalies.

(C) The defect is periumbilical.

(D) Incidence is approximately 1 in 15,000 births.

Rationale: Omphaloceles result from the failure of gut migration from the yolk sac into the abdomen. The incidence is approximately 1 in 6,000 births. The incidence of associated anomalies is approximately 40% to 60%. The defect lies within the umbilical cord. Problems associated with the defect are congenital heart disease, exstrophy of the bladder, and Beckwith-Widemann syndrome.

References: Butterworth JF IV, Mackey DC, Wasnick JD, eds. *Morgan & Mikhail's Clinical Anesthesiology*. 7th ed. New York, NY: McGraw Hill; 2022: Chapters 41-42.

Gropper MA, Cohen NH, Eriksson LI, et al, eds. *Miller's Anesthesia*. 9th ed. Philadelphia, PA: Churchill Livingstone Elsevier; 2020: Chapter 77.

89. What finding is most likely during preoperative examination of an awake and alert patient with a posterior cerebral artery aneurysm?

(A) Brown-Séquard syndrome

(B) Abnormal gaze or pupil response

(C) Decorticate posturing

(D) Hypertensive crisis

Rationale: Oculomotor palsy may result from an aneurysm in this area due to close proximity of these structures.

References: Butterworth JF IV, Mackey DC, Wasnick JD, eds. *Morgan & Mikhail's Clinical Anesthesiology*. 7th ed. New York, NY: McGraw Hill; 2022: Chapter 27.

Moore KL, Agur AMR, Dalley AF. *Moore's Essential Clinical Anatomy*. 6th ed. Philadelphia, PA: Wolters Kluwer; 2019: Chapter 8.

90. During a repeat cesarean section a term infant is delivered. One minute following delivery, the infant has a heart rate of 90, blue extremities, whimpering to stimulus, breathing regularly, and active with good muscle tone. What is the 1-minute Apgar score?

(A) 5

(B) 6

(C) 7

(D) 8

Rationale: Apgar score calculation: 2 points for regular breathing and active/good muscle tone. 1 point is given each for an HR < 100 bpm, acrocyanosis, and whimpering. Scores 0 to 4 are regarded as severely depressed; 4 to 7 mildly depressed, and 8 to 10 vigorous.

TABLE 4-5. Apgar score.

Sign	Points		
	0	1	2
Heart rate (beats/min)	Absent	<100	>100
Respiratory effort	Absent	Slow, irregular	Good, crying
Muscle tone	Flaccid	Some flexion	Active motion
Reflex irritability	No response	Grimace	Crying
Color	Blue or pale	Body pink, extremities blue	All pink

(Reproduced with permission from Butterworth JF IV, Mackey DC, Wasnick JD, eds. *Morgan & Mikhail's Clinical Anesthesiology*. 7th ed. New York: McGraw Hill; 2022.)

References: Butterworth JF IV, Mackey DC, Wasnick JD, eds. *Morgan & Mikhail's Clinical Anesthesiology*. 7th ed. New York, NY: McGraw Hill; 2022: Chapter 42.

Chestnut DH, Wong CA, Tsen LC, et al, eds. *Chestnut's Obstetric Anesthesia Principles and Practice*. 6th ed. Philadelphia, PA: Mosby Elsevier; 2020: Chapter 9.

91. Which complication is most concerning following carotid endarterectomy?

(A) Rapid emergence

(B) Hypoxemia

(C) Hypotension

(D) Delayed emergence

Rationale: Each of the complications poses challenges following carotid endarterectomy. Denervation of the carotid baroreceptor blunts the feedback loop in response to hypertension, thus postoperative hypertension is possible with carotid endarterectomy. The carotid baroreceptor is instrumental in respiratory stimulation in the presence of hypoxemia.

For a patient dependent on the hypoxic drive for ventilation (i.e., COPD or narcotic use), unchecked hypoxemia may develop.

Reference: Butterworth JF IV, Mackey DC, Wasnick JD, eds. *Morgan & Mikhail's Clinical Anesthesiology*. 7th ed. New York, NY: McGraw Hill; 2022: Chapter 22.

92. Cleft palate, micrognathia, glossoptosis, and congenital heart disease are key characteristics of which *one* of the following syndromes?

(A) Treacher Collins

(B) VATER

(C) Pierre-Robin

(D) Prader-Willi

Rationale: The listed characteristics are those of Pierre-Robin syndrome. Glossoptosis is an important characteristic as it creates a ball-valve effect in the airway that can result in asphyxiation.

References: Butterworth JF IV, Mackey DC, Wasnick JD, eds. *Morgan & Mikhail's Clinical Anesthesiology*. 7th ed. New York, NY: McGraw Hill; 2022: Chapter 19.

Cote CJ, Lerman J, Anderson BJ, eds. *A Practice of Anesthesia for Infants and Children*. 6th ed. Philadelphia, PA: Elsevier Saunders; 2019: Chapter 12.

Gropper MA, Cohen NH, Eriksson LI, et al, eds. *Miller's Anesthesia*. 9th ed. Philadelphia, PA: Churchill Livingstone Elsevier; 2020: Chapter 79.

93. Which induction agent produces effects desirable for patients with Tetralogy of Fallot?

    (A) Etomidate

    (B) Ketamine

    (C) Midazolam

    (D) Propofol

    Rationale: Tetralogy of Fallot is one of the most common cyanotic congenital heart defects. It is marked by the following four features: right ventricular outflow tract obstruction (RV), ventricular septal defect (VSD), and a rightward aortic deviation, overriding the VSD and RV.

    Due to the right ventricular outflow obstruction and coexisting VSD, patients with Tetralogy of Fallot shunt blood from right to left, ejecting deoxygenated right ventricular blood mixed with oxygenated blood into the aorta. Ketamine maintains or increases systemic vascular resistance (SVR).

    References: Butterworth JF IV, Mackey DC, Wasnick JD, eds. *Morgan & Mikhail's Clinical Anesthesiology*. 7th ed. New York, NY: McGraw Hill; 2022: Chapter 21.

    Cote CJ, Lerman J, Anderson BJ, eds. *A Practice of Anesthesia for Infants and Children*. 6th ed. Philadelphia, PA: Elsevier Saunders; 2019: Chapter 17.

    Gropper MA, Cohen NH, Eriksson LI, et al, eds. *Miller's Anesthesia*. 9th ed. Philadelphia, PA: Churchill Livingstone Elsevier; 2020: Chapter 78.

94. Which of the following is true regarding a transplanted heart?

    (A) No response to atropine

    (B) No response to isoproterenol

    (C) No response to milrinone

    (D) No response to epinephrine

Rationale: A transplanted heart does not have autonomic innervation and thus is devoid of vagal influence. Vagolytic medications such as atropine or glycopyrrolate will have no effect on heart rate. Isoproterenol and epinephrine are the medications of choice to increase heart rate. Milrinone, a phosphodiesterase inhibitor, directly increases intracellular cAMP apart from any neuron-mediated or catecholamine-mediated process and thus will be an effective inotrope.

References: Butterworth JF IV, Mackey DC, Wasnick JD, eds. *Morgan & Mikhail's Clinical Anesthesiology*. 7th ed. New York, NY: McGraw Hill; 2022: Chapter 21.

Gropper MA, Cohen NH, Eriksson LI, et al, eds. *Miller's Anesthesia*. 9th ed. Philadelphia, PA: Churchill Livingstone Elsevier; 2020: Chapter 54.

95. Which inhalational agent is most suitable for a pediatric inhalation induction?

    (A) Isoflurane

    (B) Desflurane

    (C) Sevoflurane

    (D) Halothane

    Rationale: Sevoflurane is used for a pediatric inhalation induction. Compared to desflurane and isoflurane, sevoflurane is less pungent resulting in less coughing, breath-holding, or laryngospasm. Sevoflurane has replaced halothane as the inhalational agent of choice for children.

    References: Butterworth JF IV, Mackey DC, Wasnick JD, eds. *Morgan & Mikhail's Clinical Anesthesiology*. 7th ed. New York, NY: McGraw Hill; 2022: Chapter 42.

    Barash PG, Cullen BF, Stoelting RK, et al, eds. *Clinical Anesthesia*. 8th ed. Lippincott Williams & Wilkins; 2017: Chapter 18.

96. Which of the following variables is not associated with aging?

    (A) Increased volume of distribution for lipid soluble drugs

    (B) Reduced plasma volume

    (C) Decreased volume of distribution for lipid soluble drugs

    (D) Reduced plasma protein binding

    Rationale: Pharmacokinetics and dynamics are altered with aging. An increased volume of distribution for lipid soluble drugs, reduced plasma volume, reduced plasma protein binding, and altered liver and renal function are associated with aging.

Reference: Hines RL, Marschall KE. *Stoelting's Anesthesia and Co-existing Disease.* 7th ed. Philadelphia, PA: Elsevier Saunders; 2018: Chapter 30.

97. An elderly patient with decreased albumin and coronary artery disease is scheduled for an umbilical hernia repair. What do you expect when administering an intravenous induction dose of propofol?

    (A) Higher free drug fraction
    (B) Decreased drug effect
    (C) Lower free drug fraction
    (D) Similar drug effect

    Rationale: Plasma proteins decline with aging. Albumin levels are lower. Propofol is highly protein bound. This results in a higher free drug fraction and effect.
    Reference: Hines RL, Marschall KE. *Stoelting's Anesthesia and Co-existing Disease.* 7th ed. Philadelphia, PA: Elsevier Saunders; 2018: Chapter 30.

98. What is the effect of aging on the minimum alveolar concentration (MAC)?

    (A) MAC of volatile anesthetics increases 50% after age 60.
    (B) MAC of volatile anesthetics decreases 10% after age 50.
    (C) MAC of volatile anesthetics decreases 6% per decade after 40 years of age.
    (D) MAC of volatile anesthetics increases 4% per decade after 40 years of age.

    Rationale: Sensitivity to inhalational anesthetics is affected by aging. The MAC of inhalational anesthetics decreases progressively with advancing age.
    Reference: Hines RL, Marschall KE. *Stoelting's Anesthesia and Co-existing Disease.* 7th ed. Philadelphia, PA: Elsevier Saunders; 2018: Chapter 30.

99. What is the best induction dose for an 80-year-old weighing 100 kg?

    (A) Propofol 75 mg
    (B) Sodium pentothal 250 mg
    (C) Etomidate 40 mg
    (D) Ketamine 100 mg

    Rationale: Decrease dose requirements for the elderly by up to 50%. Propofol 1 to 1.5 mg/kg is the average adult induction dose. The induction dose of sodium pentothal is 2 to 2.5 mg/kg; ketamine 1 to 1.5 mg/kg; and etomidate 0.2 to 0.4 mg/kg. None of these doses were decreased for the 80-year-old patient.

Reference: Hines RL, Marschall KE. *Stoelting's Anesthesia and Co-existing Disease.* 7th ed. Philadelphia, PA: Elsevier Saunders; 2018: Chapter 19.

100. What is the definition of premature birth?

    (A) Birth prior to 42 weeks gestation
    (B) Birth prior to 37 weeks gestation
    (C) Birth prior to 32 weeks gestation
    (D) Birth prior to 35 weeks gestation

    Rationale: A premature birth is defined as delivery prior to 37 weeks gestation.
    Reference: Butterworth JF IV, Mackey DC, Wasnick JD, eds. *Morgan & Mikhail's Clinical Anesthesiology.* 7th ed. New York, NY: McGraw Hill; 2022: Chapter 42.

101. Which body mass index (BMI) is categorized as moderate obesity?

    (A) 18.5%
    (B) 24.9%
    (C) 29.9%
    (D) 32.1%

    Rationale: BMI is categorized as follows: 25 to 29.9 kg/m^2 (overweight); 30 to 34.9 kg/m^2 (moderate obesity); 35 to 39.9 kg/m^2 (severe obesity); 40 kg/m^2 and over (morbid obesity).
    Reference: Elisha S, Heiner JS, Nagelhout JJ. *Nurse Anesthesia.* 7th ed. St. Louis, MO: Elsevier Saunders; 2023: Chapter 48.

102. Total body water will be the largest percentage of body weight in which patient?

    (A) A preterm newborn
    (B) An infant
    (C) A toddler
    (D) A school-age child

    Rationale: Total body water as a percentage of body-weight is inversely related to age.
    References: Butterworth JF IV, Mackey DC, Wasnick JD, eds. *Morgan & Mikhail's Clinical Anesthesiology.* 7th ed. New York, NY: McGraw Hill; 2022: Chapter 42.

    Elisha S, Heiner JS, Nagelhout JJ. *Nurse Anesthesia.* 7th ed. St. Louis, MO: Elsevier Saunders; 2023: Chapter 53.

103. Which sign is associated with metabolic syndrome?

    (A) High levels of high-density lipoprotein cholesterol
    (B) Hypotension

(C) High triglyceride levels

(D) Small waist circumference

Rationale: Metabolic syndrome (Syndrome X) includes three of the following signs: large waist circumference, hypertension, low levels of high-density lipoprotein, glucose intolerance, and high triglycerides levels.

Reference: Hines RL, Marschall KE. *Stoelting's Anesthesia and Co-existing Disease.* 7th ed. Philadelphia, PA: Elsevier Saunders; 2018: Chapter 19.

104. The patient is undergoing a latissimus dorsi myocutaneous flap for breast reconstruction. What is the desired mean arterial pressure?

(A) MAP > 55 mmHg

(B) MAP > 60 mmHg

(C) MAP > 65 mmHg

(D) MAP > 70 mmHg

Rationale: A MAP > 70 mmHg facilitates flap perfusion.

Reference: Macksey LF. *Surgical Procedures and Anesthetic Implications.* 2nd ed. Sudbury, MA: Jones & Bartlett Learning; 2018: Chapter 13.

105. Which patient appropriately fasted for an anesthetic to begin at 1000?

(A) A child who had cereal at 0800

(B) A child who had clear liquids at 0900

(C) An infant who breast fed at 0500

(D) An infant who had formula at 0700

Rationale: Fasting guidelines for infants and children include 2 hours for clear liquids, 4 hours for breast milk, 6 hours for infant formula or light meal, and 8 hours for a heavy meal.

References: Butterworth JF IV, Mackey DC, Wasnick JD, eds. *Morgan & Mikhail's Clinical Anesthesiology.* 7th ed. New York, NY: McGraw Hill; 2022: Chapter 42.

Gropper MA, Cohen NH, Eriksson LI, et al, eds. *Miller's Anesthesia.* 9th ed. Philadelphia, PA: Churchill Livingstone Elsevier; 2020: Chapter 77.

106. Which dose of morphine is appropriate for intrathecal postcesarean section analgesia?

(A) 2.5 mg

(B) 50 μg

(C) 0.2 mg

(D) 100 μg

Rationale: The intrathecal dose of morphine for analgesia is 0.1 to 0.2 mg. The epidural dose of morphine for analgesia is 2.5 to 5.0 mg. Fentanyl 50 to 100 μg is given via the epidural route and 10 to 20 μg via the intrathecal route.

Reference: Longnecker DE, Mackey SC, Newman MF, Sandberg WS, Zapol WM, eds. *Anesthesiology.* 3rd ed. McGraw Hill; 2018: Chapter 57.

TABLE 4-6. Opioids for neuraxial use in obstetrics

Opioid	Epidural Dose	Spinal Dose	Duration (hours)	Comments
Morphine	2.5-5 mg	0.1-0.2 mg	18-24	Useful primarily for postcesarean section analgesia
Fentanyl	50-100 μg	10-20 μg	3-4	Useful as labor and operative adjuvant
Sufentanil	10-20 μg	5-10 μg	3-4	Useful as labor and operative adjuvant
Meperidine	25 mg		2-3	
Hydromorphone	1 mg	100 μg	12	
Methadone	4-5 mg		5-6	
Diamorphine	2.5-5 mg		5-15	Not available in the United States

(Reproduced with permission from Longnecker DE, Mackey SC, Newman MF, Sandberg WS, Zapol WM, eds. *Anesthesiology.* 3rd ed. New York: McGraw Hill; 2018.)

107. When is it best to avoid teratogenic drugs?

(A) 1 to 2 weeks gestation

(B) 3 to 10 weeks gestation

(C) 12 to 15 weeks gestation

(D) 20 to 25 weeks gestation

Rationale: The period of greatest fetal development occurs during the third to tenth week of pregnancy or broadly, 5 to 55 days of gestation. Avoiding teratogenic drugs and chemicals is essential during this period of fetal development.

Reference: Longnecker DE, Mackey SC, Newman MF, Sandberg WS, Zapol WM, eds. *Anesthesiology.* 3rd ed. McGraw Hill; 2018: Chapter 57.

108. Which variable is not linked to postdural puncture headache following placement of a spinal anesthetic for cesarean section?

(A) 26 g needle

(B) Cutting needles

(C) 20 g needle

(D) Beveled needles

Rationale: Smaller gauged noncutting, nonbeveled needles are associated with a lower incidence of postdural puncture headache than larger gauged, cutting, beveled needles.

Reference: Longnecker DE, Mackey SC, Newman MF, Sandberg WS, Zapol WM, eds. *Anesthesiology*. 3rd ed. McGraw Hill; 2018: Chapter 42.

109. Which symptoms are associated with pregnant patients in the supine position?

(A) Hypotension, nausea

(B) Nausea, hypertension

(C) Normotension, nausea

(D) Hypertension, vomiting

Rationale: Supine hypotension syndrome results from compression of the gravid uterus on the inferior vena cava and aorta. Decreased venous return results in decreased cardiac output. Symptoms include hypotension, nausea, vomiting, tachycardia, sweating, and pallor. The syndrome is relieved by tilting the patient to displace the gravid uterus.

Reference: Longnecker DE, Mackey SC, Newman MF, Sandberg WS, Zapol WM, eds. *Anesthesiology*. 3rd ed. McGraw Hill; 2018: Chapter 57.

110. Which of the following physiologic changes occur during pregnancy?

(A) Hypocoagulation

(B) Plasma volume decreases

(C) Hypercoagulation

(D) Red cell mass decreases

Rationale: Hematologic changes in pregnancy include increased plasma volume and increased red cell mass. Red cell mass increase is less than plasma volume resulting in dilutional anemia. Coagulation factors increase except for factors XI and XIII. Pregnant patients are considered hypercoagulable.

References: Butterworth JF IV, Mackey DC, Wasnick JD, eds *Morgan & Mikhail's Clinical Anesthesiology*. 7th ed. New York, NY: McGraw Hill; 2022: Chapter 40.

Longnecker DE, Mackey SC, Newman MF, Sandberg WS, Zapol WM, eds. *Anesthesiology*. 3rd ed. McGraw Hill; 2018: Chapter 57.

111. The patient requests an epidural for abdominal hysterectomy. Which sensory level is needed for epidural anesthesia?

(A) T-12

(B) T-10

(C) T-8

(D) T-6

Rationale: Intraabdominal surgery requires a T_4–T_6 sensory block. Blocks below T-6 are inadequate for pain control during intraabdominal surgery.

Reference: Longnecker DE, Mackey SC, Newman MF, Sandberg WS, Zapol WM, eds. *Anesthesiology*. 3rd ed. McGraw Hill; 2018: Chapter 57.

112. The patient is scheduled for a laparoscopic cholecystectomy. Which of the following is true?

(A) Central venous pressure decreases.

(B) Lung compliance increases.

(C) Intraabdominal pressure decreases.

(D) Functional residual capacity decreases.

Rationale: Laparoscopic procedures require insufflation of carbon dioxide increasing Intraabdominal pressure. Cardiovascular effects include increased central venous pressure, stroke volume, and blood pressure. Respiratory effects include decreased functional residual capacity, increased airway pressure, and decreased lung compliance. Hypoxemia may ensue.

Reference: Longnecker DE, Mackey SC, Newman MF, Sandberg WS, Zapol WM, eds. *Anesthesiology*. 3rd ed. McGraw Hill; 2018: Chapter 51.

113. During a laparoscopic hernia repair, you notice a sudden drop in blood pressure and oxygen saturation and decreased end-tidal carbon dioxide. What is the most likely cause?

(A) CO_2 embolus

(B) Tension pneumothorax

(C) Hemorrhage

(D) Pneumomediastinum

Rationale: Insufflation of carbon dioxide gas during laparoscopy carries a risk including tension pneumothorax, hemorrhage, and pneumomediastinum. The signs and symptoms of carbon dioxide embolus include a sudden blood pressure, oxygen saturation, and notable drop in end tidal CO_2. Cardiovascular collapse and death quickly follow without prompt recognition and treatment.

Reference: Longnecker DE, Mackey SC, Newman MF, Sandberg WS, Zapol WM, eds. *Anesthesiology*. 3rd ed. McGraw Hill; 2018: Chapter 51.

114. Which of the following is true about the infant airway?

(A) The tongue is small in relation to the mandible.

(B) The larynx is located at the C_2–C_3 vertebrae.

(C)   The epiglottis is stiff and flat.

(D)   The larynx is located at C_5–C_6.

Rationale: Infants airways differ significantly from older children and adults. The tongue is large in relation to the mandible. The epiglottis is floppy, and omega shaped. Location of the larynx is at the C_2–C_3 vertebrae as compared to adults whose larynx is located at C_5–C_6.

References: Butterworth JF IV, Mackey DC, Wasnick JD, eds. *Morgan & Mikhail's Clinical Anesthesiology.* 7th ed. New York, NY: McGraw Hill; 2022: Chapter 40.

Longnecker DE, Mackey SC, Newman MF, Sandberg WS, Zapol WM, eds. *Anesthesiology.* 3rd ed. McGraw Hill; 2018: Chapter 32.

115. While reversing heparin, the anesthetist notes that the blood pressure has dropped precipitously to 42/23 mmHg. What will you do first?

(A)   Administer 100 mcg of epinephrine IV.

(B)   Administer 100 mcg of epinephrine IV.

(C)   Administer 50 mg of Benadryl and 125 mg of methylprednisolone IV.

(D)   Begin chest compressions.

Rationale: Heparin is reversed with protamine. Protamine reactions are immunologic (anaphylactic or anaphylactoid) in nature. It is accompanied by severe pulmonary artery vasoconstriction, myocardial depression, and severe systemic hypotension. First line treatment for an anaphylactic/anaphylactoid reaction is epinephrine. After administration of epinephrine and hemodynamic improvement (chest compressions may be necessary for epinephrine to travel to heart), then the other treatments may be initiated including small doses of phenylephrine.

Reference: Butterworth JF IV, Mackey DC, Wasnick JD, eds. *Morgan & Mikhail's Clinical Anesthesiology.* 7th ed. New York, NY: McGraw Hill; 2022: Chapter 22.

116. By how much are neuraxial requirements for cesarean section decreased?

(A)   60%

(B)   40%

(C)   30%

(D)   50%

Rationale: Due to increased sensitivity to local anesthetics by pregnant patients, local anesthetic dosages should be decreased by up to 30%.

Reference: Butterworth JF IV, Mackey DC, Wasnick JD, eds. *Morgan & Mikhail's Clinical Anesthesiology.* 7th ed. New York, NY: McGraw Hill; 2022: Chapter 40.

117. Which of the following is not a normal physiological change associated with pregnancy?

(A)   MAC decreases by 20%.

(B)   Functional residual capacity decreases by 20%.

(C)   Hemoglobin decreases by 20%.

(D)   Plasma volume increases by 55%.

Rationale: Minimum alveolar concentration (MAC) decreases by 30% to 40%. The respiratory rate increases by 15% and hemoglobin decreases by 20%.

Reference: Butterworth JF IV, Mackey DC, Wasnick JD, eds. *Morgan & Mikhail's Clinical Anesthesiology.* 7th ed. New York, NY: McGraw Hill; 2022: Chapter 40.

TABLE 4-7. Average maximum physiological changes associated with pregnancy.

Parameter	Change
Neurological	−40%
MAC	
Respiratory	
Oxygen consumption	+20 to 50%
Airway resistance	−35%
FRC	−20%
Minute ventilation	+50%
Tidal volume	+40%
Respiratory rate	+15%
PaO_2	+10%
$PaCO_2$	−15%
HCO_3	−15%
Cardiovascular	
Blood volume	+35%
Plasma volume	+55%
Cardiac output	+40%
Stroke volume	+30%
Heart rate	+20%
Systolic blood pressure	−5%
Diastolic blood pressure	−15%
Peripheral resistance	−15%
Pulmonary resistance	−30%
Hematological	
Hemoglobin	−20%
Platelets	−10%
Clotting factors[1]	+30 to 250%
Renal	
GFR	+50%

[1]Varies with each factor.
FRC, functional residual capacity; GFR, glomerular filtration rate; MAC, minimum alveolar concentration.
(Reproduced with permission from Butterworth JF IV, Mackey DC, Wasnick JD, eds. *Morgan & Mikhail's Clinical Anesthesiology.* 7th ed. New York: McGraw Hill; 2022.)

118. What is the best size endotracheal tube used for a patient undergoing general anesthesia for cesarean section?

(A) 5.5 mm

(B) 6.5 mm

(C) 7.5 mm

(D) 8.5 mm

Rationale: Due to the changes during pregnancy, the airway becomes swollen, friable, and visualization of airway structure is difficult. A 6- to 6.5-mm endotracheal tube facilitates intubation.

Reference: Butterworth JF IV, Mackey DC, Wasnick JD, eds. *Morgan & Mikhail's Clinical Anesthesiology*. 7th ed. New York, NY: McGraw Hill; 2022: Chapter 41.

119. How does propofol affect uterine blood flow (UBF)?

(A) Decreases UBF

(B) No change on UBF

(C) Dose-related increase in UBF

(D) Dose-related decrease in UBF

Rationale: Propofol has little or no effect on UBF. Medications with alpha adrenergic activity as well as endogenous catecholamines cause vasoconstriction decreasing UBF.

Reference: Butterworth JF IV, Mackey DC, Wasnick JD, eds. *Morgan & Mikhail's Clinical Anesthesiology*. 7th ed. New York, NY: McGraw Hill; 2022: Chapter 40.

120. What statement is false regarding the use of metoclopramide in pregnant patients?

(A) Speeds gastric emptying

(B) Increases pH

(C) Decreases gastric volume

(D) Increases lower esophageal sphincter tone

Rationale: Metoclopramide has no effect on gastric pH.

Reference: Butterworth JF IV, Mackey DC, Wasnick JD, eds. *Morgan & Mikhail's Clinical Anesthesiology*. 7th ed. New York, NY: McGraw Hill; 2022: Chapters 17 and 41.

121. A patient is scheduled for a radical neck dissection. History includes neck radiation. How will you manage this patient's airway?

(A) Standard IV induction

(B) Rapid sequence induction

(C) Laryngeal mask airway

(D) Awake fiberoptic intubation

Rationale: Radiation to the neck may cause anatomical changes that pose challenges for intubation. The best approach is to use an awake fiberoptic intubation or fiberoptic approach following inhaled anesthetic whereby the patient maintains spontaneous ventilation.

References: Butterworth JF IV, Mackey DC, Wasnick JD, eds. *Morgan & Mikhail's Clinical Anesthesiology*. 7th ed. New York, NY: McGraw Hill; 2022: Chapter 37.

Elisha S, Heiner JS, Nagelhout JJ. *Nurse Anesthesia*. 7th ed. St. Louis, MO: Elsevier Saunders; 2023: Chapter 43.

122. Less than 1 minute following an epidural test dose, the patient complains of heavy legs. What is the most likely cause?

(A) Intravascular injection

(B) Incomplete epidural analgesia

(C) Unintentional intrathecal block

(D) Local anesthetic toxicity

Rationale: Motor blocks following an epidural test dose may lead to inadvertent intrathecal injection. The onset of the motor block occurs 3 to 5 minutes following the test dose. Preceding the motor block, signs and symptoms of a sensory block will occur.

Reference: Butterworth JF IV, Mackey DC, Wasnick JD, eds. *Morgan & Mikhail's Clinical Anesthesiology*. 7th ed. New York, NY: McGraw Hill; 2022: Chapter 41.

123. The patient is receiving echothiophate eye drops for glaucoma. You plan to use succinylcholine. What should you expect?

(A) Shortened onset of action

(B) Shortened duration of action

(C) Prolonged duration of action

(D) Prolonged onset of action

Rationale: Use of echothiophate decreases plasma cholinesterase activity. For this reason, there may be prolonged action of succinylcholine.

References: Butterworth JF IV, Mackey DC, Wasnick JD, eds. *Morgan & Mikhail's Clinical Anesthesiology*. 7th ed. New York, NY: McGraw Hill; 2022: Chapter 36.

Elisha S, Heiner JS, Nagelhout JJ. *Nurse Anesthesia*. 7th ed. St. Louis, MO: Elsevier Saunders; 2023: Chapter 44.

124. The patient has severe preeclampsia. When will you avoid regional anesthesia?

(A) Platelet count 100,000/uL

(B) Platelet count 150,000/uL

(C) Platelet count 125,000/uL

(D) Platelet count 75,000/uL

Rationale: Before starting regional anesthesia for a parturient with severe preeclampsia, obtain a platelet count. Platelet counts greater than 100,000/uL are considered acceptable. While there are exceptions, platelet counts less than 100,000/uL require additional testing and patient assessment.

Reference: Butterworth JF IV, Mackey DC, Wasnick JD, eds. *Morgan & Mikhail's Clinical Anesthesiology.* 7th ed. New York, NY: McGraw Hill; 2022: Chapter 41.

125. What fetal monitoring pattern is associated with umbilical cord compression?

(A) Variable decelerations

(B) Late decelerations

(C) Early decelerations

(D) Increased variability

Rationale: Umbilical cord compression evidenced by variable deceleration. Early deceleration is associated with head compression. Late decelerations evidence fetal compromise including uteroplacental insufficiency.

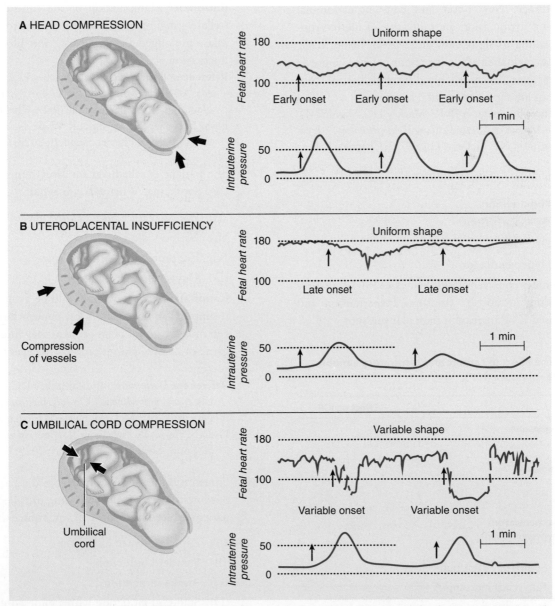

FIG. 4-4. Periodic changes in fetal heart rate related to uterine contraction. **A:** Early (type I) decelerations. **B:** Late (type II) decelerations. **C:** Variable (type III) decelerations. (Reproduced with permission from Danforth DN, Scott JR. *Obstetrics and Gynecology.* 5th ed. Philadelphia, PA: Lippincott Williams & Wilkins; 1986.)

Reference: Butterworth JF IV, Mackey DC, Wasnick JD, eds. *Morgan & Mikhail's Clinical Anesthesiology*. 7th ed. New York, NY: McGraw Hill; 2022: Chapter 41.

126. During labor the patient experiences an abrupt onset of constant abdominal pain accompanied by hypotension. What is the most likely cause?

    (A) Uterine rupture
    (B) Placenta previa
    (C) Placenta abruption
    (D) Hemorrhage

    Rationale: Uterine rupture, placenta previa, and placenta abruption are the main causes of maternal hemorrhage. New onset and constant abdominal pain and hypotension are indicative of uterine rupture leading to significant antepartum hemorrhage. Painless vaginal bleeding is present in placenta previa whereas painful vaginal bleeding with uterine contractions are signs of placental abruption.

    Reference: Butterworth JF IV, Mackey DC, Wasnick JD, eds. *Morgan & Mikhail's Clinical Anesthesiology*. 7th ed. New York, NY: McGraw Hill; 2022: Chapter 41.

127. Which of the following increases intraocular pressure?

    (A) Hypotension
    (B) Hypoventilation
    (C) Decreased CVP
    (D) Hyperventilation

    Rationale: Hypoventilation increases $PaCO_2$ thereby increasing intraocular pressure. Hypertension and increased CVP increase intraocular pressure.

TABLE 4-8. The effect of cardiac and respiratory variables on intraocular pressure (IOP).[1]

Variable	Effect on IOP
Central venous pressure	
Increase	↑↑↑
Decrease	↓↓↓
Arterial blood pressure	
Increase	↑
Decrease	↓
$PaCO_2$	
Increase (hypoventilation)	↑↑
Decrease (hyperventilation)	↓↓
PaO_2	
Increase	0
Decrease	↑

[1]↓, decrease (mild, moderate, marked); ↑, increase (mild, moderate, marked); 0, no effect.
(Reproduced with permission from Butterworth JF IV, Mackey DC, Wasnick JD, eds. *Morgan & Mikhail's Clinical Anesthesiology*. 7th ed. New York: McGraw Hill; 2022.)

References: Butterworth JF IV, Mackey DC, Wasnick JD, eds. *Morgan & Mikhail's Clinical Anesthesiology*. 7th ed. New York, NY: McGraw Hill; 2022: Chapter 36.
Elisha S, Heiner JS, Nagelhout JJ. *Nurse Anesthesia*. 7th ed. St. Louis, MO: Elsevier Saunders; 2023: Chapter 44.

128. During radical neck dissection you observe new onset bradycardia, arrhythmias, and prolonged QT intervals. What is the most likely cause of these symptoms?

    (A) Denervation of carotid sinus
    (B) Manipulation of the carotid sinus
    (C) Venous air embolism
    (D) Denervation of carotid bodies.

    Rationale: Manipulation of the carotid sinus and stellate ganglion may lead to bradycardia, arrhythmias, prolonged QT intervals, and blood pressure fluctuation.

    References: Butterworth JF IV, Mackey DC, Wasnick JD, eds. *Morgan & Mikhail's Clinical Anesthesiology*. 7th ed. New York, NY: McGraw Hill; 2022: Chapter 37.
    Elisha S, Heiner JS, Nagelhout JJ. *Nurse Anesthesia*. 7th ed. St. Louis, MO: Elsevier Saunders; 2023: Chapter 43.

129. The patient is scheduled for laser removal of vocal cord papilloma. What will you avoid?

    (A) Eye protection with colored glasses
    (B) Nitrous oxide
    (C) Eye protection with wet gauze
    (D) Oxygen and air mixture

    Rationale: Nitrous oxide should be avoided because it supports combustion. A low concentration of oxygen mixed with air helps avoid airway fire. Using wet gauze or colored glasses protects the eyes during laser surgery.

    References: Butterworth JF IV, Mackey DC, Wasnick JD, eds. *Morgan & Mikhail's Clinical Anesthesiology*. 7th ed. New York, NY: McGraw Hill; 2022: Chapter 37.
    Elisha S, Heiner JS, Nagelhout JJ. *Nurse Anesthesia*. 7th ed. St. Louis, MO: Elsevier Saunders; 2023: Chapter 43.

130. Fifteen minutes ago you transported a patient to the postanesthesia care unit following tonsillectomy. The patient is bleeding. How will you induce this patient?

    (A) Rapid sequence induction
    (B) Standard induction
    (C) Awake intubation
    (D) Standard induction with a glidescope

Rationale: Patients who experience post-tonsillectomy bleeding are considered to have a full stomach. A rapid sequence induction is indicated. Depending on the extent of the bleeding, awake intubation may be needed.

References: Butterworth JF IV, Mackey DC, Wasnick JD, eds. *Morgan & Mikhail's Clinical Anesthesiology.* 7th ed. New York, NY: McGraw Hill; 2022: Chapter 37.

Elisha S, Heiner JS, Nagelhout JJ. *Nurse Anesthesia.* 7th ed. St. Louis, MO: Elsevier Saunders; 2023: Chapter 43.

131. Which of the following is not associated with a peribulbar block?

(A) Intraconal procedure
(B) When 5 to 8 mL local anesthetic is used
(C) Extraconal procedure
(D) When patient gaze is straight ahead

Rationale: Because the peribulbar block is extraconal, it is considered a safer block than a retrobulbar block. The patient's gaze is straight ahead. In a retrobulbar block, 2 to 4 mL of local anesthetic is used.

References: Butterworth JF IV, Mackey DC, Wasnick JD, eds. *Morgan & Mikhail's Clinical Anesthesiology.* 7th ed. New York, NY: McGraw Hill; 2022: Chapter 37.

Elisha S, Heiner JS, Nagelhout JJ. *Nurse Anesthesia.* 7th ed. St. Louis, MO: Elsevier Saunders; 2023: Chapter 44.

132. Which statement is true regarding the use of inhalational agents during pregnancy?

(A) Uterine blood flow is increased.
(B) Uteroplacental blood flow is increased.
(C) Uteroplacental blood flow is decreased.
(D) Uterine blood flow is unchanged.

Rationale: Inhalational agents cause a dose-related decrease in blood pressure thereby decreasing uterine blood flow and blood flow through the placenta. The recommendation is to use less than 1 MAC to minimize the neonatal effects.

Reference: Butterworth JF IV, Mackey DC, Wasnick JD, eds. *Morgan & Mikhail's Clinical Anesthesiology.* 7th ed. New York, NY: McGraw Hill; 2022: Chapter 40.

133. The patient is scheduled for endoscopic sinus surgery. Which of the following will not minimize blood loss?

(A) Head-up position
(B) Cocaine 4%
(C) Supine position
(D) Hypotensive technique

Rationale: The head-up position rather than the supine position assists with minimizing blood loss. Cocaine 4 or 10% or epinephrine-soaked pledgets minimize blood loss. In some cases, hypotensive techniques are used.

Reference: Butterworth JF IV, Mackey DC, Wasnick JD, eds. *Morgan & Mikhail's Clinical Anesthesiology.* 7th ed. New York, NY: McGraw Hill; 2022: Chapter 37.

134. A patient is scheduled for surgery involving a LeFort II fracture. During the preoperative interview, periorbital edema and raccoon eyes hematoma are noted. What is your main anesthetic concern?

(A) Securing the airway
(B) Bleeding
(C) Emergence with a wired jaw
(D) Postoperative respiratory compromise

Rationale: Each of the options poses challenges for surgery involving a LeFort II fracture. Securing the airway may be problematic due to the nature of the fracture. Nasal endotracheal tubes are commonly used in dental reconstruction. However, care should be taken with a LeFort II or III fracture due to the possibility of additional skull fractures, brain damage, or meningitis.

Reference: Butterworth JF IV, Mackey DC, Wasnick JD, eds. *Morgan & Mikhail's Clinical Anesthesiology.* 7th ed. New York, NY: McGraw Hill; 2022: Chapter 37.

135. Which of the following is not a clinical sign of hyperthyroidism?

(A) Polyuria
(B) Weight loss
(C) Muscle fatigue
(D) Hypoactive reflexes

Rationale: Weight gain, cold intolerance, hypoactive reflexes, muscle fatigue lethargy, and depression are signs of hypothyroidism. Signs and symptoms associated with hyperparathyroidism include weight loss, bone pain and muscle weakness, heat intolerance, gastrointestinal and cognitive disturbances, and altered renal function. Exophthalmos, goiter, and tremors may be present.

References: Butterworth JF IV, Mackey DC, Wasnick JD, eds. *Morgan & Mikhail's Clinical Anesthesiology.* 7th ed. New York, NY: McGraw Hill; 2022: Chapter 35.

Elisha S, Heiner JS, Nagelhout JJ. *Nurse Anesthesia.* 7th ed. St. Louis, MO: Elsevier Saunders; 2023: Chapter 37.

136. What is the anesthetic priority for management of an unrepaired aortic dissection?

(A) Decrease blood pressure with arterial vasodilators to decrease risk of rupture or further dissection.

(B) Increase blood pressure to ensure adequate perfusion distal to the aneurysm.

(C) Decrease shear force on the aneurysm using beta-blockers to decrease risk of rupture of further dissection.

(D) Decrease heart rate with medications to decrease myocardial oxygen demand.

Rationale: Aortic dissections grow due to hemodynamic shear forces related to the rate of rise of blood pressure (dP/dt). Management of an unrepaired aortic aneurysm is focused on avoiding propagation of dissection and avoiding rupture. Hemodynamic management focuses on decreasing shear forces related to quick changes in blood pressure on systole. This is accomplished by reducing systolic pressure (arterial vasodilators) and decreasing the strength of contraction (beta-blockers). Arterial vasodilators alone may increase the shear force by decreasing the resistance against systolic ejection.
Reference: Butterworth JF IV, Mackey DC, Wasnick JD, eds. *Morgan & Mikhail's Clinical Anesthesiology.* 7th ed. New York, NY: McGraw Hill; 2022: Chapter 35.

137. The patient is scheduled for a laryngeal endoscopy. Jet ventilation is planned. What statement is false regarding jet ventilation?

(A) High-pressure (30-50 psi) is used.

(B) FiO_2 of 30% or less is used.

(C) End-tidal CO_2 is accurate.

(D) Expiration is passive.

Rationale: Due to the high frequency of injected gas (80-300 times per minute) a dilution of alveolar gas results in variable CO_2 readings.
References: Butterworth JF IV, Mackey DC, Wasnick JD, eds. *Morgan & Mikhail's Clinical Anesthesiology.* 7th ed. New York, NY: McGraw Hill; 2022: Chapter 37.
Elisha S, Heiner JS, Nagelhout JJ. *Nurse Anesthesia.* 7th ed. St. Louis, MO: Elsevier Saunders; 2023: Chapter 24.

138. A patient undergoing repair of a descending thoracic aortic aneurysm is found postoperatively to exhibit loss of lower extremity motor function bilaterally. What is the most likely cause?

(A) Blood flow to the motor cortex of the brain was decreased during cross-clamp.

(B) Blood flow to the anterior spinal cord was damaged during the surgery.

(C) Blood flow to the posterior spinal cord was damaged during the surgery.

(D) This is a normal occurrence when blood flow to the lower extremities has been restricted as in aortic cross-clamping.

Rationale: The patient has experienced anterior spinal cord ischemia and is experiencing anterior spinal artery syndrome. The artery of Adamkiewicz along with many other smaller vessels may be covered or ligated during aortic repair. If the degree of flow impairment is large, the patient may develop anterior spinal artery syndrome secondary to spinal cord ischemia. Classic symptoms of this syndrome include loss of motor function, loss of pinprick sensation, but retained vibration sensation and proprioception.
Reference: Butterworth JF IV, Mackey DC, Wasnick JD, eds. *Morgan & Mikhail's Clinical Anesthesiology.* 7th ed. New York, NY: McGraw Hill; 2022: Chapter 22.

139. The patient is undergoing a mediastinoscopy. What will you consider for this patient?

(A) Blood pressure in the left arm

(B) Small bore IV

(C) Blood pressure in the right arm

(D) Tachycardia

Rationale: Hemorrhage, air embolism, cerebral ischemia, injury to the recurrent laryngeal and phrenic nerves, pneumothorax, and reflex bradycardia may result during mediastinoscopy. The blood pressure is taken in the left arm because of possible compression of the innominate artery.
References: Butterworth JF IV, Mackey DC, Wasnick JD, eds. *Morgan & Mikhail's Clinical Anesthesiology.* 7th ed. New York, NY: McGraw Hill; 2022: Chapter 22.
Elisha S, Heiner JS, Nagelhout JJ. *Nurse Anesthesia.* 7th ed. St. Louis, MO: Elsevier Saunders; 2023: Chapters 29-30.

140. What statement is true regarding cardioversion?

(A) 50 to 100 Joules are used initially for atrial flutter.

(B) 200 to 300 Joules are used initially to convert atrial flutter.

(C) Electrical shock is asynchronous.

(D) Electrical shock is synchronized with the "Q" wave.

Rationale: Conversion of atrial rhythms begins at 50 to 100 Joules but may increase incrementally when needed. Shocks are given synchronously with the "R" wave of the QRS complex.

Reference: Butterworth JF IV, Mackey DC, Wasnick JD, eds. *Morgan & Mikhail's Clinical Anesthesiology*. 7th ed. New York, NY: McGraw Hill; 2022: Chapter 55.

141. What do you anticipate with distention of the bowel during colonoscopy?

    (A) Tachycardia
    (B) Hypertension
    (C) Bradycardia
    (D) EKG changes

Rationale: Vagal stimulation is likely with insufflation of the bowel during colonoscopy. Bradycardia, hypotension, and arrhythmias may occur.

Reference: Gropper MA, Cohen NH, Eriksson LI, et al, eds. *Miller's Anesthesia*. 9th ed. Philadelphia, PA: Churchill Livingstone Elsevier; 2020: Chapter 73.

142. The patient is scheduled for computerized tomography (CT) scan with intravenous contrast media (ICM). What is your main concern?

    (A) Patient must not move during the CT
    (B) Patient anxiety
    (C) Hypothermia
    (D) Allergic reaction

Rationale: ICM causes anaphylactic and anaphylactoid reactions. Renal dysfunction is possible. Patients at risk for reaction to ICM include asthmatics, those with numerous comorbidities and history of allergic reaction.

Reference: Elisha S, Heiner JS, Nagelhout JJ. *Nurse Anesthesia*. 7th ed. St. Louis, MO: Elsevier Saunders; 2023: Chapter 58.

143. A patient is scheduled for electroconvulsive therapy (ECT). What is your main anesthetic concern when calculating dosages for induction agents?

    (A) Anterograde amnesia
    (B) Seizure quality
    (C) Parasympathetic stimulation
    (D) Sympathetic stimulation

Rationale: Patients undergoing ECT experience initial bradycardia and secretions (parasympathetic) followed by tachycardia and hypertension (sympathetic surge) and anterograde amnesia. The quality

of the seizure is considered key to the treatment. Induction agents including propofol increase the seizure threshold and decrease the duration of the seizure. Therefore, lower dosages improve the likelihood that the seizure will result in the quality necessary for effective treatment.

Reference: Butterworth JF IV, Mackey DC, Wasnick JD, eds. *Morgan & Mikhail's Clinical Anesthesiology*. 7th ed. New York, NY: McGraw Hill; 2022: Chapter 28.

144. A patient with an intestinal obstruction is scheduled for surgery. The patient's history includes pancreatitis and gastroesophageal reflux disease (GERD). What is the best approach to airway management?

    (A) Awake fiberoptic intubation
    (B) Endotracheal intubation
    (C) LMA
    (D) Intubating LMA

Rationale: Protecting the airway is required for patients with intestinal obstruction and GERD. There is no indication for an awake fiberoptic intubation.

Reference: Elisha S, Heiner JS, Nagelhout JJ. *Nurse Anesthesia*. 7th ed. St. Louis, MO: Elsevier Saunders; 2023: Chapters 20 and 24.

145. When is cardiac output the greatest?

    (A) Immediately following delivery
    (B) Third trimester
    (C) Second trimester
    (D) First trimester

Rationale: Cardiac output increases progressively during pregnancy. During the third trimester there is a 45% increase in cardiac output. The greatest increase is immediately following delivery.

Reference: Butterworth JF IV, Mackey DC, Wasnick JD, eds. *Morgan & Mikhail's Clinical Anesthesiology*. 7th ed. New York, NY: McGraw Hill; 2022: Chapter 40.

146. Which of the following would be the most appropriate induction technique for a patient undergoing drainage of a severe cardiac tamponade via subxiphoid approach or pericardiocentesis?

    (A) Propofol, high-dose fentanyl, succinylcholine, and intubate. Maintain with light sevoflurane and positive pressure ventilation.
    (B) Ketamine, high-dose fentanyl, succinylcholine, and intubate. Maintain with light sevoflurane.

(C) Inhalational induction, LMA insertion, light maintenance with sevoflurane, ketamine supplementation.

(D) High-dose fentanyl, midazolam, and mask ventilate patient.

Rationale: The cardiac output is heart rate–dependent, and the blood pressure is dependent on arterial vasoconstriction. The anesthetic technique should ensure that sympathetic tone is maintained. High-dose fentanyl would be contraindicated. Positive pressure ventilation should be avoided if possible as it will decrease venous return, severely reducing cardiac output. Ketamine is a choice agent for induction and maintenance. Consider epinephrine use as well, as it will increase both heart rate and arterial vasoconstriction.

Reference: Butterworth JF IV, Mackey DC, Wasnick JD, eds. *Morgan & Mikhail's Clinical Anesthesiology.* 7th ed. New York, NY: McGraw Hill; 2022: Chapter 21.

147. A sedated patient experiences headache, nausea, and vomiting during stereotactic Gamma Knife surgery. What is the most likely cause?

(A) Hemorrhage

(B) Perforated aneurysm

(C) Radiocontrast reaction

(D) Embolization

Rationale: Each of the causes is possible with GammaKnife surgery. Hemorrhage is the most likely cause.

Reference: Elisha S, Heiner JS, Nagelhout JJ. *Nurse Anesthesia.* 7th ed. St. Louis, MO: Elsevier Saunders; 2023: Chapter 31.

148. Which of the following medications shortens the duration of a seizure during electroconvulsive therapy (ECT)?

(A) Caffeine

(B) Etomidate

(C) Ketamine

(D) Propofol

Rationale: Propofol when given in low doses does not affect the seizure activity with ECT. In higher doses >1.5 mg/kg, seizure threshold is increased, and seizure duration is decreased.

Reference: Butterworth JF IV, Mackey DC, Wasnick JD, eds. *Morgan & Mikhail's Clinical Anesthesiology.* 7th ed. New York, NY: McGraw Hill; 2022: Chapter 28.

149. The patient is undergoing a mastectomy. During surgery, isosulfan blue dye is injected. What do you expect?

(A) Tachycardia

(B) Increased oxygen saturation

(C) Bradycardia

(D) Decrease or minimal change in oxygen saturation

Rationale: Isosulfan blue dye may cause up to a 3% decrease in oxygen saturation.

Reference: Gropper MA, Cohen NH, Eriksson LI, et al, eds. *Miller's Anesthesia.* 9th ed. Philadelphia, PA: Churchill Livingstone Elsevier; 2020: Chapter 41.

150. Following cystoscopy the patient's blood pressure falls. What is the most likely cause?

(A) Sympathectomy

(B) Blood loss

(C) Vasoconstriction due to spinal anesthesia

(D) Lowering legs from lithotomy position

Rationale: Lithotomy position is frequently used for patients undergoing cystoscopy. When the patient's legs are lowered following the procedure, venous return and cardiac output decrease resulting in hypotension.

References: Butterworth JF IV, Mackey DC, Wasnick JD, eds. *Morgan & Mikhail's Clinical Anesthesiology.* 7th ed. New York, NY: McGraw Hill; 2022: Chapter 32.
Elisha S, Heiner JS, Nagelhout JJ. *Nurse Anesthesia.* 7th ed. St. Louis, MO: Elsevier Saunders; 2023: Chapter 23.

151. Pain relief during the second stage of labor requires neural blockade at what sensory level?

(A) T_{10} to T_{12}

(B) T_{12} to S_1

(C) T_{10} to S_1

(D) T_{10} to S_4

Rationale: During the first stage of labor neural blockade of sensory fibers T_{10} to L_1 is needed. The second stage of labor requires neural blockade of sensory fibers that extend to S_4.

References: Butterworth JF IV, Mackey DC, Wasnick JD, eds. *Morgan & Mikhail's Clinical Anesthesiology.* 7th ed. New York, NY: McGraw Hill; 2022: Chapter 41.
Chestnut DH, Wong CA, Tsen LC, et al, eds. *Chestnut's Obstetric Anesthesia Principles and Practice.* 6th ed. Philadelphia, PA: Mosby Elsevier; 2020: Chapter 20.

152. Which condition benefits most from epidural steroid injections?

(A) Radiculopathy

(B) Intractable cancer pain

(C) Intraabdominal neoplasms

(D) Phantom limb pain

Rationale: Patients with nerve root compression benefit from epidural steroid injections. Conditions that benefit from epidural steroids include chronic low back and neck pain, rheumatoid arthritis, and herpetic neuralgia. Neurolytic blocks are used for patients with intractable cancer pain including intraabdominal and pelvic neoplasms, and rib metastases. Patients with phantom limb pain benefit from spinal cord stimulation.

Reference: Butterworth JF IV, Mackey DC, Wasnick JD, eds. *Morgan & Mikhail's Clinical Anesthesiology.* 7th ed. New York, NY: McGraw Hill; 2022: Chapter 47.

153. Which drug has mainly analgesic and antipyretic properties?

(A) Acetaminophen

(B) Ketorolac

(C) Fentanyl

(D) Codeine

Rationale: The nonselective COX inhibitor Ketorolac possesses anti-inflammatory, antipyretic, and analgesic properties. Opioids including fentanyl and morphine are analgesics.

References: Butterworth JF IV, Mackey DC, Wasnick JD, eds. *Morgan & Mikhail's Clinical Anesthesiology.* 7th ed. New York, NY: McGraw Hill; 2022: Chapter 47.

Elisha S, Heiner JS, Nagelhout JJ. *Nurse Anesthesia.* 7th ed. St. Louis, MO: Elsevier Saunders; 2023: Chapter 11.

154. Which statement regarding the use of epidural analgesia and anesthesia for preeclamptic patients is true?

(A) Circulating catecholamines are decreased.

(B) Decreases intervillous blood flow.

(C) Epidural block should be avoided.

(D) Epidural blocks are difficult to place.

Rationale: Epidural blocks are suitable for patients with preeclampsia. The block decreases circulating catecholamines and improves intervillous blood flow. The epidural block also allows for control of systemic blood pressure.

Reference: Longnecker DE, Mackey SC, Newman MF, Sandberg WS, Zapol WM, eds. *Anesthesiology.* 3rd ed. McGraw Hill; 2018: Chapters 18 and 57.

155. A patient taking duloxetine and fluoxetine for chronic neuropathic pain complains of fever, agitation, sweating, and anxiety. What is the most likely cause?

(A) Duloxetine overdose

(B) Fluoxetine sensitivity

(C) Combined use of fluoxetine and duloxetine

(D) Allergic reaction to duloxetine

Rationale: Using selective serotonin reuptake inhibitors and selective serotonin-norepinephrine reuptake inhibitors in combination may lead to serotonin syndrome. Toxic levels of serotonin cause symptoms listed above but also delirium, seizures, hyperdynamic states, hyperreflexia, muscle rigidity, and myoclonus.

Reference: Butterworth JF IV, Mackey DC, Wasnick JD, eds. *Morgan & Mikhail's Clinical Anesthesiology.* 7th ed. New York, NY: McGraw Hill; 2022: Chapter 28.

156. A patient is receiving tocolytic therapy for preterm labor. Which of the following is most concerning for this patient?

(A) Hyperkalemia

(B) Hypoglycemia

(C) Pulmonary Edema

(D) Increased systemic vascular resistance

Rationale: Tocolytic therapy that includes terbutaline and ritodrine is associated with hypokalemia, hyperglycemia, and decreased systemic vascular resistance. Pulmonary edema leads to maternal death.

Reference: Longnecker DE, Mackey SC, Newman MF, Sandberg WS, Zapol WM, eds. *Anesthesiology.* 3rd ed. McGraw Hill; 2018: Chapters 18 and 57.

157. Which of the following is a systemic effect of hydrocortisone?

(A) Adrenal-pituitary insufficiency

(B) Hypoglycemia

(C) Hypotension

(D) Sodium depletion

Rationale: Corticosteroids affect multiple body systems. Sodium and water are retained. Hypertension develops as well as the potential for congestive heart failure and cardiomyopathy. Musculoskeletal effects include truncal obesity, muscle, and bone weakness as well as fractures. Hyperglycemia, dermatologic, gastrointestinal, and neurologic or psychological effects are also prevalent. Long-term use of steroids rather than a single injection such as epidural administration fosters the systemic effects.

Reference: Elisha S, Heiner JS, Nagelhout JJ. *Nurse Anesthesia.* 7th ed. St. Louis, MO: Elsevier Saunders; 2023: Chapter 33.

158. How is the renal system affected by pregnancy?

    (A) Renal plasma flow decreases
    (B) Glomerular filtration rate increases
    (C) Tubular absorption of glucose increases
    (D) Renal blood flow decreases

    Rationale: The absorption of glucose via the proximal tubules decreases. This results in normal glucosuria. Renal blood flow increases early in pregnancy by 50% to 80%.
    Reference: Butterworth JF IV, Mackey DC, Wasnick JD, eds. *Morgan & Mikhail's Clinical Anesthesiology.* 7th ed. New York, NY: McGraw Hill; 2022: Chapter 40.

159. When giving epidural steroid injections what dose will you use to avoid systemic effects?

    (A) Methylprednisolone acetate 40 mg
    (B) Triamcinolone diacetate 100 mg
    (C) Methylprednisolone acetate 20 mg
    (D) Triamcinolone diacetate 120 mg

    Rationale: The effective dose for epidural steroid injection is 40 to 80 mg for each drug. Exceeding the doses increases the likelihood of systemic effects. Decreasing the dose lessens the likelihood of effective treatment.
    Reference: Butterworth JF IV, Mackey DC, Wasnick JD, eds. *Morgan & Mikhail's Clinical Anesthesiology.* 7th ed. New York, NY: McGraw Hill; 2022: Chapter 47.

160. The patient is scheduled for in vitro fertilization (IVF). Which medication is considered safe for this patient?

    (A) Morphine
    (B) Fentanyl
    (C) Isoflurane
    (D) NSAIDs

    Rationale: Morphine may affect fertilization. NSAIDs may affect implantation of the embryo. Isoflurane decreases the number of embryos.
    Reference: Elisha S, Heiner JS, Nagelhout JJ. *Nurse Anesthesia.* 7th ed. St. Louis, MO: Elsevier Saunders; 2023: Chapter 52.

161. Which statement is false regarding open breast biopsy?

    (A) Postoperative nausea and vomiting increases.
    (B) Smooth emergence minimizes hematoma formation.
    (C) Monitor the EKG for ST-segment changes when local anesthetic with epinephrine is used.
    (D) The blood pressure cuff is placed on the nonoperative arm and IV placed on the operative side.

    Rationale: The blood pressure cuff and IV are placed on the nonoperative side.
    Reference: Macksey LF. *Surgical Procedures and Anesthetic Implications.* 2nd ed. Sudbury, MA: Jones & Bartlett Learning; 2018: Chapter 13.

162. The patient is undergoing a modified radical mastectomy. When planning the general anesthetic, why would you check with the surgeon?

    (A) Determine the patient's risk for postoperative nausea and vomiting
    (B) To type and cross-match preoperatively
    (C) Determine what if any neuromuscular blockers will be used
    (D) Determine when to give antiemetics

    Rationale: Nerve injury is possible with this surgery. The surgeon may prefer that no neuromuscular blockers are used.
    Reference: Macksey LF. *Surgical Procedures and Anesthetic Implications.* 2nd ed. Sudbury, MA: Jones & Bartlett Learning; 2018: Chapter 13.

163. What is your primary concern when caring for a patient undergoing hysteroscopy?

    (A) Vasovagal response to uterine traction
    (B) Postoperative pain
    (C) Lithotomy positioning
    (D) Absorption of glycine or saline solution

    Rationale: Each of the items poses anesthetic concerns for this patient. Absorption of glycine or saline solutions predisposes the patient to fluid overload as well as electrolyte imbalance. Electrolyte testing should be done preoperatively.
    Reference: Macksey LF. *Surgical Procedures and Anesthetic Implications.* 2nd ed. Sudbury, MA: Jones & Bartlett Learning; 2018: Chapter 20.

164. The patient is scheduled for a total abdominal hysterectomy. Why is the patient most likely to become hypotensive following induction?

    (A) Bowel prep
    (B) Chronic bleeding
    (C) Anemia
    (D) Position changes

Rationale: Dehydration following a bowel prep is common for these patients. These patients may also be anemic due to chronic bleeding.

Reference: Macksey LF. *Surgical Procedures and Anesthetic Implications*. 2nd ed. Sudbury, MA: Jones & Bartlett Learning; 2018: Chapter 20.

165. During a cystoscopy, the patient becomes diaphoretic and complains of upper abdominal pain and nausea. What is the most likely cause?

    (A) Bladder perforation
    (B) Stent placement
    (C) Biopsy
    (D) Stone removal

Rationale: Stent placement, biopsy, and stone removal may be performed with cystoscopy. The symptomology in an awake patient is consistent with bladder or ureteral perforation. Other symptoms include referred pain (diaphragmatic or shoulder) or hemodynamic changes.

Reference: Macksey LF. *Surgical Procedures and Anesthetic Implications*. 2nd ed. Sudbury, MA: Jones & Bartlett Learning; 2018: Chapter 19.

166. What medication(s) should be immediately available for penile surgery?

    (A) Midazolam
    (B) Propofol
    (C) Fentanyl
    (D) Glycopyrrolate

Rationale: For procedures involving the penis and testes, manipulation may result in profound bradycardia due to vagal stimulation. Atropine or glycopyrrolate should be immediately available.

Reference: Macksey LF. *Surgical Procedures and Anesthetic Implications*. 2nd ed. Sudbury, MA: Jones & Bartlett Learning; 2018: Chapter 19.

167. What is a primary intraoperative concern for patients undergoing rectal surgery?

    (A) Postoperative pain
    (B) Relaxation of the anal sphincter
    (C) Fluid and electrolyte balance
    (D) Postoperative nausea and vomiting

Rationale: Each of the items poses concerns for the patient. The patients are often dehydrated due to the bowel prep. Fluid and electrolyte balance may exist.

Reference: Macksey LF. *Surgical Procedures and Anesthetic Implications*. 2nd ed. Sudbury, MA: Jones & Bartlett Learning; 2018: Chapter 16.

168. During total knee arthroplasty with spinal anesthesia the patient develops hypotension, arrhythmias and loses consciousness. What is the most likely rationale?

    (A) Hemorrhage
    (B) Fluid imbalance
    (C) Tourniquet pain
    (D) Methyl methacrylate

Rationale: Bone cement (methyl methacrylate) is used during total joint procedures to cement the prosthetic components. In addition to the symptoms for this patient, hypoxia, pulmonary hypertension, and decreased cardiac output occur. A decreased end-tidal CO_2 is the first sign of bone cement implantation syndrome for patients undergoing joint replacement with general anesthesia.

References: Butterworth JF IV, Mackey DC, Wasnick JD, eds. *Morgan & Mikhail's Clinical Anesthesiology*. 7th ed. New York, NY: McGraw Hill; 2022: Chapter 38.
Elisha S, Heiner JS, Nagelhout JJ. *Nurse Anesthesia*. 7th ed. St. Louis, MO: Elsevier Saunders; 2023: Chapter 45.

169. Which is the preferred method of airway management in a child with acute epiglottitis?

    (A) Rapid sequence induction followed by laryngoscopy
    (B) Awake laryngoscopy
    (C) Inhalation induction maintaining spontaneous respiration
    (D) Urgent tracheostomy

Rationale: Spontaneously breathing inhalation induction is the preferred method.

References: Butterworth JF IV, Mackey DC, Wasnick JD, eds. *Morgan & Mikhail's Clinical Anesthesiology*. 7th ed. New York, NY: McGraw Hill; 2022: Chapter 42.
Gropper MA, Cohen NH, Eriksson LI, et al, eds. *Miller's Anesthesia*. 9th ed. Philadelphia, PA: Churchill Livingstone Elsevier; 2020: Chapter 77.

170. Which factor does not contribute to decreased uterine blood flow?

    (A) Systemic hypotension
    (B) Uterine vasoconstriction
    (C) Uterine contractions
    (D) Uterine vasodilation

Rationale: Decreased uterine blood flow is caused by factors including hypotension, uterine vasoconstriction and uterine contractions, sympathetic block, hypovolemia, supine hypotensive syndrome, and vasoconstrictors. Maternal conditions including preeclampsia, hypertension, use of cocaine, and abruptio placenta also decrease uterine blood flow.

Reference: Butterworth JF IV, Mackey DC, Wasnick JD, eds. *Morgan & Mikhail's Clinical Anesthesiology.* 7th ed. New York, NY: McGraw Hill; 2022: Chapter 40.

171. Which of the following physiologic changes occur with limb tourniquets?

(A) Cellular acidosis

(B) Metabolic alkalosis

(C) Cellular alkalosis

(D) Metabolic acidosis

Rationale: Limb tourniquets produce cellular acidosis secondary to ischemia. Hypoxia develops within 2 minutes of inflation. Endothelial capillary leak occurs with inflation of 2 hours or more.

References: Butterworth JF IV, Mackey DC, Wasnick JD, eds. *Morgan & Mikhail's Clinical Anesthesiology.* 7th ed. New York, NY: McGraw Hill; 2022: Chapter 38.

Elisha S, Heiner JS, Nagelhout JJ. *Nurse Anesthesia.* 7th ed. St. Louis, MO: Elsevier Saunders; 2023: Chapter 45.

172. While undergoing a shoulder arthroscopy with regional anesthesia the patient exhibits tachycardia, agitation, diaphoresis, hypotension, and jugular vein distention. What is the most likely cause?

(A) Tension pneumothorax

(B) Subcutaneous emphysema

(C) Pneumomediastinum

(D) Failed regional block

Rationale: Each of the items may occur during shoulder arthroscopy. The symptoms are consistent with tension pneumothorax. Other signs include absence of breath sounds on the affected side, hypoxemia, increased central venous pressure, cyanosis, and increased airway pressure (general anesthesia).

References: Butterworth JF IV, Mackey DC, Wasnick JD, eds. *Morgan & Mikhail's Clinical Anesthesiology.* 7th ed. New York, NY: McGraw Hill; 2022: Chapter 38.

Elisha S, Heiner JS, Nagelhout JJ. *Nurse Anesthesia.* 7th ed. St. Louis, MO: Elsevier Saunders; 2023: Chapter 45.

173. Which of the following risk factors is not linked to postoperative vision loss (POVL)?

(A) Thin

(B) Obese

(C) Male

(D) <18 years

Rationale: Postoperative vision loss may occur in all patients. Risk factors include male, obesity, <18 and >65 years, spinal surgery (prone position), prolonged surgery, large blood loss, and hypotension.

Reference: Elisha S, Heiner JS, Nagelhout JJ. *Nurse Anesthesia.* 7th ed. St. Louis, MO: Elsevier Saunders; 2023: Chapters 23 and 44.

174. The patient is scheduled for total hip arthroplasty. Which of the following is not an anesthetic concerns?

(A) Hemorrhage

(B) Thromboembolism

(C) Tourniquet pain

(D) Bone cement implantation syndrome

Rationale: Tourniquets are not used for total hip replacement. Reaming the femur results in significant blood loss. Bone cement (Methyl methacrylate) induces an exothermic reaction that results in vasodilation and decreased systemic vascular resistance. Pulmonary or thromboembolism due to venous stasis may result in patients undergoing lower extremity surgery. Postoperative pain is concerning but is not a life-threatening event as are the other options.

References: Butterworth JF IV, Mackey DC, Wasnick JD, eds. *Morgan & Mikhail's Clinical Anesthesiology.* 7th ed. New York, NY: McGraw Hill; 2022: Chapter 38.

Elisha S, Heiner JS, Nagelhout JJ. *Nurse Anesthesia.* 7th ed. St. Louis, MO: Elsevier Saunders; 2023: Chapter 45.

175. How are hypotensive bradycardic episodes (HBEs) that occur during shoulder surgery defined?

(A) Heart rate <50 bpm and systolic blood pressure <90 mmHg

(B) Systolic blood pressure >90 mmHg

(C) Heart rate decreases 30 bpm in 3 minutes

(D) Heart rate decreases 20 bpm in 5 minutes

Rationale: In addition to (A) and (B), a heart rate decrease of 50 bpm in 5 minutes defines HBEs.
Reference: Elisha S, Heiner JS, Nagelhout JJ. *Nurse Anesthesia.* 7th ed. St. Louis, MO: Elsevier Saunders; 2023: Chapter 45.

176. Your patient is undergoing an elective coronary artery bypass graft (CABG). The patient was managed on heparin therapy for 5 days preoperatively. The patient is now on cardiopulmonary bypass and the perfusionist is having difficulty maintaining total heparinization. What is the most likely cause?

   (A) Antithrombin deficiency
   (B) Factor V deficiency
   (C) Factor VIII deficiency
   (D) Factor IV deficiency

Rationale: Patients who have recently been managed on heparin therapy may become "heparin resistant," thus, requiring higher than usual doses to obtain therapeutic anticoagulation on bypass.
References: Butterworth JF IV, Mackey DC, Wasnick JD, eds. *Morgan & Mikhail's Clinical Anesthesiology.* 7th ed. New York, NY: McGraw Hill; 2022: Chapter 22.
Elisha S, Heiner JS, Nagelhout JJ. *Nurse Anesthesia.* 7th ed. St. Louis, MO: Elsevier Saunders; 2023: Chapter 26.

177. Which condition is associated with carbamazepine taken during pregnancy?

   (A) Spina bifida
   (B) Pyloric stenosis
   (C) Biliary atresia
   (D) Hypospadias

Rationale: Antiepileptic drugs taken during pregnancy are associated with ventricular septal defects, mid face, mouth abnormalities, and digital or nail-bed hypoplasia. Carbamazepine is specifically associated with spina bifida.
Reference: Flood P, Rathmell JP, Urbam RD, eds. *Stoelting's Pharmacology & Physiology in Anesthetic Practice.* 6th ed. Philadelphia, PA: Wolters Kluwer; 2022: Chapter 13.

178. A patient is undergoing an elective abdominal aortic aneurysm (AAA) repair. What drug are you most likely to administer after aortic clamping?

   (A) Nitroglycerin
   (B) Phenylephrine
   (C) Milrinone
   (D) Dopamine

Rationale: Because of the acute hypertension that develops above the clamp, a vasodilator infusion is often necessary to prevent excessive increases in blood pressure.
References: Butterworth JF IV, Mackey DC, Wasnick JD, eds. *Morgan & Mikhail's Clinical Anesthesiology.* 7th ed. New York, NY: McGraw Hill; 2022: Chapter 22.
Elisha S, Heiner JS, Nagelhout JJ. *Nurse Anesthesia.* 7th ed. St. Louis, MO: Elsevier Saunders; 2023: Chapter 28.

179. A 5-year-old requires endotracheal intubation for an exploratory laparotomy. What size ETT will you select?

   (A) 6
   (B) 5
   (C) 4
   (D) 3

Rationale: To determine the oral tracheal tube size use the equation: 4 plus the child's age/4.

TABLE 4-9. Oral endotracheal tube size guidelines.

Age	Internal Diameter (mm)	Cut Length (cm)
Full-term infant	3.5	12
Child	$4 + \dfrac{Age}{4}$	12 + Age/2
Adult		
Female	7.0-7.5	24
Male	7.5-9.0	24

(Reproduced with permission from Butterworth JF IV, Mackey DC, Wasnick JD, eds. *Morgan & Mikhail's Clinical Anesthesiology.* 7th ed. New York: McGraw Hill; 2022.)

References: Butterworth JF IV, Mackey DC, Wasnick JD, eds. *Morgan & Mikhail's Clinical Anesthesiology.* 7th ed. New York, NY: McGraw Hill; 2022: Chapter 19.
Elisha S, Heiner JS, Nagelhout JJ. *Nurse Anesthesia.* 7th ed. St. Louis, MO: Elsevier Saunders; 2023: Chapter 53.

180. Which of the following is linked to late deceleration?

   (A) Fetal head compression
   (B) Begins 10 to 30 seconds following the peak of a contraction
   (C) Begin with the contraction
   (D) Umbilical cord compression

Rationale: Variable decelerations are associated with umbilical cord compression and occur abruptly. Early deceleration occurs at the beginning of a contraction and is associated with head compression. Late deceleration occurs just after the peak of the contraction and is associated with uteroplacental insufficiency.

Reference: Butterworth JF IV, Mackey DC, Wasnick JD, eds. *Morgan & Mikhail's Clinical Anesthesiology.* 7th ed. New York, NY: McGraw Hill; 2022: Chapter 41.

Chestnut DH, Wong CA, Tsen LC, et al, eds. *Chestnut's Obstetric Anesthesia Principles and Practice.* 6th ed. Philadelphia, PA: Mosby Elsevier; 2020: Chapters 6 and 8.

181. Which neurosurgical procedure places the patient at highest risk for postoperative diabetes insipidus?

    (A) Resection of intracranial aneurysm in the anterior circle of Willis

    (B) Stereotactic biopsy of a lesion in the parietal lobe

    (C) Tumor resection within the posterior fossa

    (D) Transsphenoidal hypophysectomy

    Rationale: Diabetes insipidus is a known postoperative complication of pituitary resection.

    References: Butterworth JF IV, Mackey DC, Wasnick JD, eds. *Morgan & Mikhail's Clinical Anesthesiology.* 7th ed. New York, NY: McGraw Hill; 2022: Chapter 28.

    Jaffe RA, ed. *Anesthesiologist's Manual of Surgical Procedures.* 6th ed. Lippincott Williams & Wilkins; 2020: Chapter 1.1.

182. Which of the following agents will cause the greatest decrease in preload?

    (A) Verapamil

    (B) Nicardipine

    (C) Metoprolol

    (D) Nitroglycerine

    Rationale: Nitroglycerine is a nitrate that causes arterial and venodilation. Nicardipine is a calcium-channel blocking agent which is very selective for arterial vascular smooth muscle, decreasing afterload but not preload. Verapamil is a calcium-channel blocker more selective for cardiac than vascular smooth muscle. Metoprolol, a beta-blocker, will have negligible effects on preload. Nitroglycerine is the only agent on the list that will cause decreased preload secondary to venous vasodilation.

    Reference: Butterworth JF IV, Mackey DC, Wasnick JD, eds. *Morgan & Mikhail's Clinical Anesthesiology.* 7th ed. New York, NY: McGraw Hill; 2022: Chapter 21.

183. What is the correct placement of a precordial Doppler to monitor for venous air embolism?

    (A) Midclavicular line at the first intercostal space

    (B) Right sternal border at the third intercostal space

    (C) Right midaxillary line at the fifth intercostal space

    (D) Left sternal border at the fifth intercostal space

    Rationale: Correct placement is third intercostal space and right of the sternum.

    References: Butterworth JF IV, Mackey DC, Wasnick JD, eds. *Morgan & Mikhail's Clinical Anesthesiology.* 7th ed. New York, NY: McGraw Hill; 2022: Chapter 27.

    Pardo MC Jr, ed. *Basics of Anesthesia.* 8th ed. Philadelphia, PA: Elsevier Saunders; 2023: Chapter 30.

184. What is average total cerebral blood flow?

    (A) 550 mL/min

    (B) 650 mL/min

    (C) 750 mL/min

    (D) 950 mL/min

    Rationale: Cerebral blood flow can be estimated as 15% of cardiac output or 50 mL/min/100 g; both total approximately 750 mL/min.

    References: Butterworth JF IV, Mackey DC, Wasnick JD, eds. *Morgan & Mikhail's Clinical Anesthesiology.* 7th ed. New York, NY: McGraw Hill; 2022: Chapter 26.

    Hall JE. *Guyton and Hall Textbook of Medical Physiology.* 14th ed. Philadelphia, PA: Saunders Elsevier; 2021: Chapter 62.

185. How is minimum alveolar concentration (MAC) affected for inhaled anesthetics during pregnancy?

    (A) MAC is increased by 30%.

    (B) MAC is decreased by 15%.

    (C) MAC is increased by 25%.

    (D) MAC is decreased by 40%.

    Rationale: MAC is decreased to 40% for all inhalational agents during pregnancy.

    Reference: Longnecker DE, Mackey SC, Newman MF, Sandberg WS, Zapol WM, eds. *Anesthesiology.* 3rd ed. McGraw Hill; 2018: Chapter 18.

186. Calculate cerebral perfusion pressure (CPP) using the information provided and correctly interpret the result. Blood pressure is 130/90 mmHg, intracranial pressure is 12 mmHg, and central venous pressure is 6 mmHg.

    (A) CPP = 110 mmHg, high

    (B) CPP = 97 mmHg, normal

    (C) CPP = 105 mmHg, high

    (D) CPP = 91 mmHg, normal

    Rationale: Cerebral perfusion pressure is estimated by subtracting either intracranial pressure or central venous pressure, the greater value of the two, from the mean arterial pressure. The normal range is 80 to 100 mmHg.

References: Butterworth JF IV, Mackey DC, Wasnick JD, eds. *Morgan & Mikhail's Clinical Anesthesiology.* 7th ed. New York, NY: McGraw Hill; 2022: Chapter 26.
Pardo MC Jr, ed. *Basics of Anesthesia.* 8th ed. Philadelphia, PA: Elsevier Saunders; 2023: Chapter 30.

187. Inhalational anesthetic agents have what effects on cardiac conduction?

    (A) Decrease AV node refractoriness

    (B) Suppress SA node automaticity

    (C) Increases pacing thresholds

    (D) All of the above

    Rationale: Inhalational agents depress AV node automaticity. This can be observed in everyday practice both by a reduction of heart rate during anesthesia and the frequency of junctional rhythm during anesthesia. Inhalational agents mildly increase AV node refractoriness. They have no effect reported on pacing thresholds.

    Reference: Butterworth JF IV, Mackey DC, Wasnick JD, eds. *Morgan & Mikhail's Clinical Anesthesiology.* 7th ed. New York, NY: McGraw Hill; 2022: Chapter 20.

188. For Frank-Starling's law what do the x-axis and y-axis represent?

    (A) Heart rate; cardiac output

    (B) Ventricular end-diastolic volume; cardiac output

    (C) Cardiac output; ventricular end-diastolic volume

    (D) Afterload; systemic vascular resistance

    Rationale: Frank-Starling's law relates preload (ventricular end-diastolic volume) with stroke volume (or cardiac output) when heart rate and contractility remain constant. With increasing preload, cardiac output will rise until a maximum ability for the heart chamber to respond is reached. After this excessive point is reached, increasing end-diastolic volume will not increase cardiac output, and may even decrease it.

    Reference: Butterworth JF IV, Mackey DC, Wasnick JD, eds. *Morgan & Mikhail's Clinical Anesthesiology.* 7th ed. New York, NY: McGraw Hill; 2022: Chapter 20.

189. The fetal scalp pH is 7.25. How would you interpret this value?

    (A) Normal infant pH

    (B) Abnormal infant pH

    (C) Needs to be repeated to ensure accuracy

    (D) Requires neonatal resuscitation

    Rationale: A fetal scalp pH > 7.25 is considered normal. A pH of 7.20 is marginal so should be repeated to ensure accuracy. A pH < 7.20 indicates neonatal depression.

    Reference: Butterworth JF IV, Mackey DC, Wasnick JD, eds. *Morgan & Mikhail's Clinical Anesthesiology.* 7th ed. New York, NY: McGraw Hill; 2022: Chapter 41.

190. What does the formula,
    $$\frac{\text{(end-diastolic volume)} - \text{(end-systolic volume)}}{\text{end-diastolic volume}}, \text{represent?}$$

    (A) Stroke volume

    (B) Cardiac index

    (C) Cardiac output

    (D) Ejection fraction

    Rationale: Ejection fraction is defined by the proportion of ventricular blood ejected during systole. Therefore, ejection fraction is calculated as the volume of blood ejected during systole (end-diastolic volume minus end-systolic volume) is divided by volume of blood present prior to systole (end-diastolic volume). Clinically, ejection fraction can be obtained using echocardiography and is a valuable indication of systolic function.

    Reference: Butterworth JF IV, Mackey DC, Wasnick JD, eds. *Morgan & Mikhail's Clinical Anesthesiology.* 7th ed. New York, NY: McGraw Hill; 2022: Chapter 20.

191. A pacemaker is placed in a patient with symptomatic sinus bradycardia with a normally functioning atrioventricular node. What settings would be most appropriate?

    (A) AAI

    (B) AOO

    (C) DDD

    (D) DDI

    Rationale: Since the AV node is functioning normally, the atrial signal will be conducted to the ventricles normally. The pacemaker only needs to ensure an adequate ventricular rate. Therefore, dual pacing is unnecessary. AOO is inappropriate as that would be asynchronous pacing of the atrium, pacing which occurs regardless of the intrinsic atrial rate. AAI is appropriate because in this demand mode the atrium is sensed, the atrium will be paced if needed, and the pacemaker will be inhibited (i.e., not pace) if the patient's own atrial signal is detected.

Reference: Butterworth JF IV, Mackey DC, Wasnick JD, eds. *Morgan & Mikhail's Clinical Anesthesiology.* 7th ed. New York, NY: McGraw Hill; 2022: Chapter 21.

192. Which of the following agents possesses combined alpha- and beta-adrenergic blocking effects?

(A) Metoprolol

(B) Esmolol

(C) Atenolol

(D) Labetalol

Rationale: Labetalol has both alpha- and beta-blocking properties. The other agents are beta-blocking agents without direct effects on alpha receptors.

TABLE 4-10. Classification of pacemakers.

Chamber Paced	Chamber Sensed	Response to Sensing	Programmability	Antitachyarrhythmia Function
O = none	O = none	O = none	O = none	O = none
A = atrium	A = atrium	T = triggered	P = simple	P = pacing
V = ventricle	V = ventricle	I = inhibited	M = multi-programmable	S = shock
D = dual (atrium and ventricle)	D = dual (atrium and ventricle)	D = dual (triggered and inhibited)	C = communicating	D = dual (pacing and shock)
			R = rate modulation	

(Reproduced with permission from Butterworth JF IV, Mackey DC, Wasnick JD, eds. *Morgan & Mikhail's Clinical Anesthesiology.* 7th ed. New York: McGraw Hill; 2022.)

TABLE 4-11. Comparison of β-adrenergic blocking agents.

Agent	β₁-Receptor Selectivity	Half-Life	Sympathomimetic	α-Receptor Blockade	Membrane Stabilizing
Acebutolol	+	2-4 hours	+		+
Atenolol	++	5-9 hours			
Betaxolol	++	14-22 hours			
Esmolol	++	9 minutes			
Metoprolol	++	3-4 hours			±
Bisoprolol	+	9-12 hours			
Oxprenolol		1-2 hours	+		+
Alprenolol		2-3 hours	+		+
Pindolol		3-4 hours	++		±
Penbutolol		5 hours	+		+
Carteolol		6 hours	+		
Labetalol		4-8 hours		+	±
Propranolol		3-6 hours			++
Timolol		3-5 hours			
Sotalol[1]		5-13 hours			
Nadolol		10-24 hours			
Carvedilol		6-8 hours		+	±

[1]Also possesses unique antiarrhythmic properties.
(Reproduced with permission from Butterworth JF IV, Mackey DC, Wasnick JD, eds. *Morgan & Mikhail's Clinical Anesthesiology.* 7th ed. New York: McGraw Hill; 2022.)

Reference: Butterworth JF IV, Mackey DC, Wasnick JD, eds. *Morgan & Mikhail's Clinical Anesthesiology.* 7th ed. New York, NY: McGraw Hill; 2022: Chapter 21.

193. Which anesthesia-induction technique would be appropriate for a severely hypertensive patient with coronary artery disease and moderate ventricular dysfunction?

(A) Inhalational induction with sevoflurane

(B) Inhalational induction with desflurane

(C) Intravenous induction with ketamine

(D) Intravenous induction with propofol

Rationale: An inhalational induction with desflurane will likely cause catecholamine release, further increasing blood pressure and heart rate. Ketamine alone may cause severe hypertension. Ketamine can be combined with other agents such as propofol to make an appropriate induction agent. Propofol alone in a severely hypertensive patient will likely cause severe hypotension in a dose large enough to attenuate a hypertensive response to laryngoscopy. Inhalational induction with sevoflurane will allow a general anesthetic depth of anesthesia, minimizing hypertension with laryngoscopy, and without the quick and profound hypotension associated with propofol induction.

Reference: Butterworth JF IV, Mackey DC, Wasnick JD, eds. *Morgan & Mikhail's Clinical Anesthesiology.* 7th ed. New York, NY: McGraw Hill; 2022: Chapter 21.

194. Which arrhythmia is best treated with magnesium sulfate?

   (A) Ventricular fibrillation
   (B) Polymorphic ventricular tachycardia in the presence of prolonged QT syndrome
   (C) Atrioventricular nodal reentrant tachycardia
   (D) Polymorphic ventricular tachycardia in the absence of prolonged QT syndrome

Rationale: Polymorphic ventricular tachycardia in the presence of prolonged QT syndrome is also known as torsade de pointes. Torsade de pointes typically responds best to magnesium or pacing. Polymorphic ventricular tachycardias in the absence of long QT interval typically respond to conventional antiarrhythmics.

Reference: Butterworth JF IV, Mackey DC, Wasnick JD, eds. *Morgan & Mikhail's Clinical Anesthesiology.* 7th ed. New York, NY: McGraw Hill; 2022: Chapter 21.

195. What is the goal of hemodynamic management for the patient with severe mitral valve regurgitation?

   (A) Aggressive volume resuscitation
   (B) Inotropic support
   (C) Afterload reduction
   (D) Maintenance of moderate bradycardia

Rationale: Mitral regurgitation results in retrograde flow into the left atrium on systole. This results in decreased forward stroke volume. Hemodynamic management should focus on maintaining forward blood flow, accomplished by reducing afterload. Increases in afterload will increase retrograde flow and should be avoided. Bradycardia and volume overload will increase left-ventricular end-diastolic volume which can exacerbate regurgitation through mitral annular dilation.

Reference: Butterworth JF IV, Mackey DC, Wasnick JD, eds. *Morgan & Mikhail's Clinical Anesthesiology.* 7th ed. New York, NY: McGraw Hill; 2022: Chapter 21.

196. Which patient is most at risk for catastrophic bleeding upon midline sternotomy?

   (A) Patient with ischemic cardiomyopathy on multiple vasopressor therapies undergoing aortic valve replacement
   (B) Patient with heparin-induced thrombocytopenia to be treated with argatroban for cardiopulmonary bypass undergoing coronary artery bypass grafts
   (C) Patient with previous coronary artery bypass grafting undergoing mitral valve repair
   (D) Obese patient with severe aortic stenosis undergoing aortic valve replacement

Rationale: In patients with previous sternotomy, right ventricle surface or grafts (if present) may be attached to the sternum. The pericardium has been removed and scar tissue may develop adhering cardiac structures to the posterior sternum. This is often referred to as a "redo." The anesthetist should have blood immediately available and be aware that the "redo" sternotomy may enter the heart or coronary structures, leading to massive bleeding necessitating emergent transfusion and repair.

Reference: Butterworth JF IV, Mackey DC, Wasnick JD, eds. *Morgan & Mikhail's Clinical Anesthesiology.* 7th ed. New York, NY: McGraw Hill; 2022: Chapter 21.

197. What is the approximate mean arterial blood pressure for the patient whose pressure reads 115/70 mmHg?

   (A) 100 mmHg
   (B) 85 mmHg
   (C) 92.5 mmHg
   (D) 80 mmHg

Rationale: Mean arterial pressure is the average pressure. The most accurate way to measure this is to determine that area under a pressure wave is divided by the time over which that wave occurred. This can generally be estimated by the formula,

$$MAP = Diastolic\ Pressure + \frac{Pulse\ Pressure}{3} =$$
$$70 + \frac{115 - 70}{3} = 70 + \frac{45}{3} = 85\ mmHg.$$

Another commonly memorized form of this formula is

$$MAP = \frac{Systolic\ Pressure + 2 \times Diastolic\ Pressure}{3} =$$
$$\frac{115 + 2 \times 70}{3} = \frac{115 + 140}{3} = \frac{255}{3} = 85\ mmHg.$$

Reference: Butterworth JF IV, Mackey DC, Wasnick JD, eds. *Morgan & Mikhail's Clinical Anesthesiology.* 7th ed. New York, NY: McGraw Hill; 2022: Chapters 5 and 20.

198. In which valvular disorder is the left ventricular volume approximately normal, but left ventricular pressures are higher than normal?

(A) Mitral stenosis

(B) Aortic stenosis

(C) Mitral regurgitation

(D) Aortic regurgitation

Rationale: This question is an application of the pressure-volume loop for patients with valvular heart disease. With aortic stenosis, left ventricular pressures are elevated because of the added resistance. Left ventricular volumes are approximately normal despite hypertrophy.

Reference: Butterworth JF IV, Mackey DC, Wasnick JD, eds. *Morgan & Mikhail's Clinical Anesthesiology.* 7th ed. New York, NY: McGraw Hill; 2022: Chapter 21.

199. Measured systolic and pulse pressure will appear greatest when transduced and measured at which point?

(A) Aortic root

(B) Brachial artery

(C) Radial artery

(D) Dorsalis pedis

Rationale: Arterial blood pressure waveform is distorted as it moves distally. As the waveform moves distally the waveform becomes narrowed and heightened. Therefore, the measured systolic pressure and pulse pressure are highest at the most distal point measured. The dorsalis pedis is the most distal artery among the selections.

Reference: Butterworth JF IV, Mackey DC, Wasnick JD, eds. *Morgan & Mikhail's Clinical Anesthesiology.* 7th ed. New York, NY: McGraw Hill; 2022: Chapter 21.

200. Which of the following is a relative contraindication to pulmonary artery catheter placement?

(A) Atrial fibrillation

(B) Left bundle branch block

(C) Complete heart block

(D) First degree block

Rationale: The pulmonary artery catheter passes through the right ventricle and can lead to arrhythmias or right bundle branch block. In the presence of left bundle branch block, an additional right bundle branch block will lead to complete heart block. A patient in complete heart block or atrial fibrillation may make placement technically difficult, but placement is not contraindicated.

Reference: Butterworth JF IV, Mackey DC, Wasnick JD, eds. *Morgan & Mikhail's Clinical Anesthesiology.* 7th ed. New York, NY: McGraw Hill; 2022: Chapter 21.

201. Which of the following is not associated with rhabdomyolysis?

(A) Compartment syndrome

(B) Renal failure

(C) Increased muscle enzymes

(D) Decreased muscle enzymes

Rationale: Rhabdomyolysis may lead to compartment syndrome and renal failure. The muscle necrosis results in myoglobinuria that is destructive to the kidneys. Findings include increased muscle enzymes, hyperkalemia, hyperphosphatemia, and brown urine.

Reference: Macksey LF. *Surgical Procedures and Anesthetic Implications.* 2nd ed. Sudbury, MA: Jones & Bartlett Learning; 2018: Chapter 21.

202. Which law explains the effect of post-intubation airway edema in children?

(A) Poiseuille's equation

(B) Dalton's law

(C) The ideal gas law

(D) Avogadro's number

Rationale: Poiseuille's equation describes the direct relationship between flow and the radius of the tube raised to the fourth power. This principle can be applied to illustrate the effect of edema on small neonatal and pediatric airways.

References: Butterworth JF IV, Mackey DC, Wasnick JD, eds. *Morgan & Mikhail's Clinical Anesthesiology.* 7th ed. New York, NY: McGraw Hill; 2022: Chapter 42.

Shubert D, Leyba J, Niemann S. *Chemistry and Physics for Nurse Anesthesia: A Student-Centered Approach.* 3rd ed. New York, NY: Springer Publishing Company; 2017: Chapter 5.

203. Which medication used for preeclampsia may extend the duration of rocuronium?

(A) Nitroglycerin

(B) Hydralazine

(C) Labetalol

(D) Magnesium

Rationale: Nitroglycerin, hydralazine, and labetalol are commonly used to control high blood pressure associated with preeclampsia. Magnesium is also used to control high blood pressure and seizures in preeclampsia and may extend the duration of muscle relaxants. For this reason, the dose of muscle relaxants should be decreased.

Reference: Longnecker DE, Mackey SC, Newman MF, Sandberg WS, Zapol WM, eds. *Anesthesiology*. 3rd ed. McGraw Hill; 2018: Chapters 18 and 57.

204. What is the normal fetal heart rate?

(A) 80 to 100

(B) 100 to 110

(C) 110 to 160

(D) >160

Rationale: The normal fetal heart rate is 110 to 160.

References: Butterworth JF IV, Mackey DC, Wasnick JD, eds. *Morgan & Mikhail's Clinical Anesthesiology*. 7th ed. New York, NY: McGraw Hill; 2022: Chapter 41.

Chestnut DH, Wong CA, Tsen LC, et al, eds. *Chestnut's Obstetric Anesthesia Principles and Practice*. 6th ed. Philadelphia, PA: Mosby Elsevier; 2020: Chapters 6 and 8.

205. What is the best intervention to improve hypotension resulting from aortocaval compression?

(A) Give oxygen via facemask

(B) Turn the patient on their side

(C) Give ephedrine

(D) Give neosynephrine

Rationale: Each of the choices will improve hypotension; however, the first measure is to reposition the patient. Turning the patient on their side will relieve the compression of the gravid uterus on the inferior vena cava. Venous return improves.

References: Butterworth JF IV, Mackey DC, Wasnick JD, eds. *Morgan & Mikhail's Clinical Anesthesiology*. 7th ed. New York, NY: McGraw Hill; 2022: Chapter 40.

Suresh MS, Segal BS, Preston RL, Fernando R, Mason CL, eds. *Shnider and Levinson's Anesthesia for Obstetrics*. 5th ed. Philadelphia, PA: Lippincott Williams & Wilkins; 2013: Chapter 1.

206. Which opioid causes the greatest respiration depression in newborns?

(A) Demerol

(B) Morphine

(C) Fentanyl

(D) Remifentanil

Rationale: Most opioids cross the placenta and may produce respiratory depression. Neonates are most sensitive to morphine followed by Demerol. Fentanyl has minimal effect on neonatal respiration when using low doses.

References: Butterworth JF IV, Mackey DC, Wasnick JD, eds. *Morgan & Mikhail's Clinical Anesthesiology*. 7th ed. New York, NY: McGraw Hill; 2022: Chapter 41.

Suresh MS, Segal BS, Preston RL, Fernando R, Mason CL, eds. *Shnider and Levinson's Anesthesia for Obstetrics*. 5th ed. Philadelphia, PA: Lippincott Williams & Wilkins; 2013: Chapter 2.

207. The patient is scheduled for a parathyroidectomy. How might neuromuscular blockade (NMB) affect hyperparathyroidism?

(A) May require decreasing the NMB dose

(B) May require careful titration

(C) Effect of NMB not significant

(D) No change in the response to NMB

Rationale: Patient's with hyperparathyroid disease experience muscle weakness and atrophy. Response to neuromuscular blockade is variable. For this reason, titrate nondepolarizing neuromuscular blocking agents carefully using a peripheral nerve stimulator.

References: Butterworth JF IV, Mackey DC, Wasnick JD, eds. *Morgan & Mikhail's Clinical Anesthesiology*. 7th ed. New York, NY: McGraw Hill; 2022: Chapter 34.

Elisha S, Heiner JS, Nagelhout JJ. *Nurse Anesthesia*. 7th ed. St. Louis, MO: Elsevier Saunders; 2023: Chapter 37.

208. A patient undergoes bronchoscopy for removal of a foreign body. What neuromuscular blocker (NMB) is the best choice for this procedure?

(A) Succinylcholine

(B) Vecuronicum

(C) Cis-Atracurium

(D) Atracurium

Rationale: A short-acting NMB is the best choice.

Reference: Butterworth JF IV, Mackey DC, Wasnick JD, eds. *Morgan & Mikhail's Clinical Anesthesiology*. 7th ed. New York, NY: McGraw Hill; 2022: Chapter 25.

209. What increases stroke volume?

(A) Increased ventricular end-diastolic volume

(B) Increased pulmonary vascular resistance

(C) Increased heart rate

(D) Mitral regurgitation

Rationale: Stroke volume is defined by $SV = \dfrac{CO}{HR}$ (this is just an algebraic manipulation of the formula $CO = SV \times HR$ the blood that moves retrograde in the atria is not included in the commonly understood definition of stroke volume. Thus "ventricular end-diastolic volume" is the most appropriate answer.

Reference: Butterworth JF IV, Mackey DC, Wasnick JD, eds. *Morgan & Mikhail's Clinical Anesthesiology.* 7th ed. New York, NY: McGraw Hill; 2022: Chapter 20.

210. Which inhaled agent is most associated with emergence delirium in children?

   (A) Sevoflurane
   (B) Isoflurane
   (C) Desflurane
   (D) Nitrous oxide

Rationale: As compared to adults, emergence delirium is commonly associated with sevoflurane in children.

References: Barash PG, Cullen BF, Stoelting RK, et al, eds. *Clinical Anesthesia.* 8th ed. Lippincott Williams & Wilkins; 2017: Chapter 43.

Gropper MA, Cohen NH, Eriksson LI, et al, eds. *Miller's Anesthesia.* 9th ed. Philadelphia, PA: Churchill Livingstone Elsevier; 2020: Chapter 77.

211. When does blood volume return to pre-pregnancy levels?

   (A) 7 to 14 days after delivery
   (B) 24 hours after delivery
   (C) 36 hours after delivery
   (D) 21 days after delivery

Rationale: Blood volume returns to pre-pregnancy levels approximately 1 to 2 weeks following delivery.

Reference: Longnecker DE, Mackey SC, Newman MF, Sandberg WS, Zapol WM, eds. *Anesthesiology.* 3rd ed. McGraw Hill; 2018: Chapter 18.

212. An octogenarian is scheduled for a laparoscopic cholecystectomy. You plan to adjust the dosage of neuromuscular blockers. What is your rationale for this decision?

   (A) Renal function declines with aging
   (B) Renal clearance increases with aging

   (C) Hepatic blood flow increases with aging
   (D) Total body water increases by 10% to 15% with aging

Rationale: Calculating drug dosages for the elderly requires adjustment based upon changes in physiology. Renal function declines with a reduction in clearance of about 30% to 40%. Hepatic blood flow and total body water also decrease.

Reference: Hines RL, Marschall KE. *Stoelting's Anesthesia and Co-existing Disease.* 7th ed. Philadelphia, PA: Elsevier Saunders; 2018: Chapter 30.

213. Which of the following is not associated with retinopathy of prematurity?

   (A) High oxygen tension in vessels of the retina
   (B) Low oxygen tension in vessels of the retina
   (C) Wide swings in oxygen tension
   (D) Ventilated premature infants with sepsis

Rationale: Retinopathy of prematurity (ROP) may result in permanent vision loss. High oxygen tension of the vessels of the retina as well as wide swings in oxygen tension place premature infants at risk. Ventilated premature infants with a variety of conditions including sepsis are also at risk for ROP.

References: Butterworth JF IV, Mackey DC, Wasnick JD, eds. *Morgan & Mikhail's Clinical Anesthesiology.* 7th ed. New York, NY: McGraw Hill; 2022: Chapter 42.

Pardo MC Jr, ed. *Basics of Anesthesia.* 8th ed. Philadelphia, PA: Elsevier Saunders; 2023: Chapter 34.

214. Which of the following is not a concern for the anesthetists when caring for patients with omphalocele and gastroschisis?

   (A) Severe dehydration
   (B) Fluid loss
   (C) Heat loss
   (D) Low abdominal pressure with closure

Rationale: Because the defects result in exposed viscera, patients with omphalocele and gastroschisis are prone to dehydration, fluid, and heat loss. Following closure of the defect, high abdominal pressure is a concern.

Reference: Gropper MA, Cohen NH, Eriksson LI, et al, eds. *Miller's Anesthesia.* 9th ed. Philadelphia, PA: Churchill Livingstone Elsevier; 2020: Chapter 77.

215. Which of the following is not an anesthetic goal when caring for patients with Tetralogy of Fallot?

(A) Increase systemic vascular resistance (SVR)

(B) Avoid acidosis

(C) Maintain intravascular volume

(D) Maintain SVR

Rationale: Avoiding increases in peripheral vascular resistance, SVR and intravascular volume lessen cardiac shunting.

TABLE 4-12. Classification of congenital heart disease.

Lesions causing outflow obstruction
Left ventricle
   Coarctation of the aorta
   Aortic stenosis
Right ventricle
   Pulmonic valve stenosis
Lesions causing left-to-right shunting
Ventricular septal defect
Patent ductus arteriosus
Atrial septal defect
Endocardial cushion defect
Partial anomalous pulmonary venous return
Lesions causing right-to-left shunting
With decreased pulmonary blood flow
   Tetralogy of Fallot
   Pulmonary atresia
   Tricuspid atresia
With increased pulmonary blood flow
   Transposition of the great vessels
   Truncus arteriosus
   Single ventricle
   Double-outlet right ventricle
   Total anomalous pulmonary venous return
   Hypoplastic left heart

(Reproduced with permission from Butterworth JF IV, Mackey DC, Wasnick JD, eds. *Morgan & Mikhail's Clinical Anesthesiology.* 7th ed. New York: McGraw Hill; 2022.)

Reference: Butterworth JF IV, Mackey DC, Wasnick JD, eds. *Morgan & Mikhail's Clinical Anesthesiology.* 7th ed. New York, NY: McGraw Hill; 2022: Chapter 21.

216. Which feature is not associated with dementia?

(A) Acute onset

(B) Memory impairment

(C) Disorientation

(D) Slow onset

Rationale: Dementia is associated with memory impairment, disorientation, agitation and is slow, progressive, and chronic. In contrast, delirium is acute, fluctuates with levels of consciousness.

Reference: Hines RL, Marschall KE. *Stoelting's Anesthesia and Co-existing Disease.* 7th ed. Philadelphia, PA: Elsevier Saunders; 2018: Chapter 30.

217. Why is there an initial plasma concentration increase following intravenous induction in geriatric patients?

(A) Total body water increase

(B) Increased central compartment volume

(C) Total body water decreases

(D) Body fat decreases

Rationale: Because total body water and central compartment volume decreases in the elderly, the initial plasma concentration increases.

Reference: Hines RL, Marschall KE. *Stoelting's Anesthesia and Co-existing Disease.* 7th ed. Philadelphia, PA: Elsevier Saunders; 2018: Chapter 30.

218. Which of the following anesthetic implications is not concerning when caring for obese patients?

(A) Caution when administering respiratory depressants

(B) Low gastric volume

(C) High gastric volume

(D) Low pH

Rationale: Obesity affects all body systems. Anesthetic implications include minimizing risk of severe pneumonitis secondary to aspiration. Higher gastric volumes with a lower pH should be considered. Respiratory depressant effects of medications for this population should be considered.

Reference: Barash PG, Cullen BF, Stoelting RK, et al, eds. *Clinical Anesthesia.* 8th ed. Lippincott Williams & Wilkins; 2017: Chapter 45.

219. Which of the following guidelines for management of patients with obstructive sleep apnea is false?

(A) Consider regional techniques.

(B) Consider nonsteroidal anti-inflammatory agents to reduce opioid requirements.

(C) Standard use of opioids should be considered when using regional techniques.

(D) Consider the risks and benefits of using opioids in combination with regional techniques.

Rationale: Providing adequate postoperative analgesia and early mobilization are key goals for patients with obstructive sleep apnea. Patients with OSA require careful consideration in the type and amount of opioid used to ensure the key goals are achieved.

Reference: Barash PG, Cullen BF, Stoelting RK, et al, eds. *Clinical Anesthesia*. 8th ed. Lippincott Williams & Wilkins; 2017: Chapter 45.

220. Which of the following is an advantage of the sitting position for orthopedic surgery?

    (A) Risk of injury to the brachial plexus and forearm neuropathies decreases.

    (B) Risk of injury to the brachial plexus and forearm neuropathies increases.

    (C) Arm weight distorts the shoulder joint anatomy.

    (D) Arm weight distorts the intra-articular anatomy.

Rationale: Advantages of the sitting position for orthopedic surgery provides less distortion of anatomy as well as lessening the risk of brachial plexus injury and forearm neuropathy.

Reference: Macksey LF. *Surgical Procedures and Anesthetic Implications*. 2nd ed. Sudbury, MA: Jones & Bartlett Learning; 2018: Chapter 21.

Index